Handbook for

BRUNNER & SUDDARTH'S

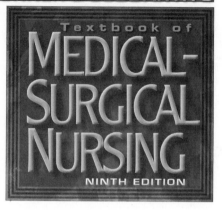

Textbook of
MEDICAL-
SURGICAL
NURSING

NINTH EDITION

Handbook for

BRUNNER & SUDDARTH'S

Textbook of

MEDICAL-SURGICAL NURSING

NINTH EDITION

Joyce Y. Johnson, RN, PhD

Registry Nurse
Crawford Long Hospital of Emory University
Adjunct Faculty
Georgia State University
School of Nursing
President, Johnson Consulting Firm
Atlanta, Georgia

Lippincott

Philadelphia • New York • Baltimore

Acquisitions Editor: Lisa Stead
Assistant Editor: Claudia Vaughn
Senior Project Editor: Sandra Cherrey Scheinin
Senior Production Manager: Helen Ewan

Senior Production Coordinator: Michael Carcel
Assistant Art Director: Doug Smock
Indexer: Nancy Newman

9 8 7 6 5 4 3 2 1

Library of Congress Cataloging-in-Publication Data
Johnson, Joyce Young.
    Handbook for Brunner and Suddarth's textbook of medical-surgical nursing / Joyce Y. Johnson.—9th ed.
    p. cm.
    Includes index.
    ISBN 0-7817-2091-5 (alk. paper)
    1. Nursing—Handbooks, manuals, etc. 2. Surgical nursing—Handbooks, manuals, etc.
I. Title: Textbook of medical-surgical nursing. II. Baughman, Diane C. Handbook for Brunner and Suddarth's textbook of medical-surgical nursing.
    [DNLM: 1. Nursing care 2. Perioperative Nursing WY49 2000]
RT41 .J56 2000
610.73 21; aa05 10-06—dc99   99-047902

Care has been taken to confirm the accuracy of the information presented and to describe generally accepted practices. However, the authors, editors, and publisher are not responsible for errors or omissions or for any consequences from application of the information in this book and make no warranty, express or implied, with respect to the contents of the publication.

The authors, editors and publisher have exerted every effort to ensure that drug selection and dosage set forth in this text are in accordance with current recommendations and practice at the time of publication. However, in view of ongoing research, changes in government regulations, and the constant flow of information relating to drug therapy and drug reactions, the reader is urged to check the package insert for each drug for any change in indications and dosage and for added warnings and precautions. This is particularly important when the recommended agent is a new or infrequently employed drug.

Some drugs and medical devices presented in this publication have Food and Drug Administration (FDA) clearance for limited use in restricted research settings. It is the responsibility of the health care provider to ascertain the FDA status of each drug or device planned for use in their clinical practice.

All praises, honor, and glory to the Lord!

To my husband, Larry, and my children, Virginia and Larry Jr.,
who are my joy and inspiration. To my family and friends,
who are my support and strength.

To my students, past and future, who are my
hope for nursing's future.

Preface

This *Handbook for Brunner & Suddarth's Textbook of Medical-Surgical Nursing* is a comprehensive yet concise clinical reference designed for use by students and nurses. Perfect for both the hospital and community settings, it presents need-to-know information on the most commonly seen diseases and disorders in an easy-to-use outline format. Each entry is formatted consistently for quick access to vital information on:

A general overview of the disease process
Most common clinical manifestations
Main diagnostic evaluation methods
Medical management
Nursing management including a detailed format: Assessment, major nursing diagnoses and collaborative problems, goals, nursing interventions, and major expected outcomes or an abbreviated format for some conditions that includes key nursing interventions.

For readers requiring more in-depth information, the *Handbook* is completely cross-referenced to *Brunner and Suddarth's Textbook of Medical-Surgical Nursing, 9th edition,* by Smeltzer and Bare, the leading comprehensive medical-surgical textbook.

SPECIAL FEATURES

Because of the revolution in health care and the increasing emphasis on home care, many entries include a separate section entitled "Promoting Home and Community-Based Care." This section focuses on information vital to nurses in the home and community settings, who play an increasingly independent role as patient care providers. Patient and family teaching information is included in these sections.

"Gerontologic Considerations" provide an understanding of specific issues related to the care of older adults, and help today's nurses and nursing students deal with this growing population.

"Nursing Alerts" call the reader's attention to priority care issues and highlight potential life-threatening situations.

"Expected Outcomes" promote outcome-based care, which has become an increasingly important strategy in health care delivery.

The *Handbook's* convenient pocket size and A-to-Z organization allow the user to reference pertinent information quickly and easily wherever care is being given.

This text has been written with an eye to providing content that, as nurses, we need to know. I hope it will provide a valuable guide to assist you in your education and nursing practice.

Joyce Y. Johnson, RN, PhD

Acknowledgments

I would like to thank Lisa Stead, Aquisitions Editor, and Claudia Vaughn, Assistant Editor, at Lippincott Williams & Wilkins for their invaluable support and guidance in this project. Special thanks to Clemmie Riggins for her clerical skills that helped this book come to completion and to Lynette Johnson for her invaluable assistance.

Contents

C

D

E

R

S

T

U

V

ACNE VULGARIS

Acne vulgaris is a common follicular disorder affecting susceptible pilosebaceous follicles (hair follicles) most commonly found on the face, neck, and upper trunk. It is the most often encountered skin condition in adolescents and young adults between the ages of 12 and 35 years, becoming more marked at puberty and adolescence. The etiology of acne appears to stem from an interplay of genetic, hormonal, and bacterial factors. Diagnosis is most often made based on signs and symptoms.

Clinical Manifestations
- Closed comedones (whiteheads)
- Open comedones (blackheads)
- Erythematous papules (inflammatory condition)
- Inflammatory pustules
- Inflammatory cysts

Medical Management
The goals of medical management are to reduce bacterial colonies, decrease sebaceous gland activity, prevent the follicles from becoming plugged, reduce inflammation, combat secondary infection, minimize scarring, and eliminate factors that predispose the patient to acne.

Nutritional Management
The patient should eliminate from the diet foods associated with acne flare-up, such as chocolate, colas, fried food, and milk products.

Skin Hygiene
- In mild cases, wash at least two times daily with cleansing soap.
- Discourage use of oil-based cosmetics or creams.

Topical Pharmacotherapy
- Benzoyl peroxide preparation
- Vitamin A acid (tretinoin)
- Topical antibiotics (eg, tetracycline, erythromycin)

Systemic Therapy
- Systemic antibiotics (eg, tetracycline, minocycline [Minocin])
- Oral retinoids (eg, vitamin A, isotretinoin [Accutane])
- Hormone therapy (eg, progesterone-estrogen preparations)

Surgical Management
- Comedo extraction
- Injections of steroids into the inflamed lesions
- Incision and drainage
- Cryosurgery
- Dermabrasion

Nursing Management

Assessment
- Observe and listen to how the patient perceives skin condition.
- Approach the patient with empathy and compassion.
- Inspect lesions by gently stretching the skin. Closed comedones appear as small, slightly elevated papules. Open comedones appear flat or slightly raised with a central follicular impaction.
- Document the presence of inflammatory lesions.

Major Nursing Diagnoses
- Ineffective management of therapeutic regimen related to insufficient knowledge about the condition and its causes, course, prevention, treatment, and skin care

- Body image disturbance related to embarrassment and frustration over appearance

Collaborative Problems/Potential Complications
- Scarring
- Infection

Planning and Goals
The major goals may include understanding the condition to enhance compliance with prescribed therapy, development of self-acceptance, and absence of complications.

Nursing Interventions
INCREASING TREATMENT COMPLIANCE
AND UNDERSTANDING
- Counsel and assure the patient that problem is not related to uncleanliness, dietary indiscretions, masturbation, sexual activity, or other misconceptions.
- Reinforce the concept that acne arises from many factors.
- Teach the rationale for using oral and topical medications.
- Explain actions and side effects of medications; encourage frequent blood tests.
- Encourage consistent treatment every day.

PROMOTING SELF-ACCEPTANCE
- Make the patient a partner in therapy; take problems seriously; give understanding, reassurance, and support.
- Consider all aspects of emotional factors.
- Assist with stress-reduction techniques as needed.

MONITORING AND MANAGING
POTENTIAL COMPLICATIONS
- Scarring: caution against manipulation of lesions; inform patient of potential scarring from surgical intervention; caution patient that discontinuing medications can result in increased chance of scarring.

- Infection: advise patient to watch for signs and symptoms of oral or vaginal candidiasis when on long-term antibiotic therapy with tetracycline.

🏠 Promoting Home and Community-Based Care

Teaching Patients Self-Care

- Instruct patient to wash face with mild soap and water twice a day.
- Advise patient to use prescribed mild abrasive soaps but to avoid all forms of excessive friction and trauma to the face; to avoid cosmetics, shaving creams, and lotions; to follow a nutritious diet; to keep hands away from face; to refrain from squeezing pimples and blackheads.
- Counsel patient on need to be consistent with treatment and use of recommended cleansing products.
- Reassure patient that most acne medications cause some drying and peeling of the skin.
- Teach patient about the disease process.
- Advise patient that treatment may take 8 to 12 weeks or longer for results.
- Teach women of childbearing age to continue contraceptive measures during treatment and for 4 to 6 weeks thereafter.
- Caution patient not to take vitamin A supplements during treatment to avoid additive toxic effects.

For more information, see Chapter 52 in Smeltzer and Bare: *Brunner and Suddarth's Textbook of Medical-Surgical Nursing*, 9th edition. Philadelphia: Lippincott Williams & Wilkins, 2000.

ACQUIRED IMMUNODEFICIENCY SYNDROME

Acquired immunodeficiency syndrome (AIDS) is defined as the most severe form of a continuum of illnesses associated with human immunodeficiency virus (HIV) infection. HIV, a retrovirus, is transmitted through bodily fluids by high-risk behaviors such as male homosexual relations, injection drug use, and heterosexual intercourse with an HIV-infected partner. Also at risk are people who received transfusions of blood or blood products contaminated with HIV, children born to mothers with HIV infection, breast-fed infants of HIV-infected mothers, and health care workers exposed to needle-stick injury associated with an infected patient.

Clinical Manifestations

Symptoms are widespread and may affect any organ system. Manifestations range from mild abnormalities in immune response without overt signs and symptoms to profound immunosuppression, life-threatening infection, malignancy, and the direct effect of HIV on body tissues.

Respiratory

- Shortness of breath, dyspnea, cough, chest pain, and fever are associated with opportunistic infections.
- *Pneumocystis carinii* pneumonia (PCP) is the most common infection.
- *Mycobacterium avium* complex (MAC) disease is a leading bacterial infection in AIDS patients.
- HIV-associated tuberculosis occurs early in the course of HIV infection, often preceding a diagnosis of AIDS. If diagnosed early, HIV-associated tuberculosis responds well to antituberculosis therapy.

Gastrointestinal

- Loss of appetite
- Nausea and vomiting

- Oral and esophageal candidiasis (white patches, painful swallowing, retrosternal pain, and possibly oral lesions)
- Chronic diarrhea, possibly with devastating effects (eg, weight loss, fluid and electrolyte imbalances, perianal skin excoriation, weakness, and inability to perform the activities of daily living)

Wasting Syndrome (Cachexia)
- Multifactorial protein-energy malnutrition
- Profound involuntary weight loss exceeding 10% of baseline body weight
- Presents with chronic diarrhea, chronic weakness, and documented intermittent or constant fever with no concurrent illness
- Anorexia, diarrhea, gastrointestinal malabsorption, lack of nutrition, and for some patients, a hypermetabolic state

Oncologic
- Higher than usual incidence of cancer, including Kaposi's sarcoma (KS), B-cell lymphomas, and carcinomas of cervix, skin, stomach, pancreas, rectum, and bladder

Neurologic
Neurologic complications involve central, peripheral, and anatomic functions.

- Encephalopathy (AIDS dementia complex [ADC]) occurs in two thirds of patients with AIDS (symptoms include memory deficits, headache, lack of concentration, progressive confusion, psychomotor slowing, apathy and ataxia, and in later stages, global cognitive impairments, delayed verbal responses, spastic paraparesis, hyperreflexia, psychosis, seizures, incontinence, and death.
- *Cryptococcus neoformans* and fungal infection (fever, stiff neck, nausea and vomiting, seizures) are also seen.
- Progressive multifocal leukoencephalopathy (PML), a central nervous system demyelinating disorder, can occur.

- Other neurologic disorders include *Toxoplasma gondii*, cytomegalovirus, and *Mycobacterium tuberculosis* infection, with symptoms ranging from confusion to blindness, aphasia, paresis, and death.

Integumentary
- KS, herpes simplex and herpes zoster viruses, and various forms of dermatitis associated with painful vesicles.
- Folliculitis, associated with dry flaking skin or atopic dermatitis

Gynecologic
- Persistent recurrent vaginal candidiasis may be the first sign of HIV infection.
- Ulcerative sexually transmitted diseases, such as chancroid, syphilis, and herpes, are more severe in women with HIV.
- Venereal warts and cervical cancer may be noted.
- Women with HIV have a higher incidence of menstrual abnormalities (amenorrhea or bleeding between periods).

Chronic Illness
- Early diagnosis and treatment of opportunistic diseases and antiviral therapy has led HIV infection to become a chronic illness.
- Also seen are fatigue, headache, profuse night sweats, unexplained weight loss, dry cough, shortness of breath, extreme weakness, diarrhea, decreased endurance, edema, blindness, and swallowing difficulties, and possible neurologic involvement resulting in dementia, hemiplegia, spastic paraparesis, painful neuropathies, proximal and distal muscle weakness, and persistent lymphadenopathy.

Depressive
- Depressive symptoms have multiple causes, including preexisting mental illness, neuropsychiatric disturbances, and psychosocial factors.

- Patients may experience irrational guilt, shame, loss of self-esteem, helplessness, worthlessness, and suicidal ideation.

Diagnostic Evaluation
Confirm the presence of HIV antibodies: enzyme-linked immunosorbent assay (ELISA) test, Western blot assay, and indirect immunofluorescence assay (IFA).

Medical Management
Goals of treatment include treatment of HIV-associated infections and malignancies, arresting of HIV growth and replication through antiviral agents, and augmentation and restoration of the immune system through the use of immunomodulators.

Antiretroviral Agents
A triple drug regimen has been used effectively.

- Zidovudine (ZDV), formerly azidothymidine (AZT)
- Dideoxyinosine (ddI)
- Dideoxycytidine (ddC)

Medications for HIV-Related Infections
- PCP: trimethoprim-sulfamethoxazole (TMP-SMZ) and antibacterial agents, such as dapsone; alternatively, pentamidine, an antiprotozoa agent
- MAC: treatment not clearly established; involves multidrug regimens (two to five agents) administered over a prolonged period
- Cryptococcal meningitis: intravenous amphotericin B with or without antifungal agents, such as fluconazole or flucytosine
- Cytomegalovirus retinitis: ganciclovir, foscavir, or cidofovir
- Encephalitis: pyrimethamine (Daraprim) and sulfadiazine or clindamycin (Cleosin)
- Candidiasis: clotrimazole (Mycelex), ketoconazole, or fluconazole

Malignancies
- KS: alpha-interferon, surgical excision of lesions, liquid nitrogen to lesions, vinblastine injected into intraoral lesions, interferon; chemotherapy with doxorubicin (Adriamycin), bleomycin, and vincristine (ABV); radiation
- Lymphomas: limited successful treatment; chemotherapy and radiation therapy may be used

Immunomodulators
- Alpha-interferon
- Other substances under evaluation (eg, interleukin-2, lentinan, granulocyte-macrophage colony-stimulating factor)

Antidepressant Therapy
Psychotherapy is integrated with pharmacology (tofranil, imipramine [Norpramin], fluoxetine [Prozac], methylphenidate [Ritalin], electroconvulsive therapy if depression is severe).

Antidiarrheal Therapy
- Octreotide acetate (Sandostatin)

Appetite Stimulants
- Megestrol acetate (Megace); dronabinol (Marinol)

Vaccines
Research continues to work on development of a vaccine for HIV.

Supportive Care and Alternative Therapies
- Spiritual: laughter, hypnosis, faith healing, guided imagery, positive affirmations
- Nutritional: vegetarian and macrobiotic diets, vitamin C or beta-carotene supplements, tumeric (curcumin), Chinese herbs
- Drug and biologic: medicines not approved by the Food and Drug Administration; oxygen, ozone, and urine therapy

- Physical forces and devices: acupuncture, acupressure, massage therapy, yoga, therapeutic touch, reflexology, crystals
- Provide assistance for obtaining or preparing meals, as needed
- Parenteral feeding (total parenteral nutrition), if necessary
- Intravenous fluid and electrolyte replacement to treat imbalances

Nursing Management
Assessment
- Identify potential risk factors, including sexual practices and injection drug use history.
- Assess physical and psychological status.
- Thoroughly explore factors affecting immune system functioning.

NUTRITIONAL STATUS
- Obtain a dietary history.
- Identify factors that may interfere with oral intake, such as anorexia, nausea, vomiting, oral pain, or difficulty swallowing.
- Assess the patient's ability to purchase and prepare food.
- Measure nutritional status by weight, anthropometric measurements (triceps skin-fold measurement), and blood urea nitrogen, serum protein, albumin, and transferrin levels.

SKIN AND MUCOUS MEMBRANES
- Inspect daily for breakdown, ulceration, and infection.
- Monitor the oral cavity for redness, ulcerations, and creamy-white patches (candidiasis).
- Assess the perianal area for excoriation and infection.
- Obtain wound cultures to identify infectious organisms.

RESPIRATORY STATUS
- Monitor for cough, sputum production, shortness of breath, orthopnea, tachypnea, and chest pain; assess breath sounds.

- Assess other parameters of pulmonary function (chest radiographs, arterial blood gases, and pulmonary function tests).

NEUROLOGIC STATUS
- Assess mental status as early as possible to provide a baseline (eg, note level of consciousness and orientation to person, place, and time and the occurrence of memory lapses).
- Observe for sensory deficits, such as visual changes, headache, and numbness and tingling in the extremities.
- Observe for motor impairments, such as altered gait and paresis.
- Observe for seizure activity.

FLUID AND ELECTROLYTE STATUS
- Examine the skin and mucous membranes for turgor and dryness.
- Assess for dehydration by observing for increased thirst, decreased urine output, low blood pressure, weak rapid pulse, or urine specific gravity.
- Monitor electrolyte imbalances (laboratory studies).
- Assess for signs and symptoms of electrolyte depletion, including decreased mental status, muscle twitching, muscle cramps, irregular pulse, nausea and vomiting, and shallow respirations.

LEVEL OF KNOWLEDGE
- Evaluate the patient's knowledge of disease and transmission.
- Assess the level of knowledge of family and friends.
- Explore the patient's reaction to the diagnosis of AIDS.
- Explore how the patient has dealt with illness and major life stressors in the past.
- Identify the patient's resources for support.

USE OF ALTERNATIVE THERAPIES
- Question the patient about use of alternative therapies.
- Encourage the patient to report any use of alternative therapies to the primary health care provider.

- Become familiar with the potential side effects of alternative therapies; if side effect is suspected to result from alternative therapies, discuss with the patient and the primary and alternative health care providers.
- View alternative therapies with an open mind, and try to understand the importance of the treatment to the patient.

Major Nursing Diagnoses
- Impaired skin integrity related to cutaneous manifestations of HIV infection, excoriation, and diarrhea.
- Risk for infection related to immunodeficiency.
- Activity intolerance related to weakness, fatigue, malnutrition, impaired fluid and electrolyte balance, and hypoxia associated with pulmonary infections.
- Altered thought processes related to shortened attention span, impaired memory, confusion, and disorientation (HIV encephalopathy).
- Ineffective airway clearance related to PCP, increased bronchial secretions, and decreased ability to cough related to weakness and fatigue.
- Altered nutrition: less than body requirements related to decreased oral intake.
- Diarrhea related to enteric pathogens or HIV infection.
- Pain related to impaired perianal skin integrity secondary to diarrhea, KS, and peripheral neuropathy.
- Social isolation related to stigma of the disease, withdrawal of support systems, isolation procedures, and fear of infecting others.
- Anticipatory grieving related to changes in lifestyle and roles to unfavorable prognosis.
- Knowledge deficit related to means of preventing HIV transmission and self-care.

Collaborative Problems/Potential Complications
- Opportunistic infections
- Impaired breathing or respiratory failure
- Wasting syndrome and fluid and electrolyte imbalance
- Adverse reaction to medications

Planning and Goals

Goals include achievement and maintenance of skin integrity, resumption of usual bowel habits, absence of infection, improved activity tolerance, improved thought processes, improved airway clearance, increased comfort, improved nutritional status, increased socialization, expression of grief, increased knowledge regarding disease prevention and self-care, and absence of complications.

Nursing Interventions

PROMOTING SKIN INTEGRITY

- Assess skin and oral mucosa for changes in appearance, location and size of lesions, and evidence of infection and breakdown; encourage regular oral care.
- Encourage the patient to balance rest and mobility whenever possible; assist immobile patients to change position every 2 hours.
- Use devices, such as alternating-pressure mattresses and low-air-loss beds.
- Encourage patients to avoid scratching, to use nonabrasive and nondrying soaps, and to use nonperfumed skin moisturizers on dry skin; administer antipruritics, antibiotics, analgesics, medicated lotions, ointments, and dressings as prescribed; avoid excessive use of tape.
- Keep bed linen free of wrinkles, and avoid tight or restrictive clothing to reduce friction to the skin.
- Advise patients with foot lesions to wear white cotton socks and shoes that do not cause the feet to perspire.

MAINTAINING PERIANAL SKIN INTEGRITY

- Assess perianal region for impaired skin integrity and infection.
- Instruct patient to keep the area as clean as possible, to cleanse after each bowel movement, to use sitz bath or irrigation, and to dry the area thoroughly after cleaning.
- Assist debilitated patient in maintaining hygienic practices.
- Promote healing with prescribed topical ointments and lotions.
- Culture wounds if infection is suspected.

PROMOTING USUAL BOWEL HABITS

- Assess bowel patterns for the occurrence of diarrhea (frequency and consistency of stool, report of pain or cramping with bowel movements).
- Assess factors that exacerbate the frequency of diarrhea.
- Measure and document the volume of liquid stool as fluid volume loss; obtain stool cultures.
- Counsel the patient about ways to decrease diarrhea, such as to rest the bowel, then avoid foods that act as bowel irritants, including raw fruits and vegetables; encourage small, frequent meals.
- Administer prescribed medications, such as anticholinergic antispasmodics or opiates, antibiotics, and antifungal agents.

PREVENTING INFECTION

- Instruct patient and caregivers to monitor for signs and symptoms of infection.
- Monitor laboratory values that indicate the presence of infection, such as white blood cell count and differential blood cell count; assist in obtaining culture specimens as ordered.
- Advise on strategies to avoid infection.
- Strongly urge patients and sexual partners to avoid exposure to body fluids and to use condoms for any sexual activities.
- Strongly discourage injection drug use because of risk to the patient of other infections and transmission of HIV infection.
- Maintain strict aseptic technique for invasive procedures.
- Observe universal precautions in all patient care.

IMPROVING ACTIVITY TOLERANCE

- Monitor ability to ambulate and perform daily activities.
- Assist in planning daily routines to maintain a balance between activity and rest.
- Instruct patient in energy conservation techniques (eg, sitting while washing or preparing a meal).

- Decrease anxiety that contributes to weakness and fatigue by using measures such as relaxation and guided imagery.
- Strategize with other health care team members to uncover and address factors associated with fatigue (such as epoetin alfa [Epogen] for fatigue related to anemia).

MAINTAINING THOUGHT PROCESSES
- Assess for alterations in mental status.
- Reorient to person, place, and time as necessary; maintain and post a regular daily schedule.
- Give instructions, and instruct family to speak to patient, in a slow, simple, and clear manner.
- Provide night lights for the patient's bedroom and bathroom, and plan safe leisure activities that the patient has previously enjoyed.
- Provide around-the-clock supervision as necessary for patients with HIV encephalopathy.

IMPROVING AIRWAY CLEARANCE
- At least daily, assess respiratory status, mental status, and skin color.
- Note and document presence of cough and quantity and characteristics of sputum; send specimen for analysis as ordered.
- Encourage adequate rest to maximize patient's energy expenditure and prevent fatigue.
- Provide pulmonary therapy, such as coughing, deep breathing, postural drainage, percussion, and vibration, every 2 hours to prevent stasis of secretions and promote airway clearance.
- Assist the patient in attaining a position (high- or semi-Fowler's) that facilitates breathing and airway clearance.
- Evaluate fluid volume status; encourage intake of 3 to 4 liters daily.
- Provide humidified oxygen, suctioning, intubation, and mechanical ventilation as necessary.

RELIEVING PAIN AND DISCOMFORT

- Assess patient for the quality and severity of pain associated with impaired perianal skin integrity, lesions of KS, and peripheral neuropathy.
- Explore the effects of pain on elimination, nutrition, sleep, affect, and communication along with exacerbating and relieving factors.
- Encourage patient to use soft cushions or foam pads while sitting; topical anesthetics or ointments as prescribed.
- Instruct patient to avoid irritating foods and to use antispasmotics and antidiarrheal preparations if necessary.
- Administer nonsteroidal antiinflammatory agents, opiates, and nonpharmacologic approaches, such as relaxation techniques.
- Tricyclic antidepressants and elastic stockings may be helpful for neuropathic pain.

IMPROVING NUTRITIONAL STATUS

- Assess weight, dietary intake, anthropometric measurements, serum albumin, blood urea nitrogen, protein, and transferrin levels.
- Instruct patient about ways to supplement nutritional value of meals (eg, add eggs, butter, milk).
- Based on an assessment of factors interfering with oral intake, implement specific measures to facilitate oral intake; consult the dietitian to determine nutritional requirements.
- Control nausea and vomiting; encourage patient to eat easy-to-swallow foods; encourage oral hygiene before and after meals.
- Encourage rest before meals; do not schedule meals after painful or unpleasant procedures.
- Provide enteral or parenteral feedings to maintain nutritional status, as indicated.

DECREASING THE SENSE OF SOCIAL ISOLATION

- Provide an atmosphere of acceptance and understanding of AIDS patients, their families, and partners.

- Assess the patient's usual level of social interaction early to provide a baseline for monitoring changes in behavior.
- Encourage the patient to express feelings of isolation and aloneness; assure the patient that these feelings are not unique or abnormal.
- Assure patients, family, and friends that AIDS is not spread through casual contact.

COPING WITH GRIEF
- Help patients explore and identify resources for support and mechanisms for coping.
- Encourage the patient to maintain contact with family, friends, and coworkers and to continue usual activities whenever possible.
- Encourage the patient to use local or national AIDS support groups and hotlines and to identify losses and deal with them when possible.

MONITORING AND MANAGING COMPLICATIONS
- Respiratory failure and impaired breathing: monitor arterial blood gas values, oxygen saturation, respiratory rate and pattern, and breath sounds; provide suctioning and oxygen therapy; assist patient on mechanical ventilation to cope with associated stress.
- Inform the patient that signs and symptoms of opportunistic infections include fever, malaise, difficulty breathing, nausea or vomiting, diarrhea, difficulty swallowing, and any occurrences of swelling or discharge; these symptoms should be reported to the health care provider immediately.
- Wasting syndrome and fluid and electrolyte disturbances: monitor weight gains or losses, skin turgor and dryness, ferritin levels, hemoglobin and hematocrit, and electrolytes. Assist in selecting foods that replenish electrolytes. Initiate measures to control diarrhea; provide intravenous fluids and electrolytes as prescribed.
- Side effects of medications: provide information about purpose, administration, side effects (those reportable to

physician), and strategies to manage or prevent side effects of medications. Carefully monitor laboratory test values.

🏠 Promoting Home and Community-Based Care

Teaching Patients Self-Care

- Thoroughly discuss the disease and all fears and misconceptions; instruct patient, family, and friends about the transmission of AIDs.
- Discuss precautions to prevent transmission of HIV: use of condoms during vaginal or anal intercourse; using dental dam or avoiding oral contact with the penis, vagina, or rectum; avoiding sexual practices that might cut or tear the lining of the rectum, vagina, or penis; and avoiding sexual contact with multiple partners, those known to be HIV positive, those who use illicit injectable drugs, and those who are sexual partners of people who inject drugs.
- Teach how to prevent disease transmission, including hand washing and methods of safely handling items soiled with bodily fluids.
- Instruct patients to not donate blood.
- Emphasize the importance of taking medication as prescribed, and assist patient and caregivers in fitting the medication regimen into their lives.
- Teach medication administration, including intravenous preparations.
- Teach guidelines about infection, follow-up care, diet, rest, and activities.
- Instruct patients and families in how to administer enteral or parenteral feedings, if applicable.
- Give support and guidance in coping with this disease.

Continuing Care

- Refer patient and family for home care nursing or hospice for physical and emotional support.
- Assist families or caregivers in providing supportive care.

- Assist in the administration of parenteral antibiotics, chemotherapy, nutrition, complicated wound care, and respiratory care.
- Provide emotional support to patients and families.
- Refer patients to community programs, housekeeping assistance, meals, transportation, shopping, individual and group therapy, support for caregivers, telephone networks for the homebound, and legal and financial assistance.
- Encourage the patient and family to discuss end-of-life decisions.

Evaluation

EXPECTED OUTCOMES
- Maintains skin integrity
- Resumes usual bowel habits
- Experiences no infections
- Maintains adequate level of activity tolerance
- Maintains usual level of thought processes
- Maintains effective airway clearance
- Experiences increased sense of comfort, less pain
- Maintains adequate nutritional status
- Experiences decreased sense of social isolation
- Progresses through grieving process
- Reports increased understanding of AIDS and participates in self-care activities as possible
- Remains free of complications

NURSING ALERT: PREVENTING HIV TRANSMISSION

- Teach health care workers to apply Standard Precautions to blood and all body fluids, secretions, and excretions except sweat (ie, cerebrospinal fluid; synovial, pleural, peritoneal, pericardial, amniotic, and vaginal fluids; and semen).
- Consider all body fluids to be potentially hazardous in emergency circumstances when differentiation between fluid types is difficult.

For more information, see Chapter 48 in Smeltzer and Bare: *Brunner and Suddarth's Textbook of Medical-Surgical Nursing,* 9th edition. Philadelphia: Lippincott Williams & Wilkins, 2000.

ACUTE RESPIRATORY DISTRESS SYNDROME

Acute respiratory distress syndrome (ARDS; noncardiogenic pulmonary edema) is a clinical syndrome characterized by sudden and progressive edema, increasing bilateral infiltrates, reduced lung compliance, and hypoxemia refractory to oxygen supplementation. ARDS results from an inflammatory "trigger" that causes injury to the alveolar capillary membrane. People at risk for ARDS are those experiencing direct injury to the lungs (eg, aspiration, smoke inhalation, or localized infection) or indirect insult to the lungs (eg, shock or hematologic disorders). The mortality rate of ARDS may be as high as 50% to 60%.

Clinical Manifestations
- Rapid onset of severe dyspnea, usually 12 to 48 hours after an initiating event
- Labored breathing and tachypnea

Diagnostic Evaluation
- Based on clinical criteria: history of risk factors, acute onset of respiratory distress, bilateral pulmonary infiltrates, absence of left heart failure, and severe refractory hypoxemia

Medical Management
- Identify and treat the underlying condition; ensure early detection; use aggressive supportive therapy treatment; prevent infection.
- Provide adequate ventilation initially; as disease progresses, use positive end-expiratory pressure (PEEP).

- Monitor arterial blood gas values, pulse oximetry, and pulmonary function testing.
- Provide circulatory support; treat hypovolemia carefully; and avoid overload.
- Provide adequate fluid management; administer intravenous solutions.
- Provide nutritional support (35 to 45 kcal/kg daily).
- Pharmacologic therapy may include human recombinant interleukin-1 receptor antagonist, neutrophil inhibitors, pulmonary-specific vasodilators, surfactant replacement therapy, antioxidant therapy, and corticosteroids (late in the course of ARDS).

Nursing Management

Assessment

Monitor the patient closely, because ARDS can quickly progress to a life-threatening situation.

Major Nursing Diagnoses

- Impaired gas exchange related to congestion
- Anxiety related to fear of death

Planning and Goals

The goals of patient care may include achieving adequate spontaneous, nonlabored ventilation; maintaining arterial blood gas value within normal limits for patient without ventilator assistance; and ensuring that the patient experiences minimal anxiety.

Nursing Interventions

PROMOTING ADEQUATE VENTILATION

- Facilitate respiratory management: position the patient to maximize respiration, oxygen, endotracheal intubation, tracheostomy, suctioning, and mechanical ventilation with sedation and paralytics as needed.
- Provide safety interventions related to ventilator care.
- Encourage rest.
- Encourage oral fluid intake if patient is not ventilated.

MINIMIZING ANXIETY
- Provide emotional support and reduce patient anxiety.
- Explain all procedures and deliver care in calm, reassuring manner.

Evaluation

EXPECTED OUTCOMES
- Unlabored spontaneous patient respirations
- Arterial blood gases, pulse oximetry, and pulmonary function tests within normal limits

---

For more information, see Chapter 21 in Smeltzer and Bare: *Brunner and Suddarth's Textbook of Medical-Surgical Nursing,* 9th edition. Philadelphia: Lippincott Williams & Wilkins, 2000.

ADDISON'S DISEASE (CHRONIC PRIMARY ADRENOCORTICAL INSUFFICIENCY)

Addison's disease is caused by a deficiency of cortical hormones. It results when the adrenal cortex function is inadequate to meet the patient's need for cortical hormones. Autoimmune or idiopathic atrophy of the adrenal glands is responsible for 80% of cases. Other causes include surgical removal of both adrenal glands or infection (tuberculosis or histoplasmosis) of the adrenal glands. Inadequate secretion of adrenocorticotropic hormone (ACTH) from the primary pituitary gland results in adrenal insufficiency. Symptoms may also result from sudden cessation of exogenous adrenocortical hormonal therapy.

Clinical Manifestations
- The chief clinical manifestations include muscular weakness, anorexia, gastrointestinal symptoms, fatigue, emaciation, dark pigmentation of the skin and mucous membranes, hypotension, low blood glucose, low serum sodium, and high serum potassium.

- Mental changes (depression, emotional lability, apathy, and confusion) are present in 60% to 80% of patients.
- In severe cases, disturbance of sodium and potassium may be marked by depletion of sodium and water and severe, chronic dehydration.

Addisonian Crisis

This medical emergency develops as the disease progresses.

- Cyanosis, fever, and classic signs of shock: pallor, apprehension, rapid and weak pulse, rapid respirations, and low blood pressure
- Complaints of headache, nausea, abdominal pain, diarrhea, signs of confusion, and restlessness
- Slight overexertion, exposure to cold, and acute infections decrease salt intake and may lead to circulatory collapse, shock, and death
- Stress of surgery or dehydration from preparation for diagnostic tests or surgery may precipitate addisonian or hypotensive crisis

Diagnostic Evaluation

Definitive diagnosis is confirmed by low levels of adrenocortical hormones in blood or urine (decreased serum cortisol levels).

Medical Management

Immediate treatment is directed toward combating shock.

- Restore blood circulation, administer fluids, monitor vital signs, and place patient in a recumbent position with legs elevated.
- Administer intravenous hydrocortisone, followed by 5% dextrose in normal saline.
- Vasopressor amines may be required if hypotension persists.
- Antibiotics may be prescribed for infection.
- Oral intake may be initiated as soon as tolerated.
- If the adrenal gland does not regain function, lifelong replacement of corticosteroids and mineralocorticoids is required.

- Dietary intake should be supplemented with salt during times of gastrointestinal losses of fluids through vomiting and diarrhea.

Nursing Management
Assessment
FOCUSING ON FLUID IMBALANCE AND STRESS
- Check blood pressure from a lying to standing position; check pulse rate.
- Assess skin color and turgor.
- Assess history of weight changes, muscle weakness, and fatigue.
- Ask patient and family members about onset of illness or increased stress that may have precipitated crisis.

Major Nursing Diagnoses
- Fluid volume deficit related to inadequate fluid intake and to fluid loss secondary to inadequate adrenal hormone secretion
- Knowledge deficit about the need for hormone replacement and dietary modification

Collaborative Problems/Potential Complications
- Addisonian crisis

Planning and Goals
Goals may include improving fluid balance, improving response to activity, decreasing stress, increasing knowledge about the need for hormone replacement and dietary modifications, and ensuring absence of complications.

Nursing Interventions
RESTORING FLUID BALANCE
- Record weight changes daily.
- Assess skin turgor and mucous membranes.
- Instruct patient to report increased thirst.
- Monitor lying, sitting, and standing blood pressures frequently.

- Assist the patient in selecting, and encourage the patient to consume, food and fluids that assist in restoring and maintaining fluid and electrolyte balance (eg, foods high in sodium during gastrointestinal disturbances and very hot weather). Include a dietitian for added guidance.
- Assist patient and family in learning to administer hormone replacement and to modify dosage during illness and stressful occasions.
- Provide patient with written and verbal instructions about mineralocorticoid and glucocorticoid therapy.

IMPROVING ACTIVITY TOLERANCE
- Take precautions to avoid unnecessary activities and stress that might precipitate a hypotensive episode.
- Detect signs of infection or presence of stressors that may have triggered the crisis.
- Provide a quiet, nonstressful environment during acute crises; all activities are carried out for the patients.
- Explain all procedures to reduce fear and anxiety.
- Explain the rationale for minimizing stress during acute crisis.

MONITORING AND MANAGING COMPLICATIONS (ADDISONIAN CRISIS)
- Assess for signs and symptoms of crisis: circulatory collapse and shock.
- Avoid physical and psychological stress, including exposure to cold, overexertion, infection, and emotional distress.
- Initiate immediate treatment with intravenous fluid, glucose, and electrolytes, especially sodium; corticosteroid supplements; and vasopressors.
- Avoid patient exertion; anticipate and take measures to meet patient's needs.
- Monitor symptoms, vital signs, weight, and fluid and electrolyte balance to evaluate patient's progress to precrisis state.
- Identify factors that led to crisis episode.

🏠 Promoting Home and Community-Based Care

Teaching Patients Self-Care

- Give patient and family members explicit verbal and written instructions about the rationale for replacement therapy and proper dosage.
- Teach the patient and family how to modify the drug dosage and increase salt in times of illness, very hot weather, and stressful situations.
- Instruct patient to modify diet and fluid intake to maintain fluid and electrolyte balance.
- Provide the patient and family with a syringe and vial of injectable steroid (Solu-Cortef) for emergency use and instruct when and how to use.
- Advise patient to inform health care providers (eg, dentists) of receiving steroids, and wear a medical alert bracelet.
- Teach patient and family the signs of excessive or insufficient hormone replacement.
- Instruct patient regarding modification of diet (sodium) for illness and hot weather to maintain fluid and electrolyte balance.

Continuing Care

- Encourage patients to weigh themselves daily and detect significant changes in weight that indicate fluid loss (due to too much hormone) or retention (due to too little hormone).
- If the patient is unable to return to work and family responsibilities after hospital discharge, refer to home health care nurse.
- Assess recovery, monitor hormone replacement, and assess stress in the home.
- Assess patient's plans for follow-up visits to the clinic or a physician's office.

For more information, see Chapter 38 in Smeltzer and Bare: *Brunner and Suddarth's Textbook of Medical-Surgical Nursing*, 9th edition. Philadelphia: Lippincott Williams & Wilkins, 2000.

ALZHEIMER'S DISEASE

Alzheimer's disease (AD) is one of the three most common nonreversible dementias. Dementia is an acquired syndrome in which progressive deterioration in global intellectual abilities occurs, which interferes with the person's customary occupational and social performance. Specific neuropathologic and biochemical changes are noted with AD that result in decreased brain size and decreased acetylcholine production. This degenerative neurologic disease begins insidiously and is characterized by gradual loss of cognitive and functional abilities and disturbances in behavior and affect. Family history and the presence of Down's syndrome are two risk factors for AD. In addition, genetic studies have linked familial Alzheimer's disease (FAD) to chromosomes 21, 14, and 1 as well as to the apolipoprotein E gene locus on chromosome 19 that is linked with either an increased risk for late-onset AD (after 65 years of age) or protection against this risk. Death occurs as a result of a complicating condition such as pneumonia, malnutrition, or dehydration.

Clinical Manifestations

Symptoms are highly variable:

- Early in disease, forgetfulness and subtle memory loss occur.
- Social skills and behavior patterns remain intact (early).
- Forgetfulness is manifested in many daily actions with progression of the disease (eg, the patient gets lost in a familiar environment or repeats the same stories).
- The ability to formulate concepts and think abstractly disappears.
- The patient may exhibit inappropriate impulsive behavior.
- Personality changes are negative; the patient may become depressed, suspicious, paranoid, hostile, and even combative.

- Speaking skills deteriorate to nonsense syllables; agitation and physical activity increase.
- Voracious appetite may develop from high activity level; dysphagia is noted with disease progression.
- Eventually the patient requires help with all aspects of daily living, including toileting because incontinence occurs.
- The terminal stage may last for months.

Diagnostic Evaluation

The diagnosis is one of exclusion and is confirmed by autopsy.

- Clinical symptoms found through health history, including physical findings
- Electroencephalography (EEG)
- Computed tomography (CT) scan
- Magnetic resonance imaging (MRI)
- Examination of laboratory tests, primarily blood and cerebrospinal fluid (CSF)

Nursing Management

Assessment

- Perform history and physical examination, noting symptoms indicating dementia; report to physician.
- Assist with diagnostic evaluation, promoting calm environment to maximize patient safety and cooperation.

Major Nursing Diagnoses

- Altered thought processes related to decline in cognitive function
- Risk for injury related to decline in cognitive function
- Anxiety related to confused thought processes
- Altered nutrition: less than body requirements related to cognitive decline
- Activity intolerance related to imbalance in activity-rest pattern
- Self-care deficit, bathing/hygiene, feeding, toileting related to cognitive decline
- Impaired social interaction related to cognitive decline

- Knowledge deficit of family/caregiver related to care for patient as cognitive function declines
- Altered family processes related to decline in patient's cognitive function

Planning and Goals

Goals may include maintenance of physical safety, reduction of anxiety, maintenance of adequate nutrition, improvement of communication, promotion of independence, management of sleep pattern disturbances, provision for patient needs for socialization and intimacy, and support and education of caregivers.

Nursing Interventions

SUPPORTING COGNITIVE FUNCTION

- Provide a calm, predictable environment.
- Minimize confusion and disorientation; give the patient a sense of security with a quiet, pleasant manner, clear simple explanations, and use of memory aids and cues.

PROMOTING PHYSICAL SAFETY

- Provide a safe environment to allow patient to move about as freely as possible and relieve family worry about safety.
- Prevent falls and other accidents by removing obvious hazards.
- Monitor the patient's intake of medications and food.
- Allow smoking only with supervision.
- Reduce wandering behavior with gentle persuasion and distraction.
- Avoid restraints because they may increase agitation.
- Secure doors leading from the house.
- Supervise all activities outside the home to protect the patient.
- Ensure that patient wears an identification bracelet or neck chain.

REDUCING ANXIETY AND AGITATION

- Give constant emotional support to reinforce a positive self-image.

- When skill losses occur, adjust goals to fit with patient's declining ability.
- Structuring activities is helpful to avoid agitation.
- Keep the environment simple, familiar, and noise free.
- Remain calm and unhurried, particularly during a combative, agitated state known as *catastrophic reaction* (overreaction to excessive stimulation).
- Promote the patient's interpretation of messages by remaining unhurried and by reducing noises and distractions.
- Use easy-to-understand sentences to convey messages.

PROMOTING ADEQUATE NUTRITION
- Keep mealtimes simple and calm without confrontations.
- Cut food into small pieces to prevent choking, and convert liquids to gelatin to ease swallowing.
- Prevent burns by serving hot food and beverages warm.
- Offer one dish at a time.

PROMOTING BALANCED ACTIVITY AND REST
- Access to the outdoors should be blocked.
- Help the patient to relax to sleep with music, warm milk, or a back rub.
- Give sufficient opportunities to participate in exercise activities to enhance nighttime sleep.
- Discourage long periods of daytime sleeping.
- Assess and address any unmet underlying physical or psychological needs that may prompt wandering or other inappropriate behavior.

PROMOTING INDEPENDENCE IN SELF-CARE ACTIVITIES
- Simplify daily activities into short achievable steps so that the patient can experience a sense of accomplishment.
- Maintain personal dignity and autonomy.
- Encourage the patient to make choices when appropriate and to participate in self-care activities as much as possible.

PROVIDING FOR SOCIALIZATION AND INTIMACY
NEEDS

- Encourage visits, letters, and phone calls (visits should be brief and nonstressful with one to two visitors at a time).
- Advise that the nonjudgmental friendliness of a pet can provide satisfying activity and an outlet for energy.
- Encourage the spouse to talk about any sexual concerns, and suggest sexual counseling if necessary.

🏠 Promoting Home and Community-Based Care

- Be sensitive to the highly emotional issues that the family is confronting.
- Refer to the Alzheimer's Association for family support groups, respite care, and adult day care.

Evaluation

EXPECTED OUTCOMES

- Patient maintains cognitive, functional, and social interaction abilities for as long as possible.
- Patient remains free of injury.
- Patient demonstrates minimal anxiety and agitation.
- Patient communicates needs.
- Patient's socialization and intimacy needs are met.
- Patient and family caregivers are knowledgeable about condition and treatment and care regimens.

For more information, see Chapter 11 in Smeltzer and Bare: *Brunner and Suddarth's Textbook of Medical-Surgical Nursing,* 9th edition. Philadelphia: Lippincott Williams & Wilkins, 2000.

AMYOTROPHIC LATERAL SCLEROSIS

Amyotrophic lateral sclerosis (ALS) is a disease of unknown cause in which there is a loss of motor neurons (nerve cells controlling muscles) in the anterior horns of the spinal cord and the motor nuclei of the lower brain stem. As these cells die, the muscle fibers that they supply undergo atrophic changes. The degeneration of the neurons may occur in both the upper and lower motor neuron systems. ALS affects more men than women, with onset occurring usually in the fifth or sixth decade of life. In the United States, it is often referred to as *Lou Gehrig's disease.* Death occurs from infection, respiratory failure, or aspiration. The average time from onset to death is about 3 years.

Clinical Manifestations

The clinical features of ALS depend on the location of the affected motor neurons. In most patients, the chief symptoms are progressive muscle weakness, atrophy, and fasciculations (twitching).

Symptoms of Patients With Loss of Motor Neurons in the Anterior Horns of the Spinal Cord

- Progressive weakness and atrophy of the muscles are noted in the arms, trunk, or legs.
- Spasticity is usually present, and deep tendon stretch reflexes are brisk and overactive.
- Anal and bladder sphincters are not affected.

Symptoms of Patients With Weakness in the Musculature Supplied by the Cranial Nerves (25% of Patients in Early Stage)

- Difficulty talking, swallowing, and ultimately breathing
- Soft palate and upper esophageal weakness, causing liquids to be regurgitated through the nose
- Impaired ability to laugh, cough, or blow the nose

Symptoms of Patients With Bulbar Muscle Impairment

- Progressive difficulty in speaking, swallowing, and aspiration
- Nasal voice and unintelligible speech
- Emotional lability, but intellectual function unimpaired
- Eventually, compromised respiratory function

Diagnostic Evaluation

- Diagnosis is based on signs and symptoms because no clinical or laboratory tests are specific for this disease.
- Electromyographic (EMG) studies are beneficial.

Medical Management

No specific treatment for ALS is available.

Symptomatic Treatment and Rehabilitative Measures

- Baclofen, dantrolene sodium, or diazepam for spasticity
- Quinine for muscle cramps
- Nasogastric feedings, cervical esophagostomy, or gastrostomy for patients with aspiration or swallowing difficulties

Mechanical Ventilation

- Decision is based on patient and family's understanding of the disease, prognosis, and implications of initiating such therapy.
- Encourage patient to complete an advance directive or "living will" to preserve autonomy.

Nursing Management

The nursing care of the patient with ALS is generally the same as the basic care plan for patients with degenerative neurologic disorders (see Myasthenia Gravis).

For more information, see Chapter 59 in Smeltzer and Bare: *Brunner and Suddarth's Textbook of Medical-Surgical Nursing,* 9th edition. Philadelphia: Lippincott Williams & Wilkins, 2000.

●ANAPHYLAXIS

Anaphylaxis is a clinical response to an immediate (type I hypersensitivity) immunologic reaction between a specific antigen and an immunoglobulin E antibody. An anaphylactoid (anaphylaxis-like) reaction is clinically similar to anaphylaxis and may occur with medications, food, exercise, and cytotoxic antibody transfusions. Reactions may be local or systemic. Local anaphylactic reactions usually involve urticaria and angioedema at the site of exposure and can be severe but are rarely fatal. Systemic reactions occur in major organ systems within about 30 minutes of exposure.

Clinical Manifestations
Mild
- Peripheral tingling; a warm sensation; fullness in the mouth and throat
- Nasal congestion; periorbital swelling, pruritus; sneezing; tearing of the eyes
- Symptom onset within the first 2 hours of exposure

Moderate
- May include any of the mild symptoms plus anxiety, bronchospasm, and edema of the airways or larynx with dyspnea, cough, and wheezing
- Same onset of symptoms same as with a mild reaction

Severe
- An abrupt onset with the same signs and symptoms described above, progressing rapidly to bronchospasm, laryngeal edema, severe dyspnea, and cyanosis
- Dysphagia, abdominal cramping, vomiting, diarrhea, and seizures
- Cardiac arrest and coma, rarely

Medical Management
PREVENTION
- Obtain careful history of any sensitivities *before* administering medications.

- Venom immunotherapy may be given to people allergic to insect venom.
- Insulin-allergic diabetic patients or penicillin-sensitive patients may require desensitization.

Treatment

- Evaluate respiratory and cardiovascular function.
- Institute cardiopulmonary resuscitation (CPR) if in cardiac arrest.
- Provide oxygen in high concentrations during CPR or when cyanotic, dyspneic, or wheezing.
- Give epinephrine, antihistamines, and steroids to prevent recurrences of the reaction and for urticaria and angioedema. Aminophylline may be administered if indicated.
- Use volume expanders and vasopressor agents to maintain blood pressure and normal hemodynamic status; glucagon may be used.
- Educate patients with mild reactions about risk for potential recurrences.
- Closely observe patients with severe reactions for 12 to 14 hours.

Nursing Management

🏠 Promoting Home and Community-Based Care

Prevention is the most important aspect of anaphylaxis.

- Teach people who are sensitive to insect bites and stings, have food or medication reactions, or have idiopathic or exercise-induced anaphylactic reactions strategies to avoid exposure to allergens.
- Instruct patient to always carry an emergency kit that contains epinephrine.
- Provide verbal and written instruction about the emergency kit.
- Ensure patient's ability to demonstrate correct self-injection.

- Encourage patient to wear identification, such as MedicAlert bracelet.

For more information, see Chapter 49 in Smeltzer and Bare: *Brunner and Suddarth's Textbook of Medical-Surgical Nursing,* 9th edition. Philadelphia: Lippincott Williams & Wilkins, 2000.

ANEMIA

Anemia is a condition of lower-than-normal red blood cell (RBC) count and hemoglobin (Hgb) level. Anemia results in a diminished amount of oxygen delivery to body tissues. There are many different kinds of anemia, but all can be classified as being due to either a decrease in production of RBCs, excessive destruction of RBCs, or a loss of RBCs (bleeding). Other etiologic factors include deficits in iron and nutrients, hereditary factors, and chronic diseases. Complications of severe anemia include congestive heart failure, paresthesias and confusion, and other problems specific to the type of anemia.

Clinical Manifestations

Several factors influence the development of anemia, including its severity, speed of development (the faster the onset, the more severe the symptoms), and duration (ie, its chronicity); the patient's metabolic requirements; coexisting disorders or disabilities (eg, cardiopulmonary disease); and special complications or features of the condition that produced the anemia. Pronounced symptoms of anemia include the following:

- Dyspnea, chest pain, muscle pain or cramping, tachycardia
- Weakness, fatigue, general malaise
- Pallor of the skin and mucous membranes (sclera, oral mucosa)
- Jaundice (megaloblastic or hemolytic anemia)
- Smooth, red tongue (iron-deficiency anemia)

- Beefy-red, sore tongue (megaloblastic anemia)
- Angular cheilosis (ulceration of the corner of the mouth)
- Brittle, ridged, concave nails and pica (unusual craving for starch, dirt, ice) in patients with iron-deficiency anemia

Diagnostic Evaluation

- Complete hematologic studies (ie, Hgb, hematocrit, reticulocyte count, and RBC indices, particularly mean corpuscular volume)
- Iron studies (serum iron level, total iron-binding capacity, percentage saturation, and ferritin)
- Serum vitamin B_{12} and folate levels; haptoglobin and erythropoietin levels
- Bone marrow aspiration and biopsy
- Other studies as indicated to determine underlying illness

Medical Management

- Correct or control the cause of the anemia
- Replace lost or destroyed RBCs

Nursing Management

Assessment

- Obtain a health history, physical examination, and laboratory values
- Ask patient about the extent and type of symptoms experienced and the impact of those symptoms on the patient's lifestyle; medication history; alcohol intake; athletic endeavors.
- Ask patient about any loss of blood (eg, excessive menses or vaginal bleeding), use of iron supplements during pregnancy.
- Question family history regarding inherited anemias
- Perform nutritional assessment: ask about dietary habits resulting in nutritional deficiencies, such as iron, vitamin B_{12}, and folic acid.
- Monitor relevant laboratory test results; note changes.

- Assess cardiac status (for symptoms of increased work-load or congestive heart failure):
  - Tachycardia, palpitations, dyspnea
  - Dizziness, orthopnea, exertional dyspnea
  - Cardiomegaly, hepatomegaly, peripheral edema
- Assess for neurologic deficits:
  - Presence and extent of peripheral numbness and paresthesias
  - Ataxia and poor coordination
  - Confusion
- Assess for gastrointestinal function:
  - Nausea, vomiting
  - Diarrhea, melena or dark stools, occult blood
  - Anorexia, glossitis

Major Nursing Diagnoses

- Activity intolerance related to weakness, fatigue, and general malaise
- Altered nutrition: less than body requirements related to inadequate intake of essential nutrients
- Altered tissue perfusion related to inadequate blood volume or hematocrit
- Noncompliance with prescribed therapy

Collaborative Problems/Potential Complications

- Congestive heart failure
- Paresthesias
- Confusion

Planning and Goals

The major goals may include tolerance of normal activity, attainment or maintenance of adequate nutrition, compliance with prescribed therapy, and absence of complications.

Nursing Interventions

MANAGING FATIGUE

- Assist the patient to prioritize activities and establish a balance between activity and rest.

- Encourage the patient with chronic anemia to maintain physical activity and exercise to prevent deconditioning.
- Use safety precautions to prevent falls from poor coordination, paresthesias, and weakness.

MONITORING AND MANAGING COMPLICATIONS
- Decrease activities and stimuli that cause an increase in heart rate and cardiac output.
- Encourage patient to identify situations that precipitate palpitations and dyspnea.
- Administer oxygen; elevate head of bed for dyspnea.
- Monitor vital signs and observe for indications of fluid retention.
- Monitor for signs of paresthesia, poor coordination, ataxia, and confusion.
- Implement safety measures to prevent injury.

MAINTAINING ADEQUATE NUTRITION
- Encourage a well-balanced diet high in protein, high caloric foods, fruits, and vegetables.
- Teach patient to avoid or limit intake of alcohol and spicy (irritating) and gas-producing foods.
- Plan dietary teaching sessions for patient and family; consider cultural aspects of nutrition.
- Discuss dietary supplements (eg, vitamins, iron, folate) as prescribed.

MAINTAINING ADEQUATE PERFUSION
- Monitor vital signs closely, and adjust or withhold medications (antihypertensives) as indicated.
- Administer supplemental oxygen, transfusions, and intravenous fluids as ordered.

MONITORING AND MANAGING
POTENTIAL COMPLICATIONS
- Assess the patient with anemia for congestive heart failure.
- Obtain and record body weights in addition to intake and output.
- Administer diuretics as ordered.

- Perform a neurologic assessment: note paresthesias, signs of spinal cord damage, gait disturbance, problems with balance, mild but gradual confusion, diminished sense of position and vibration.

🏠 Promoting Home and Community-Based Care

Promoting Compliance With Prescribed Therapy
- Teach patient and family the purpose of prescribed medication, how and how long to take the medication, and how to manage side effects of therapy.
- Assist patients in developing ways to incorporate the therapeutic plan into their lifestyle.
- Inform the patient that abruptly stopping some medications may have serious consequences.
- Assist patient with obtaining needed insurance coverage or exploring alternatives for obtaining expensive medications, if needed.

🍁 Gerontologic Considerations

- Anemia is the most common hematologic condition that affects elderly people. This population typically has a decreased ability of the bone marrow to respond to the body's need for blood cells.
- The elderly person may be unable to increase blood cell production adequately in cases of increased need, seriously affecting cardiopulmonary function.
- Identify and treat the cause of anemia rather than considering it a consequence of aging.
- Elderly people with a concurrent cardiac or pulmonary problem may be unable to tolerate the anemia. A prompt, thorough evaluation of the anemia is warranted.

Evaluation
EXPECTED OUTCOMES
- Tolerates activity at level that is safe and acceptable
- Attains and maintains adequate nutrition

- Maintains adequate perfusion
- Experiences no or minimal complications

For more information, see Chapter 30 in Smeltzer and Bare: *Brunner and Suddarth's Textbook of Medical-Surgical Nursing,* 9th edition. Philadelphia: Lippincott Williams & Wilkins, 2000.

ANEMIA, APLASTIC

Aplastic anemia (hypoproliferative) is a rare disease caused by a decrease in or damage to marrow stem cells in the bone marrow and replacement of the marrow with fat. It can be congenital or acquired. It may be idiopathic, result from certain infections or from pregnancy, or be caused by medications, chemicals, or radiation damage. The most common offenders are antimicrobials (chloramphenicol), benzene, several pesticides, inorganic arsenic, anticonvulsants, phenylbutazone, sulfonamides, and gold compounds. A prompt and complete recovery may be anticipated if patient exposure is terminated early. Death is usually caused by hemorrhage or infection.

Clinical Manifestations
- Gradual onset marked by fatigue and pallor; dyspnea on exertion
- Purpura (bleeding), retinal hemorrhages are common
- Repeated throat infections with possible lymphadenopathy and splenomegaly

Diagnostic Evaluation
- Complete blood count and analysis are performed.
- Diagnosis is made by bone marrow aspirate and biopsy.

Medical Management
- Bone marrow peripheral stem cell transplantation
- Administration of immunosuppressive therapy with antithymocyte globulin (ATG) and cyclosporine

Preventive Management
- Use potentially toxic medications only when alternative therapies are not available.
- Monitor blood cell counts in patients receiving potentially bone marrow–toxic drugs, such as chloramphenicol.

Supportive Therapy
- Discontinue any offending drug.
- Prevent symptoms with transfusions of red blood cells and platelets.
- Protect patients with pronounced leukopenia from contact with people who have infections.

Nursing Management
See Nursing Management under Anemia for additional information.

- Preserve patient's energy by planning care depending on the degree of weakness and fatigue.
- Assess for signs of infection and bleeding; use meticulous care of intravenous sites or wounds and avoid trauma.
- Guard against any wound, abrasion, or ulcer of mucous membrane or skin as a potential site of infection.
- Encourage and assist with meticulous body and oral hygiene (with soft toothbrush, no floss).
- Avoid trauma when possible (including subcutaneous and intramuscular injections, padded side rails, avoidance of suctioning) when thrombocytopenia is present.

🏠 Promoting Home and Community-Based Care

- Teach patient the importance of regular atraumatic bowel movements and to use stool softeners and oral laxatives because hemorrhoids can develop and become infected or bleed.
- Protect patients with pronounced leukopenia from contact with people who have infections.

- Teach people taking toxic drugs on a long-term basis the need for periodic blood studies and symptoms that should be reported.

For more information, see Chapter 30 in Smeltzer and Bare: *Brunner and Suddarth's Textbook of Medical-Surgical Nursing,* 9th edition. Philadelphia: Lippincott Williams & Wilkins, 2000.

ANEMIA, IRON-DEFICIENCY

Iron-deficiency anemia is a condition in which the total-body iron content is decreased below a normal level and iron stores are depleted. It is the most common type of anemia in the world. It typically results when the intake of dietary iron is inadequate to maintain the level necessary for hemoglobin synthesis. For most adults, blood loss is the cause of this anemia. Risk factors include a history of ulcers, gastritis, intestinal hookworm, gastrointestinal tumors, malabsorption, or diet very high in fiber (prevents iron absorption). The most frequent cause in premenopausal women is menorrhagia. Chronic alcoholism often causes inadequate iron intake and loss of iron through blood from the gastrointestinal tract.

Clinical Manifestations
- Symptoms of anemia: fatigue, irritability, numbness, and tingling of extremities
- Symptoms in more severe cases: smooth, sore tongue; brittle and ridged nails; and angular cheilosis (mouth ulceration)
- Pica (unusual cravings, such as for clay, ice, or starch), a history of multiple pregnancy, or gastrointestinal bleeding
- Hemoglobin proportionately lower than hematocrit and red blood cell count
- Serum iron concentration low
- Total iron-binding capacity high; serum ferritin low

Diagnostic Evaluation
- Bone Marrow Aspirate
- Laboratory values, including serum ferritin levels (indicates iron stores), blood count (hemoglobin, hematocrit, red blood cell count, mean corpuscular volume), serum iron level, and total iron-binding capacity

Medical Management
- Search for the cause, which may be a curable gastrointestinal cancer or uterine fibroids.
- Test stool specimens for occult blood.
- Administer prescribed iron preparations (oral, intramuscular, or intravenous).
- Avoid tablets with enteric coating; may be poorly absorbed.
- Continue iron for a year after bleeding has been controlled.

Nursing Management
See Nursing Management under Anemia for additional information.
- Administer intramuscular or intravenous iron in some cases when oral iron is not absorbed, is poorly tolerated, or is needed in large amounts.
- Administer a small test dose before intramuscular injection to avoid risk of anaphylaxis (which is greater with intramuscular than with intravenous injections).

🏠 Providing Home and Community-Based Care

Teaching Patients Self-Care
- Advise patient to take iron supplements an hour before meals. If gastric distress occurs, suggest taking the supplement with meals and, after symptoms subside, resuming between-meal schedule for maximum absorption.
- Inform the patient that iron salts change stool to dark green or black color.
- Advise the patient to brush and floss teeth frequently because ferrous sulfate is likely to be deposited on the

teeth and gums; take liquid iron through a straw and rinse mouth with water.

- Teach preventive education because iron-deficiency anemia is common in menstruating and pregnant women.
- Educate patients regarding food sources high in iron (eg, organ and other meats, beans, leafy green vegetables, raisins, and molasses).
- Advise the patient to take iron-rich foods with vitamin C to enhance absorption.
- Inform the patient to avoid taking antacids or dairy products with iron.
- Provide nutritional counseling for those whose normal diet is inadequate.
- Encourage patient to continue iron therapy for total therapy time (6 to 12 months), even when they no longer feel fatigued.

Evaluation

EXPECTED OUTCOMES

See Nursing Management under Anemia for additional information.

For more information, see Chapter 30 in Smeltzer and Bare: *Brunner and Suddarth's Textbook of Medical-Surgical Nursing,* 9th edition. Philadelphia: Lippincott Williams & Wilkins, 2000.

ANEMIA, MEGALOBLASTIC (VITAMIN B$_{12}$ AND FOLIC ACID DEFICIENCY)

The anemias caused by deficiencies of the vitamins B$_{12}$ and folic acid show identical bone marrow and peripheral blood changes. Both vitamins are essential for DNA synthesis. The two anemias may coexist. In each case, hyperplasia of the marrow occurs, and the precursor erythroid and myeloid cells are large and bizarre. A pancytopenia develops.

Vitamin B$_{12}$ deficiency can occur from inadequate intake in strict vegetarians; faulty absorption from the gastrointestinal tract; absence of intrinsic factor (pernicious anemia); disease involving the ilium or pancreas, which impairs B_{12} absorption; and gastrectomy. People with pernicious anemia have a higher incidence of gastric cancer than the general public.

Folic acid deficiency occurs when intake of folate is deficient or the requirement is increased. People at risk include those who rarely eat uncooked vegetables or fruits—primarily elderly people living alone or people with alcoholism. Alcohol, hemolytic anemia, and pregnancy increase folic acid requirements. Patients with malabsorptive or small bowel disease may not absorb folic acid normally.

Clinical Manifestations
Symptoms are progressive and may be marked by spontaneous partial remissions and exacerbations.
- Gradual development of signs of anemia (weakness, listlessness, and pallor)
- Possible development of a smooth, sore, red tongue and mild diarrhea (pernicious anemia)
- Possible development of confusion; more often, paresthesias in the extremities and difficulty keeping balance; loses position sense
- Lack of neurologic manifestations with folic acid deficiency alone
- Vitiligo (patchy loss of skin pigmentation) and premature graying hair (often seen in pernicious anemia)
- Without treatment, patients die, usually from congestive heart failure from anemia

Diagnostic Evaluation
- Schilling test (primary diagnostic tool)
- Complete blood count
- Serum levels of folate and vitamin B_{12}

Medical Management
Vitamin B_{12} Deficiency
- Oral supplementation with vitamins or fortified soy milk (strict vegetarians)

- Intramuscular injections of vitamin B_{12} for defective absorption or absence of intrinsic factor
- Prevention of recurrence with lifetime vitamin B_{12} therapy for patient who has had pernicious anemia or noncorrectable malabsorption

Folic Acid Deficiency

- Intake of a nutritious diet and 1 mg of folic acid daily
- Intramuscular folic acid for malabsorption syndromes
- Folic acid taken orally as a separate tablet (except prenatal vitamins)
- Folic acid replacement stopped when hemoglobin returns to normal, with the exception of alcoholics, who continue replacement as long as alcohol intake is continued

Nursing Management

See Nursing Management under Anemia for additional information.

Assessment

- Assess patients at risk for megaloblastic anemia for clinical manifestation (eg, inspecting the skin, sclera, and mucous membranes for jaundice, noting vitiligo or premature graying, or smooth, red, sore tongue).
- Perform a careful neurologic assessment (eg, note gait and stability; test position and vibration sense).

🏠 Promoting Home and Community-Based Care

Teaching Patients Self-Care

- Assess the need for assistive devices (eg, canes, walkers) and the need for support and guidance in managing activities of daily living and the home environment.
- Ensure safety when position sense, coordination, and gait are affected.
- Refer for physical or occupational therapy as needed.
- When sensation is altered, instruct patient to avoid excessive heat and cold.

- Advise patients to prepare bland, soft foods and to eat small amounts frequently.
- Explain that other nutritional deficiencies, such as alcohol-induced anemia, can induce neurologic problems.
- Instruct patient in complete urine collections for the Schilling test and to enhance the patient's understanding and ability to comply with this collection.
- Teach patients about the chronicity of their disorder and the necessity for monthly vitamin B_{12} injections even when the patient has no symptoms; instruct patient to self-administer their injections, when appropriate.
- Stress the importance of ongoing medical follow-up and screening because gastric atrophy associated with pernicious anemia increases the risk of gastric carcinoma.

For more information, see Chapter 30 in Smeltzer and Bare: *Brunner and Suddarth's Textbook of Medical-Surgical Nursing,* 9th edition. Philadelphia: Lippincott Williams & Wilkins, 2000.

ANEMIA, SICKLE CELL

Sickle cell anemia is a severe hemolytic anemia resulting from the inheritance of the sickle hemoglobin gene (HbS), which causes a defective hemoglobin molecule. The molecule assumes a sickle shape when exposed to low oxygen tension. These long, rigid cells become lodged in small vessels and can obstruct blood flow to body tissue, causing ischemia and possibly necrosis ("sickling crisis"). The HbS gene is inherited with some people having the sickle cell trait (a carrier, inheriting one abnormal gene) and some having sickle cell disease (inheriting two abnormal genes). Sickled RBCs have a shortened life span, resulting in anemia. Sickle cell disease is found predominantly in people of African descent and less often in people descended from the Mediterranean countries, the Middle East, or aboriginal tribes of India.

Clinical Manifestations
- Symptoms and complications result from chronic hemolysis or thrombosis.
- Anemia with hemoglobin values in the 7 to 10 g/dL range.
- Jaundice is characteristic, most obvious in the sclera.
- Bone marrow expands in childhood, sometimes causing enlargement of bones of the face and skull.
- Tachycardia, cardiac murmurs, and often cardiomegaly are associated with chronic anemia.
- Dysrhythmias and heart failure may occur in adults.
- There is pain in various parts of the body. All tissues and organs are vulnerable and susceptible to hypoxic damage or true ischemic necrosis at any time.
- Sickle cell crisis occurs: painful crisis, aplastic crisis, or sequestration crisis.
- Acute chest syndrome occurs: rapidly falling hemoglobin level, tachycardia, fever, and bilateral infiltrates seen on chest radiographs.

Diagnostic Evaluation
- Hemoglobin and hematocrit levels, blood smear, hemoglobin electrophoresis
- Isoelectric focusing, high-performance liquid chromatography techniques
- Sickling occurs whether the patient has sickle trait or sickle cell anemia; only electrophoresis shows a distinction

Medical Management
- Many antisickling drugs are undergoing trial; currently, hydroxyurea has been shown to be effective (increases fetal hemoglobin production).
- Bone marrow transplantation is a potential cure but is limited because of lack of donors or organ damage.
- Chronic transfusions with red blood cells are done for exacerbation of anemia, for prevention of complications, or to improve response to infection.

- Pulmonary function is monitored, pulmonary hypertension is treated early, if found.
- Infections and acute chest syndrome, which predispose to crises, are treated promptly.
- Incentive spirometry is performed to prevent pulmonary complications; bronchoscopy is done to identify source of pulmonary disease.
- Fluid restriction (not addressive hydration) may be beneficial; steroids may be useful.
- Folic acid therapy is administered daily for increased marrow requirement.
- Supportive care involves pain management, oral or intravenous hydration, supplemental oxygen, physical and occupational therapy, physiotherapy, cognitive and behavioral intervention, and support groups.

Nursing Management

See Nursing Management under Anemia for additional information.

Assessment

- Question patients in crisis about factors that could have precipitated the crisis and measures used to prevent crises.
- Assess all body systems, with particular emphasis on pain, swelling, and fever (all joint areas and abdomen).
- Elicit symptoms of cerebral hypoxia by careful neurologic examination.
- Carefully assess respiratory system, including breath sounds and oxygen saturation levels.
- Assess for signs of cardiac failure (edema, increased point of maximal impulse, and cardiomegaly) by radiography.
- Assess for signs of dehydration and history of fluid intake; examine mucous membranes, skin turgor, urine output, serum creatinine, and blood urea nitrogen values.
- Assess current and past history of medical management, particularly chronic transfusion therapy, hydroxyurea use, and prior treatment for infection.

- Assess for the presence of any infectious process (examine the chest and long bones and femoral head because pneumonia and osteomyelitis are common).
- Monitor hemoglobin, hematocrit, and reticulocyte count and compare with baseline levels.
- Discuss history of alcohol intake.

Major Nursing Diagnoses
- Pain related to tissue hypoxia due to agglutination of sickled cells within blood vessels
- Risk for infection
- Powerlessness related to illness-induced helplessness
- Knowledge deficit regarding prevention of crisis

Collaborative Problems/Potential Complications
- Hypoxia, ischemia, infection, and poor wound healing leading to skin breakdown and ulcers
- Dehydration
- Cerebrovascular accident (stroke)
- Anemia
- Heart failure, pulmonary hypertension, and acute chest syndrome
- Impotence, priapism
- Renal dysfunction
- Substance abuse related to chronic pain
- Poor compliance

Planning and Goals
The major goals include relief of pain, prevention of crisis, enhanced sense of self-esteem and power, and absence of complications.

Nursing Interventions
MANAGING PAIN
- Use the patient's subjective description of pain and pain rating on a pain scale to guide the use of analgesics.
- Support and elevate any joint that is acutely swollen until the swelling diminishes.

- Teach the patient relaxation techniques, breathing exercises, and distraction to help the pain.
- When the acute painful episode has diminished, implement aggressive measures to preserve function (eg, physical therapy, whirlpool baths, and transcutaneous nerve stimulation).

PREVENTING AND MANAGING INFECTION
- Monitor the patient for signs and symptoms of infection.
- Initiate prescribed antibiotics promptly.
- Assess the patient for signs of dehydration.
- Teach the patient to take prescribed oral antibiotics at home, if indicated, emphasizing the need to complete the entire course of antibiotic therapy; assist the patient to identify a feasible administration schedule.

PROMOTING COPING SKILLS
- Enhance pain management to promote a therapeutic relationship based on mutual trust.
- Focus on the patient's strengths rather than deficits to enhance effective coping skills.
- Provide opportunities for the patient to make decisions about daily care to increase feelings of control.

Promoting Home and Community-Based Care

Minimizing Knowledge Deficit
- Teach the patient with sickle cell anemia the situations that can precipitate a sickle cell crisis and steps they can take to prevent or diminish such crises (eg, keep warm, maintain adequate hydration, avoid stressful situations).
- Arrange for group education, when possible, carried out by members of the community who are from the same ethnic group as those with the disease.

Managing Complications
Management measures for many of the potential complications are delineated in the previous sections; addi-

tional measures should be taken to address the following issues.

LEG ULCERS
- When present, carefully manage leg ulcers and protect leg from trauma and contamination.
- Use scrupulous aseptic technique to prevent nosocomial infections.

PRIAPISM LEADING TO IMPOTENCE
- Teach the patient to empty the bladder at the onset of the attack, to exercise, and then to take a warm bath.
- Inform the patient that if an episode persists more than 3 hours, medical attention is recommended.

CHRONIC PAIN AND SUBSTANCE ABUSE
- Emphasize the importance of complying with a prescribed treatment plan.
- Use a nonjudgmental attitude, and actively seek involvement from the patient in establishing a treatment plan and developing useful strategies.
- Promote trust with the patient through adequate management of acute pain during episodes of crisis.
- Suggest to the patient that receiving care from a single provider over time is much more beneficial than receiving care from rotating physicians and staff in an emergency department.
- When emergent crises do arise, the staff in the emergency department should contact the patient's primary health care provider so that optimal management is achieved.
- Promote continuity of care and establish written contracts with the patient.

Evaluation
EXPECTED OUTCOMES
- Reports control of pain
- Is free of infection
- Expresses improved sense of control

- Increases knowledge about disease process
- Experiences absence of complications

For more information, see Chapter 30 in Smeltzer and Bare: *Brunner and Suddarth's Textbook of Medical-Surgical Nursing,* 9th edition. Philadelphia: Lippincott Williams & Wilkins, 2000.

ANEURYSM, AORTIC

An aneurysm is a localized sac or dilation of an artery formed at a weak point in the vessel wall. The most common cause is atherosclerosis. Saccular and fusiform are the most common forms of aneurysm. Saccular aneurysms project from one side of the vessel only; fusiform aneurysms involve dilation of an entire arterial segment. Mycotic aneurysms are small aneurysms due to local infections. Aortic aneurysms are usually classified as thoracic, abdominal, or dissecting. Other causes include trauma to the wall of the artery, infection (pyogenic or syphilitic), and congenital defects of the artery wall. Men are affected more often than women. Rupture can lead to hemorrhage and death.

Thoracic aortic aneurysms occur most frequently in men between the ages of 40 and 70 years. The thoracic area is the most common site for the development of a dissecting aneurysm. About one third of patients die from rupture. *Abdominal aortic aneurysms* are more common among whites between the ages of 60 and 90 years. Most occur below the renal arteries. Forty percent of patients have symptoms. Risk factors include genetic predisposition, smoking, and hypertension. A *dissecting aneurysm of the aorta* is caused by rupture in the intimal layer resulting in blood dissecting the vessel layers. It is often associated with poorly controlled hypertension and is three times more common in men between 50 and 70 years of age. Early diagnosis is difficult because of a variable clinical picture.

Clinical Manifestations

Symptoms are variable and depend on how rapidly the aneurysm dilates and affects surrounding structures.

Thoracic Aortic Aneurysm

Some do not produce symptoms.

- Constant, boring pain, which may occur only when supine (prominent symptom)
- Dyspnea
- Cough (paroxysmal and brassy)
- Hoarseness
- Stridor
- Weak voice or aphonia (complete loss of voice)
- Dysphagia
- Dilated superficial veins on the chest, neck, or arms
- Edematous areas on the chest wall
- Cyanosis
- Unequal pupils

Abdominal Aortic Aneurysm

- Patients complain of "heart beating" in abdomen when lying down or a feeling of an abdominal mass or abdominal throbbing.
- "Blue-toe syndrome" (an occlusion of a digital vessel) may be noted if associated with thrombus.
- Severe back pain or abdominal pain is a sign of impending rupture.

Dissecting Aneurysm

- Sudden onset with severe and persistent pain described as "tearing" or "ripping" in the anterior chest or back, extending to shoulders, epigastric area, or abdomen (may be mistaken for an acute myocardial infarction)
- Pallor, sweating, and tachycardia
- Elevated blood pressure or markedly different from one arm to the other
- Death usually caused by external rupture of the hematoma

Diagnostic Evaluation
- Chest radiograph, angiogram, transesophageal echocardiography, and magnetic resonance imaging (MRI)
- Ultrasonography or computed tomography (CT) scan to determine the size, length, and location of the aneurysm
- In abdominal aortic aneurysms: a pulsatile mass in the middle and upper abdomen

Medical Management
Medical or surgical treatment depends on the type of aneurysm.

Medical Treatment
- Strict control of blood pressure and reduction in pulsatile flow
- Systolic pressure maintained at 100 to 120 mm Hg with antihypertensive drugs, such as nitroprusside
- Pulsatile flow reduced by medications that reduce cardiac contractility, such as propranolol

Surgical Repair
- The goal of surgery is to remove the aneurysm and restore vascular continuity with a graft (resection and bypass graft or endovascular grafting).
- Surgery is the treatment of choice for abdominal aneurysms larger than 5 cm (2 inches) in diameter or those that are enlarging.
- Intensive monitoring in the critical care unit is required.
- Prognosis for a ruptured aneurysm is poor, and surgery is performed immediately.

Nursing Management
See Preoperative and Postoperative Nursing Management for additional information.

Assessment
PREOPERATIVE
- Guide assessment by the fact that the aneurysm may rupture (signs include persistent or intermittent back or

abdominal pain that may be localized in the middle or lower abdomen or lower back).
- Establish functional capacity of all organ systems, recognizing possible cerebral, cardiovascular, pulmonary, and renal impairment due to atherosclerosis.
- Implement medical therapies to stabilize patient.

POSTOPERATIVE
- Intensely monitor the pulmonary, cardiovascular, renal, and neurologic systems.
- Monitor for complications: arterial occlusion, hemorrhage, infection, ischemic colon, renal failure, and impotence.
- Prescribe an exercise schedule after the acute recovery phase.
- Discourage prolonged sitting.

NURSING ALERT

- Constant intense back pain, falling blood pressure, and decreasing hematocrit are signs of a rupturing abdominal aortic aneurysm.
- Hematomas into the scrotum, perineum, flank, or penis indicate retroperitoneal rupture.
- Signs of heart failure or a loud bruit suggest rupture into the vena cava.
- Rupture into the peritoneal cavity is rapidly fatal.

For more information, see Chapter 28 in Smeltzer and Bare: *Brunner and Suddarth's Textbook of Medical-Surgical Nursing,* 9th edition. Philadelphia: Lippincott Williams & Wilkins, 2000.

ANEURYSM, INTRACRANIAL

An intracranial (cerebral) aneurysm is a dilation of the walls of a cerebral artery that develops as a result of weakness in the arterial wall. Its cause is unknown; it may be due to atherosclerosis, a congenital defect of the vessel walls, hypertensive vascular disease, head trauma, or advancing age. Most commonly affected are the internal carotid, anterior or posterior cerebral, anterior or posterior communicating, and middle cerebral arteries. Symptoms are produced when the aneurysm enlarges and presses on nearby cranial nerves or brain tissue, or ruptures, causing subarachnoid hemorrhage.

Clinical Manifestations
- Rupture of the aneurysm causes sudden, unusually severe headache; often, loss of consciousness for a variable period; pain and rigidity of the back of the neck and spine; and visual disturbances (visual loss, diplopia, ptosis).
- Tinnitus, dizziness, and hemiparesis may also occur. If aneurysm leaks blood and forms a clot, patient may show little neurologic deficit, or severe bleeding, resulting in cerebral damage followed rapidly by coma and death.
- Prognosis depends on the neurologic condition of the patient, age, associated diseases, and extent and location of the aneurysm.

Diagnostic Evaluation
- Computed tomography (CT) scan
- Cerebral angiography
- Lumbar puncture

Medical Management
- Allow the brain to recover from the initial insult (bleeding).
- Prevent or minimize the risk of rebleeding.
- Prevent or treat other complications: rebleeding, cerebral vasospasm, acute hydrocephalus, and seizures.

ANEURYSM, INTRACRANIAL   59

- Provide bed rest with sedation to prevent agitation and stress.
- Manage the vasospasm with calcium-channel blockers, such as nimodipine (Nimotop), verapamil (Isoptin), and nifedipine (Procardia).
- Institute surgical treatment (arterial bypass) or medical treatment to prevent rebleeding.
- Manage increased intracranial pressure (ICP):
  - Cerebral spinal fluid (CSF) drainage by lumbar puncture or ventricular catheter drainage
  - Mannitol to reduce ICP, with monitoring for signs of dehydration and rebound elevation of ICP
  - Antifibrinolytic agents to delay or prevent dissolution of the clot if surgery is delayed or contraindicated
- Manage systemic hypertension:
  - Antihypertensive therapy
  - Monitor blood pressure constantly by arterial line
  - Anticonvulsive agents administered prophylactically
  - Stool softeners to prevent straining and elevation of blood pressure
  - Analgesics for head and neck pain
  - Deep vein thrombosis prevention using graded-pressure elastic stockings

Nursing Management
Assessment

- Perform a complete neurologic assessment: level of consciousness, pupillary reaction, motor and sensory function, cranial nerve deficits (extraocular eye movements, facial droop, presence of ptosis), speech difficulties, visual disturbance or headache, and nuchal rigidity or other neurologic deficits.
- Document and report neurologic assessment findings, and reassess and report any changes in the patient's condition.
- Detect subtle changes, especially alterations of level of consciousness (earliest sign of deterioration, ie, mild drowsiness and slight slurring of speech).

Major Nursing Diagnoses
- Altered cerebral perfusion due to bleeding from the aneurysm
- Sensory-perceptual alteration due to the restrictions of subarachnoid precautions
- Anxiety due to illness or restrictions of aneurysm precautions

Collaborative Problems/Potential Complications
- Seizures
- Vasospasm
- Hydrocephalus
- Aneurysm rebleeding

Planning and Goals
Patient goals include improved cerebral tissue perfusion, relief of sensory and perceptual deprivation, relief of anxiety, and the absence of complications.

Nursing Interventions
IMPROVING CEREBRAL TISSUE PERFUSION
- Monitor closely for neurologic deterioration.
- Check blood pressure, pulse, level of responsiveness, pupillary responses, and motor function hourly; monitor respiratory status and report changes immediately.
- Implement subarachnoid precautions (immediate and absolute bed rest in a quiet, nonstressful setting; restrict visitors, except for family).
- Elevate head of bed 15 to 30 degrees or as ordered.
- Avoid any activity that suddenly increases blood pressure or obstructs venous return (eg, Valsalva maneuver), eliminate caffeine, administer all personal care, and minimize external stimuli.
- Apply elastic pressure stockings or sequential compression boots. Observe legs for signs and symptoms of deep vein thrombosis (tenderness, swelling, warmth, and positive Homans' sign).

RELIEVING SENSORY DEPRIVATION
• Keep sensory stimulation to a minimum.
• Explain restrictions to help reduce the patient's sense of isolation.

RELIEVING ANXIETY
• Inform patient of plan of care.
• Provide support and appropriate reassurance to patient and family.
• Provide reality orientation.

MONITORING AND MANAGING POTENTIAL
COMPLICATIONS (SEIZURE)
• Maintain seizure precautions.
• Maintain airway and prevent injury if a seizure occurs.
• Administer medication treatment as prescribed (phenytoin [Dilantin] is medication of choice).

MONITORING AND MANAGING
POTENTIAL COMPLICATIONS
Vasospasm
Vasospasm may occur several days after surgery or on the initiation of treatment.
• Assess for signs of possible vasospasm (intensified headaches, a decrease in level of responsiveness, or evidence of aphasia or partial paralysis); report immediately.
• Administer calcium-channel blockers or fluid-volume expanders as prescribed.

Aneurysm Rebleeding
• Monitor for symptoms and report; rebleeding occurs most often in the first 2 weeks. Symptoms include sudden severe headache, nausea, vomiting, decreased level of consciousness, and neurologic deficit.
• Administer medications to maintain blood pressure and antifibrinolytics as ordered to delay lysis of the clot.

Hydrocephalus
• Monitor for onset of symptoms, which may be acute (first 24 hours after hemorrhage), subacute (days later), or delayed (several weeks later).

- Report symptoms immediately: acute hydrocephalus is characterized by sudden stupor or coma; subacute or delayed is characterized by gradual onset of drowsiness, behavioral changes, and ataxic gait.

Evaluation

EXPECTED OUTCOMES
- Demonstrates intact neurologic status and normal vital signs and respiratory patterns
- Demonstrates normal sensory perceptions
- Exhibits reduced anxiety level
- Is free of complications

For more information, see Chapter 59 in Smeltzer and Bare: *Brunner and Suddarth's Textbook of Medical-Surgical Nursing,* 9th edition. Philadelphia: Lippincott Williams & Wilkins, 2000.

ANGINA PECTORIS

Angina pectoris is a clinical syndrome characterized by paroxysms of pain or a feeling of pressure in the anterior chest. The cause is insufficient coronary blood flow, resulting in an inadequate supply of oxygen to meet the myocardial demand. Angina is usually a result of atherosclerotic heart disease and is associated with a significant obstruction of a major coronary artery. Factors affecting anginal pain are physical exertion, exposure to cold, eating a heavy meal, stress, or any emotion-provoking situation that increases myocardial workload.

Clinical Manifestations
- Pain varies from a feeling of indigestion to a choking or heavy sensation in the upper chest to agonizing pain. The patient with diabetes mellitus may not experience severe pain with angina.
- Angina is accompanied by severe apprehension and a feeling of impending death.

- The pain is usually retrosternal, deep in the chest behind the upper or middle third of the sternum.
- Discomfort is poorly localized and may radiate to the neck, jaw, shoulders, and inner aspect of the upper extremities.
- The patient feels a tightness, choking, or strangling sensation with a viselike, insistent quality.
- Angina is accompanied by a feeling of weakness or numbness in the arms, wrists, and hands.
- An important characteristic of anginal pain is that it subsides when the precipitating cause is removed.

Diagnostic Evaluation
- Evaluation of clinical manifestations of pain and patient history
- Electrocardiogram (ECG) changes; stress testing
- Echocardiogram, nuclear scan, or invasive procedures, such as cardiac catheterization and coronary artery angiography

Medical Management
The goals of medical management are to decrease the oxygen demands of the myocardium and to increase the oxygen supply through pharmacologic therapy and risk factor control. Surgically, the goals of management are met through revascularization of the blood supply to the myocardium. Frequently, a combination of medical and surgical therapies is used.

Approaches to Revascularize the Myocardium
- Coronary artery bypass surgery or minimally invasive direct coronary artery bypass (MIDCAB)
- Percutaneous transluminal coronary angioplasty (PTCA)
- Application of intracoronary stents to enhance blood flow
- Lasers to vaporize plaques
- Percutaneous coronary endarterectomy to extract obstruction
- Rotational antherectomy

Pharmacologic Therapy

- Nitrates, the mainstay of therapy (nitroglycerin)
- Beta-adrenergic blockers (propranolol hydrochloride [Inderal])
- Calcium ion antagonists and calcium-channel blockers (nifedipine [Procardia], verapamil [Isoptin, Calan], diltiazem [Cardizem])
- Antiplatelet medications (aspirin, ticlopidine [Ticlid], or heparin)
- Oxygen therapy

Risk Factor Control

- See Modifiable Risk Factors under Coronary Artery Disease for additional information.

Nursing Management

Assessment

- Observe and record all facets, pain (location, description and intensity), and patient activities that precede and precipitate attacks of anginal pain.
- Design a logical program of prevention from patient history.

Major Nursing Diagnoses

- Altered myocardial tissue perfusion secondary to coronary artery disease as evidenced by chest pain (or equivalent symptoms)
- Anxiety related to fear of death
- Knowledge deficit about the underlying disease and methods for avoiding complications
- Ineffective management of therapeutic regimen, noncompliance related to nonacceptance of necessary lifestyle changes

Collaborative Problems/Potential Complications

Potential complications of angina include myocardial infarction and its complications.

Planning and Goals

Patient will demonstrate pain relief and absence of return of pain, reduction of anxiety, awareness of the underlying nature of the disorder, understanding of the prescribed care, and adherence to the self-care program.

Nursing Interventions

PREVENTING PAIN

- Teach patient to understand the symptom complex and avoid activities known to cause anginal pain.
  - Direct patient to stop all activities and sit or rest in bed if chest pain is sensed.
  - Teach patient to avoid sudden exertion, exposure to cold, tobacco; eat regularly but lightly, maintain prescribed weight.
  - Discourage over-the-counter drugs, such as diet pills, nasal decongestants, or drugs that increase heart rate and blood pressure.
- If patient has frequent pain or pain with minimal activity, alternate rest and activity periods.
- Assess pain, patient's vital signs, and ST segment on ECG.
- Administer oxygen.

REDUCING ANXIETY

- Explore the implications that the diagnosis has for the patient.
- Provide essential information about the illness, and explain the importance of following prescribed directives for the ambulatory patient at home.

Promoting Home and Community-Based Care

Teaching Patients Self-Care

- Educate the patient about the basic nature of the illness.
- Furnish the facts needed to reorganize living habits: to reduce the frequency and severity of anginal attacks; to delay underlying disease; to provide protection from other complications.

Continuing Care

- Prepare self-care program in collaboration with the patient, family, or friends.
- Plan activities to minimize the occurrence of angina episodes.
- Teach patient that any pain unrelieved within 30 minutes by the usual methods should be treated at the closest emergency center.

Gerontologic Considerations

- The elderly person who experiences angina may not exhibit the typical pain profile because of changes in neuroceptors.
- Pain is often manifested in the jaw, or fainting may occur. Advise patient to recognize feelings of weakness as an indication for rest or taking prescribed medications.
- During cold-temperature exposure, the elderly patient may experience anginal symptoms more quickly than younger people. Encourage the patient to dress with extra clothing.

Evaluation

EXPECTED OUTCOMES
- Reports that pain is relieved promptly
- Understands ways to avoid complications and demonstrates freedom from complications
- Demonstrates less anxiety
- Adheres to self-care program

For more information, see Chapter 25 in Smeltzer and Bare: *Brunner and Suddarth's Textbook of Medical-Surgical Nursing,* 9th edition. Philadelphia: Lippincott Williams & Wilkins, 2000.

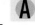

AORTIC INSUFFICIENCY (REGURGITATION)

Aortic insufficiency is the flow of blood back into the left ventricle from the aorta during diastole. The result is left ventricular dilation and hypertrophy. It may be caused by inflammatory lesions that deform the leaflets of the aortic valve. The lesions prevent complete sealing of the aortic orifice during diastole. This disorder may result from endocarditis, congenital abnormalities, or diseases such as syphilis and dissecting aneurysm that cause dilation or tearing of the ascending aorta.

Clinical Manifestations
- Develops insidiously (without symptoms in most patients).
- Earliest manifestation: increased force of heartbeat, that is, visible or palpable pulsations over the temporal arteries (head) and at the neck (carotid)
- Exertional dyspnea and easy fatigability
- Signs and symptoms of left ventricular failure (orthopnea, paroxysmal nocturnal dyspnea)
- Pulse pressure widened
- Water-hammer pulse (the pulse strikes the palpating finger with quick, sharp strokes and then suddenly collapses)

Diagnostic Evaluation
ECG, echocardiogram, and cardiac catheterization are used in the diagnosis.

Medical Management
- Antibiotic prophylaxis is used before invasive and dental procedures.
- Treatment of heart failure and dysrhythmias is undertaken.
- Treatment of choice is aortic valve replacement; surgery is recommended in the presence of left ventricular hypertrophy.

- Valve repair (valvuloplasty commissurotomy) may be performed instead of replacement. Repaired valves function longer than replaced valves, and continuous anticoagulation is not required.
- Anticoagulation is not required.

Nursing Management

See Preoperative and Postoperative Nursing Management for additional information.

- Teach patient regarding wound care, diet, activity, medication, and self-care.
- Instruct patients on the importance of antibiotic prophylaxis to prevent endocarditis.
- Reinforce all new information and self-care instructions for 4 to 8 weeks after the procedure.

For more information, see Chapter 26 in Smeltzer and Bare: *Brunner and Suddarth's Textbook of Medical-Surgical Nursing*, 9th edition. Philadelphia: Lippincott Williams & Wilkins, 2000.

AORTIC STENOSIS

Aortic valve stenosis is the narrowing of the orifice between the left ventricle and the aorta. In adults, the stenosis may be congenital, or it may be a result of rheumatic endocarditis or cusp calcification of unknown cause. There is progressive narrowing of the valve orifice over a period of several years to several decades. The heart muscle increases in size (hypertrophy) in response to all degrees of obstruction; clinical signs of heart failure occur when compensatory mechanisms of the heart fail.

Clinical Manifestations

- Exertional dyspnea
- Dizziness and fainting
- Angina pectoris
- Blood pressure possibly low but usually normal

- Low pulse pressure (30 mm Hg or less)
- Physical examination: loud, rough, systolic murmur heard over the aortic area; vibration over the base of the heart

Diagnostic Evaluation
- 12-lead ECG and echocardiogram
- Left heart catheterization

Medical Management
- Antibiotic prophylaxis is done to prevent endocarditis.
- Medications for left ventricular failure or dysrhythmia are administered as needed.
- Surgical replacement of the aortic valve is the definitive treatment favored. Uncorrected condition can lead to irreversible heart failure.

Nursing Management
See Preoperative and Postoperative Nursing Management for additional information.

For more information, see Chapter 26 in Smeltzer and Bare: *Brunner and Suddarth's Textbook of Medical-Surgical Nursing,* 9th edition. Philadelphia: Lippincott Williams & Wilkins, 2000.

APPENDICITIS

The appendix is a small, finger-like appendage attached to the cecum just below the ileocecal valve. Because it empties into the colon inefficiently and its lumen is small, it is prone to becoming obstructed and is vulnerable to infection (appendicitis). It is the most common cause of acute inflammation in the right lower quadrant of the abdominal cavity and the most common cause of emergency abdominal surgery. Males are affected more than females, teenagers more frequently than adults; the highest incidence is in those between the ages of 10 and 30 years.

Clinical Manifestations

- Lower right quadrant pain usually accompanied by low-grade fever, nausea, and sometimes vomiting
- At McBurney's point (located halfway between the umbilicus and the anterior spine of the ilium), local tenderness with pressure and some rigidity of the lower portion of the right rectus muscle
- Rebound tenderness may be present; location of appendix dictates amount of tenderness, muscle spasm, and occurrence of constipation or diarrhea
- Rovsing's sign (elicited by palpating left lower quadrant, which paradoxically causes pain in right lower quadrant)
- If appendix ruptures, pain becomes more diffuse; abdominal distention develops from paralytic ileus, and condition worsens

Diagnostic Evaluation

- Diagnosis is based on a complete physical examination and laboratory and radiologic tests.
- Leukocyte count greater than 10,000/mm^3; neutrophil count greater than 75%; abdominal radiographs and ultrasound studies reveal right lower quadrant density or localized airflow levels.

Medical Management

- Surgery is indicated if appendicitis is diagnosed and should be performed as soon as possible to decrease risk of perforation.
- Administer antibiotics and intravenous fluids until surgery is performed.
- Analgesics can be given after diagnosis is made.

Complications of Appendectomy

- The major complication is perforation of the appendix, which can lead to peritonitis or an abscess.
- Perforation generally occurs 24 hours after onset of pain (symptoms include fever, toxic appearance, and continued pain or tenderness).

Nursing Management

- Nursing goals include relieving pain, preventing fluid volume deficit, reducing anxiety, eliminating infection due to the potential or actual disruption of the gastrointestinal tract, maintaining skin integrity, and attaining optimum nutrition.
- Preoperatively: prepare for surgery, start intravenous line, antibiotic, nasogastric tube (if evidence of paralytic ileus), and ask patient to void. *Do not administer an enema or laxative (could cause perforation).*
- Postoperatively: place in semi-Fowler's position, give narcotic analgesic as ordered, administer oral fluids when tolerated, give food as desired on day of surgery (if tolerated). If dehydrated before surgery, administer intravenous fluids.
- If a drain is left in place at the area of the incision, monitor carefully for signs of intestinal obstruction, secondary hemorrhage, or secondary abscesses (eg, fever, tachycardia, and increased leukocyte count).

Promoting Home and Community-Based Care

Teaching Patients Self-Care

- Teach the patient and family to care for the wound and perform dressing changes and irrigations as prescribed.
- Reinforce need for follow-up appointment with surgeon.
- Discuss incision care and activity guidelines.
- Refer for home care nursing as indicated to assist with care and continued monitoring of complications and wound healing.

Gerontologic Considerations

In the elderly, signs and symptoms of appendicitis may vary greatly. Signs may be very vague and suggestive of bowel obstruction or another process; some patients may experience no symptoms until the appendix ruptures. The incidence of perforated appendix is higher in the elderly because many of these people do not seek health care as quickly as younger people.

For more information, see Chapter 35 in Smeltzer and Bare: *Brunner and Suddarth's Textbook of Medical-Surgical Nursing,* 9th edition. Philadelphia: Lippincott Williams & Wilkins, 2000.

ARTERIAL EMBOLISM AND ARTERIAL THROMBOSIS

Arterial emboli arise most commonly from thrombi that develop in the chambers of the heart as a result of atrial fibrillation, myocardial infarction, infective endocarditis, or chronic congestive heart failure. Arterial thrombosis is a slowly developing clot in a degenerated vessel that can itself occlude an artery. Thrombi also become detached and are carried from the left side of the heart into the arterial system, where they cause obstruction. The immediate effect is cessation of distal blood flow. Secondary vasospasm can contribute to ischemia. Emboli tend to lodge at arterial bifurcations and atherosclerotic narrowing (cerebral, mesenteric, renal, and coronary arteries). Acute thrombosis frequently occurs in patients with preexisting ischemic syndromes.

Clinical Manifestations

The symptoms of arterial emboli depend primarily on the size of the embolus, the organ involved, and the state of the collateral vessels.

- Symptoms can generally be described as the five Ps: pain, pallor, pulselessness, paresthesia, and paralysis.
- The part of limb below the occlusion is markedly colder and paler than above as a result of ischemia.

Diagnostic Evaluation

- Sudden or acute onset of symptoms is diagnostic.
- Two-dimensional echocardiography, transesophageal echocardiography, chest radiograph, electrocardiogram,

noninvasive duplex and Doppler ultrasonography, and arteriography might be used.

Medical Management

Acute Embolic Occlusion

- Emergency embolectomy is the surgical procedure of choice only if the involved extremity is viable.

Collateral Circulation

- Intravenous anticoagulation with heparin
- Intraarterial thrombolytic agents, such as streptokinase or urokinase (drug of choice); contraindications are internal bleeding, stroke, recent major surgery, uncontrolled hypertension, and pregnancy

Nursing Management

- Encourage movement of the leg to stimulate circulation and prevent stasis.
- Continue anticoagulants to prevent thrombosis of the affected artery and to diminish development of subsequent thrombi.
- Assess the surgical incision frequently for hemorrhage.

For more information, see Chapter 28 in Smeltzer and Bare: *Brunner and Suddarth's Textbook of Medical-Surgical Nursing,* 9th edition. Philadelphia: Lippincott Williams & Wilkins, 2000.

ARTERIOSCLEROSIS AND ATHEROSCLEROSIS

Arteriosclerosis, or "hardening of the arteries," is the most common disease of the arteries. It is a diffuse process whereby the muscle fibers and the endothelial lining of the walls of small arteries and arterioles become thickened. Atherosclerosis primarily affects the intima of the large and medium-sized arteries, causing changes that include the accumulation of lipids (atheromas), calcium, blood components, carbohydrates, and fibrous tissue on the intimal layer of the artery. Although the pathologic processes of arteriosclerosis and atherosclerosis differ, rarely does one occur without the other. The terms are used interchangeably. The most common direct results of atherosclerosis in the arteries include narrowing (stenosis) of the lumen, obstruction by thrombosis, aneurysm, ulceration, and rupture; ischemia and necrosis occur if the supply of blood, nutrients, and oxygen is severely and permanently disrupted. The fibrous plaques of atherosclerosis are found predominantly in the abdominal aorta and coronary, popliteal, and internal carotid arteries.

Risk Factors

Many risk factors are associated with atherosclerosis; the greater the number of risk factors, the greater the likelihood of developing the disease.

- Smoking (largest risk factor)
- High-fat (suspected risk factor, along with high serum cholesterol and blood lipid levels)
- Hypertension
- Diabetes
- Obesity, stress, and lack of exercise

Clinical Manifestations

Clinical features depend on the tissue or organ affected: heart (angina and myocardial infarction due to coronary atherosclerosis), brain (transient ischemic attacks and stroke due to cerebrovascular disease), peripheral vessels (includes hypertension and symptoms of aneurysm of the aorta, renovascular disease, atherosclerotic lesions of the extremities). See specific condition for greater detail.

Medical Management

Traditional management of atherosclerosis depends on risk factor modification, medication administration, a controlled exercise program, interventional or surgical graft procedures, and nursing measures related to the resulting diseases.

Several radiologic techniques have been shown to be important adjunctive therapies to surgical procedures, such as laser angioplasty and rotational atherectomy.

 ## Gerontologic Considerations

Atherosclerotic cardiovascular disease is found in 80% of the population older than 65 years of age and is the most common condition of the arterial system in elderly people.

For more information, see Chapter 28 in Smeltzer and Bare: *Brunner and Suddarth's Textbook of Medical-Surgical Nursing,* 9th edition. Philadelphia: Lippincott Williams & Wilkins, 2000.

ARTHRITIS, RHEUMATOID

Rheumatoid arthritis (RA) is an inflammatory disorder that primarily involves the synovial membrane of the joints. RA occurs between the ages of 30 and 50 years, with peak incidence between 40 and 60 years of age. Women are affected two to three times more frequently than men. RA is believed to be an immune response to unknown antigens. The stimulus may be viral or bacterial. There may be a predisposition to the disease.

Clinical Manifestations
- Clinical features are determined by the stage and severity of the disease.
- Joint pain, swelling, warmth, erythema, and lack of function are classic clinical features.
- Palpitation of joints reveals spongy or boggy tissue.
- Fluid can usually be aspirated from the inflamed joint.

Characteristic Pattern of Joint Involvement
- Begins with small joints in hands, wrists, and feet
- Progressively involves knees, shoulders, hips, elbows, ankles, cervical spine, and temporomandibular joints

- Symptoms are usually acute in onset, bilateral, and symmetric
- Joints may be hot, swollen, and painful; morning stiffness lasting for more than 30 minutes
- Deformities of the hands and feet are common

Extraarticular Features

- Fever, weight loss, fatigue, anemia, sensory changes, and lymph node enlargement
- Raynaud's phenomenon
- Rheumatoid nodules, nontender and movable; found in subcutaneous tissue over bony prominences
- Arteritis, neuropathy, scleritis, pericarditis, splenomegaly, and Sjögren's syndrome (dry eyes and mucous membranes)

Diagnostic Evaluation

- Several factors contribute to an RA diagnosis: rheumatoid nodules, joint inflammation, laboratory findings, extraarticular changes.
- Rheumatoid factor (RF) is present in more than 80% of patients.
- Red blood count and C_4 complement component are decreased; erythrocyte sedimentation rate is elevated.
- C-reactive protein (CRP) and antinuclear antibody (ANA) may be positive.
- Arthrocentesis and radiographs may be completed.

Medical Management

Treatment begins with education, a balance of rest and exercise, and referral to community agencies for support.

- Early RA: medication management involves therapeutic doses of salicylates or nonsteroidal antiinflammatory drugs (NSAIDs); antimalarials, gold, penicillamine, or sulfasalazine; methotrexate; biologic response modifiers and antitumor necrosis factor receptors (TNFR) are being tested; analgesics for periods of extreme pain.

A

- Moderate, erosive RA: formal program of occupational and physical therapy; an immunomodulator, like cyclosporine, may be added.
- Persistent, erosive RA: reconstructive surgery and corticosteroids are used.
- Advanced unremitting RA: immunosuppressive agents, such as methotrexate, cyclophosphamide, and azathioprine are used.
- RA patients frequently experience anorexia, weight loss, and anemia, requiring careful dietary history to identify usual eating habits and food preferences. (Corticosteroids may stimulate appetite and cause weight gain.)
- Low-dose antidepressant medications (amitriptyline) are used to reestablish adequate sleep pattern and manage pain.

Nursing Management
Assessment
- Assess the patient's self-image related to musculoskeletal changes, and determine whether the patient is experiencing unusual fatigue, weakness, pain, morning stiffness, fever, or anorexia.
- Assess the skin, hair, ear, mouth, chest, abdomen, genitalia, and cardiovascular, pulmonary, neurologic, renal, and musculoskeletal systems.
- Assess the joints by inspecting, palpating, and inquiring about tenderness, swelling, and redness in the affected joints.
- Assess joint mobility, range of motion, and muscle strength.
- Focus on identifying patient problems and factors, abilities, past experiences, preconceptions, and unknown fears.

Major Nursing Diagnoses
- Pain related to inflammation, increased disease activity, tissue damage, fatigue, and lowered tolerance level

- Fatigue related to increased disease activity, pain, inadequate rest, deconditioning, inadequate nutrition, emotional stress, depression
- Impaired physical mobility related to muscle weakness, pain on movement, lack of or improper use of ambulatory devices
- Self-care deficits (feeding, bathing, dressing, toileting) related to contractures, fatigue, or loss of motion
- Sleep pattern disturbance related to pain and fatigue
- Body image disturbance related to physical and psychological changes and dependency imposed by chronic illness
- Ineffective coping related to actual or perceived lifestyle or role changes

Collaborative Problems/Potential Complications
- Adverse effects of medications

Planning and Goals
Patient goals may include relief of pain and discomfort, relief of fatigue, obtainment of optimal functional mobility, maintenance of self-care, improved body image, achievement of an optimal and individual level of independence in activities of daily living, improved quality of sleep, increased knowledge regarding self-management, and attainment of a positive self-concept and absence of complications.

Nursing Interventions
RELIEVING PAIN AND DISCOMFORT
- Question carefully to distinguish pain from stiffness.
- After administering medication, reassess pain levels at intervals. With persistent pain, compare assessment findings with baseline pain measurements and evaluations.
- Teach and use pain management techniques for immediate short-term management (ie, use of heat and cold, joint protection and support with splints and braces, rest, and analgesics).
- Educate the patient regarding long-term pain management (ie, use of antiinflammatory medications,

establishing an exercise regimen for maintaining joint mobility, and relaxation techniques).
- Provide comfort measures while giving care.
- Set realistic expectations so that patient and significant others realize pain can be controlled depending on disease activity.

REDUCING FATIGUE
- Educate patient on biologic, psychological, social, and personal factors related to RA that cause or contribute to fatigue.
- Teach the patient how to use level of fatigue to monitor the disease and balance physical activities accordingly.
- Encourage patient to use naps, nighttime sleep, and splints for joints to provide rest to system and joints.
- A sleep-inducing routine, medication, and comfort measures may help improve the quality of sleep.

INCREASING MOBILITY
- Teach the patient to support all joints in a position of optimal function: lie on a firm mattress with feet against a footboard, only one pillow under head.
- Instruct the patient to lie prone (on the abdomen) several times daily to prevent hip flexion contracture.
- Encourage active range-of-motion exercises to prevent joint stiffness.
- Understand that deformity does not equate with disability and patient's ability to perform self-care.
- Relieve persistent pain and morning stiffness to increase patient's mobility and self-care.
- Provide assistive devices and assist the patient in learning to use them properly (cane held in hand opposite affected side, forearm-trough style crutches if disease involves the hands and wrists).

FACILITATING SELF-CARE
- Be sensitive to the patient's feelings, demonstrating acceptance and positive attitudes about using assistive devices.

- Help preserve the patient's independence in inpatient and home settings by making available adaptive equipment for eating, toileting, bathing, and dressing.

IMPROVING SLEEP
- Identify the cause of a sleep problem.
- Adjust antiinflammatory and analgesic administration times.
- Encourage and provide a sleep-inducing routine, medication, and comfort measures to help improve the quality of sleep.

IMPROVING SELF-CONCEPT
- Try to understand the patient's emotional reactions to the disease.
- Encourage communication, so that patient and family verbalize feelings, perceptions, and fears related to the disease.
- Help the patient and family identify areas in which they have some control over disease symptoms and treatment.
- Encourage patient and family to commit to the management program for more positive outcomes.

MONITORING AND MANAGING
POTENTIAL COMPLICATIONS
- Work with the physician and pharmacist to help the patient recognize and deal with side effects from medications.
- Side effects to monitor for include gastrointestinal bleeding or irritation, bone marrow suppression, kidney or liver toxicity, increased incidence of infection, mouth sores, rashes, and changes in vision. Other signs and symptoms include bruising, breathing problems, dizziness, jaundice, dark urine, black or bloody stools, diarrhea, nausea and vomiting, and headaches.
- Monitor closely for systemic and local infections, which often can be masked by high doses of corticosteroids.

INCREASING KNOWLEDGE REGARDING
DISEASE MANAGEMENT

- Tailor education to patient's previous knowledge base, interest level, degree of comfort, and social or cultural influences.
- Instruct patient on basic disease management, medications, and necessary adaptations in lifestyle.
- Encourage patient to practice new self-management skills.

Promoting Home and Community-Based Care

Teaching Patients Self-Care

- Focus patient teaching on the RA, possible changes related to the disorder, the prescribed therapeutic regimen, side effects of medications, strategies to maintain independence and function, and patient safety in the home.
- Encourage the patient and family to verbalize their concerns and ask questions.
- Address pain, fatigue, and depression before initiating a teaching program because it can interfere with the patient's ability to learn.
- Instruct the patient about basic disease management and necessary adaptations in lifestyle.

Continuing Care

- Refer for home care as warranted (eg, frail patient with significantly limited function).
- Note problems caused by RA that may interfere with treatment of a primary condition, and treatment of a primary condition may cause or increase problems related to RA.
- Identify any barriers to compliance, and make appropriate referrals.
- Assess the patient's need for assistance in the home, and supervise home health aides who may meet many of the needs of the patient with a rheumatic disease.

- Make referrals to physical and occupational therapists as problems are identified and limitations increase.
- Alert the patient and family to support services such as Meals on Wheels and local Arthritis Foundation chapters.
- Emphasize the importance of follow-up appointments to the patient and family.

Evaluation

EXPECTED OUTCOMES
- Experiences relief of pain or improved comfort level
- Experiences reduction in level of fatigue
- Increases or maintains level of mobility
- Maintains self-care activities
- Experiences improved body image
- Experiences absence of complications

For more information, see Chapter 50 in Smeltzer and Bare: *Brunner and Suddarth's Textbook of Medical-Surgical Nursing,* 9th edition. Philadelphia: Lippincott Williams & Wilkins, 2000.

ASTHMA

Asthma is a chronic inflammatory disease of the airways characterized by hyperresponsiveness, mucosal edema, and mucus production. Acute exacerbations last from minutes, to hours, to days and are interspersed with symptom-free periods.

Asthma can begin at any age and is the most common chronic disease of childhood. Risk factors for asthma include allergy (strongest factor) and chronic exposure to airway irritants on allergens (eg, grass, weed pollens, mold, dust, or animals). Common triggers for asthma symptoms and exacerbations in asthma patients include airway irritants (eg, pollutants, cold, heat, strong odors, smoke, perfumes), exertion, stress, sinusitis, and esophageal reflux.

Clinical Manifestations
- The most common symptoms of asthma are cough (with or without mucus production), dyspnea, and wheezing (first on expiration, then possibly during inspiration as well).
- Asthma attacks frequently occur at night.
- An asthma exacerbation is frequently preceded by increasing symptoms over days but may begin abruptly.
- Chest tightness and dyspnea occur.
- Expiration requires effort and becomes prolonged.
- As exacerbation progresses, central cyanosis secondary to severe hypoxia may occur.
- Additional symptoms, such as diaphoresis, tachycardia, and a widened pulse pressure, may occur.
- A severe, continuous reaction, status asthmaticus, may occur and is life-threatening.
- Eczema, urticaria, and temporary edema are allergic reactions that may be noted with asthma.

Diagnostic Evaluation
- A family environmental and occupational history is essential.
- During acute episodes, sputum and blood test, pulse oximetry, arterial blood gases (ABGs), and pulmonary function tests are performed.

Medical Management
Pharmacologic Therapy
- Beta-adrenergic agonists
- Methylxanthines
- Anticholinergics
- Corticosteroids: metered dose inhaler (MDI)
- Mast cell inhibitors

Nursing Management
Assessment
- Evaluate and identify substances that precipitate the attacks (obtain history of exacerbations, family, environment, health history).

- Monitor respiratory status for progression or resolution of asthma attack (eg, breath sounds, pulse oximetry, vital signs, peak flow).
- Obtain history of use of medical and medication allergy.

Major Nursing Diagnoses
- Ineffective airway clearance related to airway constriction and excess mucus production
- Anxiety related to fear of death
- Risk for ineffective management of treatment regimen

Planning and Goals
Patient has unlabored breathing, clear breath sounds, and pulmonary studies within normal limits. Patient demonstrates knowledge of self-care regimen for prevention and treatment of asthma exacerbations.

Nursing Interventions
PROMOTING AIRWAY CLEARANCE
- Administer prescribed therapy, and monitor patient responses.
- Administer fluids and antibiotics (if infection present).
- Assist with intubation and respiratory support as needed.

MINIMIZING ANXIETY
- Provide nursing care, using a calm approach.
- Keep the patient and family informed about procedures.

🏠 Promoting Home and Community-Based Care

Teaching Patients Self-Care
- Teach patient and family about asthma (chronic inflammatory), the purpose and action of medications, how and what triggers to avoid (eg, exposure to offending pollens—stay in air-conditioned rooms during pollen season or, if feasible, change climate zone).
- Instruct patient and family about peak-flow monitoring.

- Teach patient how to implement an action plan and how and when to seek assistance.
- Emphasize adherence to the prescribed therapy, preventive measures, and need for follow-up appointments.

Continuing Care
- Refer for home health nurse as indicated.
- Initiation of a home visit to assess for allergens may be indicated (with recurrent exacerbations).
- Encourage patient to maintain good physical and mental health because attacks may be induced by suggestion alone.
- Refer the patient to community support groups.

For more information, see Chapter 21 in Smeltzer and Bare: *Brunner and Suddarth's Textbook of Medical-Surgical Nursing,* 9th edition. Philadelphia: Lippincott Williams & Wilkins, 2000.

ASTHMA: STATUS ASTHMATICUS

Status asthmaticus is severe persistent asthma that is unresponsive to conventional therapy and can last longer than 24 hours. Infection, anxiety, nebulizer abuse, dehydration, increased adrenergic block, and nonspecific irritants may contribute to these episodes. An acute episode may be precipitated by hypersensitivity to aspirin. Two predominant pathologic problems occur: a decrease in the diameter of the bronchi and a ventilation-perfusion abnormality.

Clinical Manifestations
- Same as those seen in severe asthma
- No correlation between severity of attack and number of wheezes
- With greater obstruction, wheezing may disappear; frequently a sign of impending respiratory failure

Diagnostic Evaluation

- Primarily by pulmonary function studies and ABGs
- Respiratory alkalosis most common finding (rising pCO_2 to normal or higher) is a danger sign of impending respiratory failure)

Medical Management

- Treat initially with beta-adrenergic agonists, corticosteroids, supplemental oxygen, and intravenous fluids to hydrate.
- Start with low-flow humidified oxygen (Venturi mask or nasal catheter); the flow rate is determined by ABGs (PaO_2 65 to 85 mm Hg).
- Sedatives are contraindicated.
- Hospitalization is required if blood gas levels deteriorate or pulmonary function test results are low.
- Mechanical ventilation needed if patient is tiring or in respiratory failure or patient's condition does not respond to initial treatment.

Nursing Management

Assessment

- Assess for signs of dehydration by checking skin turgor.
- Monitor respiratory status constantly for the first 12 to 24 hours, or until status asthmaticus stops.

Major Nursing Diagnoses

- Ineffective airway clearance related to airway constriction and thick secretions
- Fluid volume deficit related to increased hydration needs associated with asthma

Planning and Goals

Patient has unlabored breathing, clear breath sounds, and pulmonary studies within normal limits. Patient demonstrates knowledge of self-care regimen for prevention and treatment of asthma exacerbations.

Nursing Interventions

PROMOTING AIRWAY CLEARANCE
- Keep room quiet and free of respiratory irritants (flowers, smoke, perfumes); use nonallergenic pillow.

PROMOTING ADEQUATE HYDRATION
- Combat dehydration with adequate fluid intake to loosen secretions and facilitate expectoration.
- Administer prescribed intravenous fluids to 3000 to 4000 mL/day unless contraindicated.

Promoting Home and Community-Based Care

Keep recurrences to a minimum with patient education. See Nursing Management under Asthma for additional information.

 NURSING ALERT

Rising pCO_2 is a danger signal of impending respiratory failure.

For more information, see Chapter 21 in Smeltzer and Bare: *Brunner and Suddarth's Textbook of Medical-Surgical Nursing,* 9th edition. Philadelphia: Lippincott Williams & Wilkins, 2000.

B

BACK PAIN, LOW

Most low back pain is caused by musculoskeletal problems (eg, acute lumbosacral strain, unstable lumbosacral ligaments and weak muscles, osteoarthritis of the spine, spinal stenosis, intervertebral disk problems, inequality of leg length). Older patients may have back pain associated with osteoporotic vertebral fractures or bone metastasis. Many other medical and psychosomatic conditions are causes of back pain. Obesity, stress, and occasionally depression may contribute to low back pain. Patients with chronic low back pain may develop a dependence on alcohol or analgesics.

Clinical Manifestations
- Patient complains of either acute back pain or chronic back pain (lasting more than 3 months without improvement) and fatigue.
- Pain radiates along a nerve root (radiculopathy; sciatica) and is accentuated by movement.
- Pain is associated with straight-leg raising (spinal root irritation).
- Paravertebral muscle spasm (greatly increased muscle tone of back postural muscles) occurs, with a loss of normal lumbar curve and possible spinal deformity.
- Back pain is aggravated by activity (usually due to musculoskeletal rather than other conditions).

Diagnostic Evaluation
- History and physical examination
- Spinal radiograph
- Computed tomography (CT) scan
- Magnetic resonance imaging (MRI) scan

- Bone scan and blood studies
- Myelogram and discogram; epidural venogram
- Electromyogram and nerve conduction studies

Medical Management

The focus is on relief of pain and discomfort, activity modification, and patient education.

Supportive
- Bed rest if pain is severe, analgesics, stress reduction, relaxation; self-limiting and resolves within 4 weeks
- Position in bed to increase lumbar flexion; elevate head 30 degrees, and flex knees slightly; avoid prone position
- Physical therapy; intermittent pelvic traction; heat or cold therapy; manipulation may be helpful in the absence of radiculopathy symptoms; diathermy; whirlpool; exercise program; low back supports and braces

Medications
- Analgesics (mild or opioids)
- Muscle relaxants
- Tranquilizers
- Antiinflammatory agents and nonsteroidal antiinflammatory drugs (NSAIDs)

Exercise Program
- Low back supports and braces

Nursing Management

Assessment
- Encourage patient to describe the discomfort (onset, location).
- Obtain history about previous pain control and how back problem is affecting lifestyle.
- Observe patient's posture, position changes, and gait.
- Assess spinal curves, pelvic crest, leg length discrepancy, and shoulder symmetry.

- Palpate the paraspinal muscles, and note spasm and tenderness.
- Note discomfort and limitations in movement when bending forward and laterally.
- Evaluate nerve involvement by assessing for abnormal sensations, muscle weakness or paralysis, and back and leg pain with straight-leg raises.
- Assess for obesity and nutritional balance.

Major Nursing Diagnoses
- Pain related to musculoskeletal problems
- Impaired physical mobility related to pain muscle spasm and decreased flexibility
- Altered nutrition: more than body requirements related to obesity
- Self-concept disturbance related to impaired mobility, chronic pain, and altered role performance
- Knowledge deficit related to back-conserving body mechanic techniques

Planning and Goals
Patient demonstrates relief of pain, improved physical mobility, improved role performance, proper use of back-conserving body mechanics, and weight reduction.

Nursing Interventions
RELIEVING PAIN
- Encourage the patient to reduce stress on the back and change position frequently.
- Modify perceived pain through behavioral therapies, such as diaphragmatic breathing, relaxation, guided imagery, and diversions (eg, reading, watching television).
- Self-applied intermittent heat or cold may reduce pain.
- Assess patient's response to each medication prescribed.

IMPROVING PHYSICAL MOBILITY
- Encourage patient to alternate lying, sitting, and walking activities and advise to avoid sitting, standing, and

walking for long periods; resume self-care activities and exercise as pain subsides.

- Rest on firm, nonsagging mattress. With severe pain, limit activity for 2 to 3 days.
- Encourage patient adherence to prescribed exercise program. Avoid twisting and jarring motions. Maintain proper posture with chest up and abdomen tucked in.

MODIFYING NUTRITION FOR WEIGHT REDUCTION
- Provide a sound nutritional plan that includes a change in eating habits to maintain desirable weight.
- Monitor weight loss, and note achievements.
- Provide encouragement and positive reinforcement, and facilitate adherence.

IMPROVING SELF-CONCEPT
- Assist patient and support people to recognize continued dependency to help patient cope with the underlying reason.
- Monitor for "low back neurosis." Help patient cope with specific stressors and control stressful situations.
- Refer for counseling or psychotherapy if needed.

PROMOTING PROPER BODY MECHANICS
- Teach patient how to stand, sit, lie, and lift properly:
  - Shift weight frequently when standing and rest one foot on a low stool; wear low heels.
  - Sit with knees and hips flexed and knees level with hips or higher. Keep feet flat on the floor; use chair with arm rests.
  - Sleep on side with knees and hips flexed or supine with knees flexed and supported; avoid sleeping prone.
  - Lift objects using thigh muscles not back, stand with wide base of support, and lift objects close to the body. Wear a back brace when lifting, and avoid lifting more than one third of own weight.
- Instruct patient to practice protective and defensive postures, positions, and body mechanics to strengthen the back and to diminish chance of recurrence of back pain.

Evaluation

EXPECTED OUTCOMES
- Experiences pain relief
- Demonstrates resumption of physical mobility
- Demonstrates back-conserving body mechanics
- Resumes role-related responsibilities
- Achieves desired weight

For more information, see Chapter 62 in Smeltzer and Bare: *Brunner and Suddarth's Textbook of Medical-Surgical Nursing,* 9th edition. Philadelphia: Lippincott Williams & Wilkins, 2000.

BELL'S PALSY

Bell's palsy (facial paralysis) is due to peripheral involvement of the seventh cranial nerve on one side, which results in weakness or paralysis of the facial muscles. The cause is unknown, but possible causes may include vascular ischemia, viral disease (herpes simplex, herpes zoster), autoimmune disease, or a combination. Bell's palsy may represent a type of pressure paralysis causing a distortion of the face, increased lacrimation (tearing), and painful sensations in the face, behind the ear, and eye. The patient may experience speech difficulties and be unable to eat on the affected side owing to weakness.

Medical Management
The objectives of management are to maintain muscle tone of the face and to prevent or minimize denervation.

Reassure patient that no stroke has occurred and that spontaneous recovery occurs within 3 to 5 weeks in most patients.

Steroid therapy may be given to reduce inflammation and edema, which reduces vascular compression and permits restoration of blood circulation to the nerve. Early steroid administration appears to diminish severity, relieve pain, and minimize denervation.

Facial pain is controlled with analgesics or heat applied to the involved side of face.

Electrical stimulation may be applied to face to prevent muscle atrophy.

Surgical exploration may be done if tumor is suspected or for surgical decompression of the facial nerve, and for surgical rehabilitation of a paralyzed face.

Nursing Management

Promoting Home and Community-Based Care

Teaching Patients Self-Care: Eye Care
- Because the blink reflex is diminished, the involved eye may not close completely and needs to be protected.
- Inform of potential complications: corneal irritation and ulceration, overflow of tears, and absence of blink reflex.
- Cover eye with a protective shield at night.
- Apply eye ointment to keep eyelids closed during sleep.
- Teach patient to close the paralyzed eyelid manually before going to sleep.
- Instruct patient to wear wrap-around sunglasses or goggles to decrease normal evaporation from the eye.

Continuing Care: Maintain Muscle Tone
- Massage face with gentle upward motion several times daily.
- Use facial exercises, such as wrinkling the forehead, blowing out the cheeks, and whistling, in an effort to prevent muscle atrophy.
- Instruct patient to avoid exposing the face to cold and drafts.

For more information, see Chapter 59 in Smeltzer and Bare: *Brunner and Suddarth's Textbook of Medical-Surgical Nursing,* 9th edition. Philadelphia: Lippincott Williams & Wilkins, 2000.

BENIGN PROSTATIC HYPERPLASIA AND PROSTATECTOMY

Benign prostatic hyperplasia (BPH) is enlargement, or hypertrophy, of the prostate. The prostate gland enlarges, extending upward into the bladder and obstructing the outflow of urine. Incomplete emptying of the bladder and urinary retention with stasis of urine may result in hydronephrosis, hydroureter, and urinary tract infections. The cause is uncertain, but evidence suggests hormonal involvement. BPH is a common occurrence in men older than 50 years of age.

Clinical Manifestations
- On examination, the prostate is large, rubbery, and nontender.
- Prostatism (obstructive and irritative symptom complex) is noted:
  - Hesitancy in starting urination, increased frequency of urination, nocturia, urgency, abdominal straining
  - Decrease in volume and force of urinary stream, interruption of urinary stream, dribbling
  - Sensation of incomplete emptying of the bladder, acute urinary retention (more than 60 mL), and recurrent urinary tract infections
- Fatigue, anorexia, nausea and vomiting, and epigastric discomfort
- Ultimately, azotemia and renal failure, with chronic urinary retention and large residual volumes

Diagnostic Evaluation
- Physical examination, including a digital rectal examination (DRE)
- Urinalysis and urodynamic studies to determine obstructive flow
- Renal function tests, including serum creatinine levels
- Complete blood studies, including clotting studies

Medical Management

The plan of treatment depends on the cause, severity of obstruction, and condition of the patient

- Immediate catheterization is necessary if patient is unable to void (a urologist may be consulted if unable to insert an ordinary catheter). A suprapubic cystostomy is sometimes necessary
- "Watchful waiting" to monitor disease progression
- Balloon dilation or alpha-1-adrenergic receptor blockers (terazosin) relax smooth muscle of the bladder neck and prostate
- Hormonal manipulation with antiandrogen (finasteride [Proscar]) decreases the size of the prostate and improves urinary flow
- Transurethral laser resection with ultrasound guidance
- Transurethral needle ablation (spares the urethra, nerves, muscles, and membranes)
- Microwave thermotherapy (using transurethral probe) applied to hypertrophied tissue, which then becomes necrotic and sloughs
- Surgery (prostatectomy) to remove the hypertrophied portion of the prostate gland
  - Transurethral resection of the prostate (TUR or TURP); urethral endoscopic procedure is most common approach
  - Suprapubic prostatectomy; abdominal incision
  - Perineal prostatectomy; perineal incision and incontinence, impotence, or rectal injury may be complications
  - Retropubic prostatectomy; low abdominal incision

Nursing Management

See Nursing Management of the patient undergoing prostatectomy under Cancer of the Prostate for additional information.

For more information, see Chapter 45 in Smeltzer and Bare: *Brunner and Suddarth's Textbook of Medical-Surgical Nursing,* 9th edition. Philadelphia: Lippincott Williams & Wilkins, 2000.

BONE TUMORS

Neoplasms of the musculoskeletal system are of a variety of types. They include osteogenic, chondrogenic, fibrogenic, muscle, and marrow cell tumors as well as nerve, vascular, and fatty cell tumors. They may be primary tumors or metastatic tumors from primary cancers elsewhere in the body (eg, breast, lung, prostate, kidney). Metastatic bone tumors are more common than primary bone tumors. Tumors weaken the bone structure, resulting in bone fracture.

Types of Bone Tumors
Benign Bone Tumors
- Slow growing and well circumscribed; present few symptoms; not a cause of death
- Benign primary neoplasms of the musculoskeletal system: osteochondroma, enchondroma, osteoid osteoma, bone cyst, rhabdomyoma, fibroma
- Benign tumors of the bone and soft tissue are more common than malignant tumors
- Bone cysts: expanding lesions within the bone (eg, aneurysmal and unicameral)
- Osteochondroma: the most common benign bone tumor, may become malignant
- Enchondroma: a common tumor of the hyaline cartilage of hand, ribs, leg, humerus, or pelvis
- Osteoid osteoma: is a painful tumor that occurs in children and young adults
- Osteoclastoma (giant cell tumors) are benign for long periods but may invade local tissue and cause destruction; may undergo malignant transformation and metastasize

Malignant Bone Tumors
- Primary malignant musculoskeletal tumors are relatively rare and arise from connective and supportive tissue cells (sarcomas) or bone marrow elements (myelomas). Soft

tissue sarcomas include liposarcoma, fibrosarcoma, and rhabdomyosarcoma. Metastasis to the lungs is common.

- Osteogenic sarcoma (osteosarcoma) is the most common and is often fatal owing to metastasis to the lungs. It is seen most frequently in rapidly growing bones (boys aged 10 to 25 years), older people with Paget's disease, and patients exposed to radiation. Common sites are distal femur, proximal tibia, and proximal humerus.
- Chondrosarcoma, the second most common primary malignant bone tumor, is a large, bulky, slow-growing tumor that affects adults (men more frequently). Tumor sites may include pelvis, ribs, femur, humerus, spine, scapula, and tibia. They may recur after treatment.

Metastatic Bone Cancer (Secondary Bone Tumor)

Metastatic bone tumors are more common than any primary malignant bone tumor. Tumors that metastasize to bone most frequently include carcinomas of the kidney, prostate, lung, breast, ovary, and thyroid. Metastatic tumors frequently attack the skull, spine, pelvis, femur, and humerus.

Clinical Manifestations

Bone tumors present with a wide range of associated problems:

- Asymptomatic or pain (mild, occasional to constant, severe)
- Varying degrees of disability; at times, obvious bone growth
- Weight loss, malaise, and fever may be present
- Pain, swelling, and limitation of motion; the bony mass may be palpable, tender, and fixed; common sites are distal femur, proximal tibia, and proximal humerus

Diagnostic Evaluation

- May be diagnosed incidentally after pathologic fracture
- Computerized tomography (CT), bone scans, myelograms, magnetic resonance imaging (MRI), arteriography, and radiographs

- Biochemical assays of the blood and urine (alkaline phosphatase frequently elevated with osteogenic sarcoma; serum acid phosphatase elevated with metastatic carcinoma of the prostate; hypercalcemia present with breast, lung, and kidney cancer bone metastasis)
- Surgical biopsy for histologic identification; staging based on tumor size, grade, location, and metastasis

Medical Management

The goal of treatment is to destroy or remove the tumor. This may be accomplished by surgical excision (ranging from local incision to amputation and disarticulation), radiation, or chemotherapy.

- Soft tissue sarcomas are treated with radiation, limb-sparing excision with grafting as needed, and adjuvant chemotherapy.
- Metastatic bone cancer treatment is palliative; therapeutic goal is to relieve pain and discomfort as much as possible.
- Internal fixation of pathologic fractures, arthroplasty, or methylmethacrylate (bone cement) minimizes associated disability and pain.

Nursing Management
Assessment

- Ask patient about onset and course of symptoms. Note patient's and family's understanding of disease, coping with the problem, and management of pain.
- Palpate mass gently on physical examination. Note size and associated soft tissue swelling, pain, and tenderness.
- Assess neurovascular status and range of motion of extremity.
- Evaluate mobility and ability to perform activities of daily living.

Major Nursing Diagnoses

- Knowledge deficit related to the disease process and the therapeutic regimen

- Pain related to pathologic process and surgery
- Risk for injury: pathologic fracture related to tumor
- Ineffective coping related to fear of the unknown, perception of disease process, and inadequate support system
- Disturbance in self-esteem related to loss of body part or alteration in role performance

Collaborative Problems/Potential Complications
- Delayed wound healing
- Nutritional deficiency
- Infection

Planning and Goals
The major goals include knowledge of disease process and treatment regimen, control of pain, absence of pathologic fractures, effective patterns of coping, improved self-esteem, and absence of complications.

Nursing Interventions
PREOPERATIVE
- Explain diagnostic test, treatments, and expected results.
- Reinforce and clarify information provided by the physician.
- Encourage independence and function as long as possible.

POSTOPERATIVE
- Monitor vital signs; assess blood loss and development of complications (eg, deep vein thrombosis, pulmonary emboli, infection, contracture, and disuse atrophy).
- Elevate affected part to control swelling; assess neurovascular status of extremity; immobilize the area by splints, casts, or elastic bandages until the bone heals.

Controlling Pain
- Use nonpharmacologic and pharmacologic pain management techniques.
- Work with patient to design the most effective pain management.

- Prepare patient and give support during painful procedures.

Preventing Pathologic Fracture
- Support affected bones, and handle gently during nursing care.
- Use external supports (eg, splints) for additional protection.
- Follow prescribed weight-bearing restrictions.
- Teach how to use ambulatory devices safely and how to strengthen unaffected extremities.

Coping Effectively
- Encourage patient and family to verbalize fears, concerns, and feelings honestly.
- Support and accept patient and family as they deal with the impact of the malignant bone tumor.
- Expect feelings of shock, despair, and grief.
- Refer to health professionals and clergy for specific psychological help.

Promoting Self-Esteem
- Support family in working through adjustments that must be made, specifically changes in body image due to surgery and possible amputation.
- Provide realistic reassurance about the future and resumption of role-related activities; encourage self-care and socialization.
- Involve patient and family throughout treatment to encourage confidence and restoration of self-concept, and promote a sense of being in control of one's life.

Monitoring and Managing Potential Problems
- Minimize pressure on wound site to promote circulation.
- Promote healing with an aseptic, nontraumatic wound dressing.
- Monitor and report laboratory findings to facilitate treatment.

- Reposition patient frequently to prevent skin breakdown; use therapeutic beds when indicated.

Achieving Adequate Nutritional Status
- Give antiemetics and provide relaxation techniques to reduce gastrointestinal reaction.
- Control stomatitis with anesthetic or antifungal mouthwash.
- Provide adequate hydration, nutritional supplements, or total parenteral nutrition.

Managing Osteomyelitis and Wound Infections
- Use prophylactic antibiotics and strict aseptic dressing techniques.
- Prevent other infections (eg, upper respiratory), so that hematogenous spread does not result in osteomyelitis.
- Monitor white blood cell count, and instruct patient to avoid contact with people who have colds or infections.

Promoting Home and Community-Based Care

- Prepare and coordinate continuing health care and direct patient education toward medications, dressings, treatment regimens, weight-bearing limitations, and physical and occupational therapy programs.
- Teach signs and symptoms of possible complications to patient and family.
- Arrange for home care, and advise patient to keep telephone numbers of contact people readily available.
- Emphasize the need for long-term health supervision to ensure cure or to detect tumor recurrence or metastasis.
- Explore end-of-life issues if the patient has metastatic disease.

For more information, see Chapter 62 in Smeltzer and Bare: *Brunner and Suddarth's Textbook of Medical-Surgical Nursing,* 9th edition. Philadelphia: Lippincott Williams & Wilkins, 2000.

BOWEL OBSTRUCTION, LARGE

Intestinal obstruction (mechanical or functional) exists when blockage prevents the flow of contents through the intestinal tract. Large bowel obstruction results in an accumulation of intestinal contents, fluid, and gas proximal to the obstruction. Obstruction in the colon can lead to severe distention and perforation unless gas and fluid can flow back through the ileal valve. Dehydration occurs more slowly than in small bowel obstruction. If the blood supply is cut off, intestinal strangulation and necrosis occur; this condition is life-threatening.

Clinical Manifestations

Symptoms develop and progress relatively slowly.

- Constipation may be the only symptom for days (obstruction in sigmoid or rectum).
- Abdomen eventually becomes markedly distended, loops of large bowel become visibly outlined through the abdominal wall, and the patient suffers from crampy lower abdominal pain.
- Fecal vomiting develops; symptoms of shock may occur.

Diagnostic Evaluation

Symptoms and radiologic studies: flat and upright abdominal radiographs; barium studies are contraindicated.

Medical Management

- Colonoscopy to untwist and decompress the bowel, if obstruction is high in the colon.
- Cecostomy may be performed for patients who are poor surgical risks and urgently need relief from the obstruction.
- Rectal tube to decompress an area that is lower in the bowel.
- Usual treatment is surgical resection to remove the obstructing lesion; a temporary or permanent colostomy

may be necessary; an ileoanal anastomosis may be performed if entire large colon must be removed.

Nursing Management

- Monitor symptoms indicating worsening intestinal obstruction.
- Provide emotional support and comfort.
- Administer intravenous fluids and electrolyte replacement.
- Prepare patient for surgery if no response to medical treatment.
- Provide preoperative teaching as the patient's condition indicates.
- Give general abdominal wound care postoperatively.
- Provide routine postoperative nursing care.

See Preoperative and Postoperative Nursing Management for additional information.

For more information, see Chapter 35 in Smeltzer and Bare: *Brunner and Suddarth's Textbook of Medical-Surgical Nursing,* 9th edition. Philadelphia: Lippincott Williams & Wilkins, 2000.

BOWEL OBSTRUCTION, SMALL

Most bowel obstructions (85%) occur in the small intestine. An accumulation of intestinal contents, fluid, and gas develops above the intestinal obstruction. Distention and retention reduce the absorption of fluids and stimulate gastric secretion. Reflux vomiting may also occur. Fluids and electrolytes are lost. Dehydration and acidosis develop because of water and sodium loss. With acute fluid losses, hypovolemic shock may occur. Increasing distention and pressure within the intestinal lumen cause a decrease in venous and arteriolar capillary pressure, resulting in edema, congestion, necrosis, and eventual rupture or perforation of the intestinal wall with resultant peritonitis. Adhesions are the most common (60%) cause of obstruction. Other causes include hernias, neoplasms, intussusception, volvulus, and paralytic ileus.

Clinical Manifestations
- The initial symptom is usually crampy pain that is wave-like and colicky; the patient may pass blood and mucus but no fecal matter or flatus; vomiting occurs.
- Peristaltic waves become extremely vigorous and assume a reverse direction, propelling intestinal contents toward the mouth, if the obstruction is complete.
- If the obstruction is in the ileum, fecal vomiting takes place.
- Dehydration results in intense thirst, drowsiness, generalized malaise, and aching.
- Tongue and mucous membranes become parched; abdomen becomes distended (the lower the obstruction in the gastrointestinal tract, the more marked the distention).
- If uncorrected, shock occurs due to dehydration and loss of plasma volume.

Diagnostic Evaluation
- Symptoms, radiologic, and laboratory studies

Medical Management
- Decompression of the bowel may be achieved through a nasogastric or small bowel tube.
- When bowel is completely obstructed, possibility of strangulation warrants surgical intervention. Surgical treatment depends on the cause of obstruction.
- Before surgery, intravenous therapy is instituted to replace water, sodium, chloride, and potassium.

Nursing Management
- Maintain the function of the nasogastric tube; assess and measure the nasogastric output; assess for fluid and electrolyte imbalance.
- Monitor nutritional status; assess for improvement in bowel function (ie, return of normal bowel sounds,

decreased abdominal distention, subjective improvement in abdominal pain and tenderness, and passage of flatus or stool).

- Report discrepancies in intake and output, worsening of pain or abdominal distention, and increased nasogastric output.
- If the patient's condition does not improve, prepares him or her for surgery.
- Provide postoperative nursing care similar to that for other abdominal surgeries (see Preoperative and Postoperative Nursing Management for additional information).

For more information, see Chapter 35 in Smeltzer and Bare: *Brunner and Suddarth's Textbook of Medical-Surgical Nursing,* 9th edition. Philadelphia: Lippincott Williams & Wilkins, 2000.

BRAIN ABSCESS

A brain abscess is a collection of infectious material within the tissue of the brain. It may occur by direct invasion of the brain from intracranial trauma or surgery, by spread of infection from nearby sites (eg, sinuses, ears, teeth), or by spread of infection from other organs (lung abscess, infective endocarditis) and can be a complication associated with some forms of meningitis. It can be a complication in patients whose immune systems have been suppressed through therapy or disease.

Clinical Manifestations
- Generally, symptoms result from edema, brain shift, infection, or the location of the abscess.
- Headache, usually worse in morning, is the most continuing symptom.
- Vomiting and focal neurologic signs (weakness of an extremity, decreasing vision, seizures) may occur depending on the site of the abscess.

- Change in mental status may occur (eg, lethargic, confused, irritable, or disoriented behavior).
- Fever may or may not be present.

Diagnostic Evaluation
- Computed tomography (CT) scan locating the site of the abscess
- Magnetic resonance imaging (MRI) to obtain images of the brain stem and posterior fossa

Medical Management
Prevention
To prevent brain abscesses, treat otitis media, mastoiditis, sinusitis, dental infections, and systemic infections promptly.

Treatment
The goal of management is to eliminate the abscess.

- Antimicrobial therapy, surgical incision, or aspiration
- Corticosteroids to reduce the inflammatory cerebral edema
- Anticonvulsant medications for prophylaxis against seizures
- Monitor abscess resolution with CT scans
- Neurologic deficits after treatment may include hemiparesis, seizures, visual defects, and cranial nerve palsies
- Relapse common, with high mortality rate

Nursing Management
Interventions are supportive of the medical treatment. See Nursing Management under associated neurologic conditions (eg, Epilepsies, Meningitis, or Increased Intracranial Pressure).

For more information, see Chapter 59 in Smeltzer and Bare: *Brunner and Suddarth's Textbook of Medical-Surgical Nursing,* 9th edition. Philadelphia: Lippincott Williams & Wilkins, 2000.

BRAIN TUMORS

A brain tumor is a localized intracranial lesion that occupies space within the skull. In adults, most brain tumors originate in glial cells. The highest incidence of brain tumors in adults occurs between the fifth and seventh decades, with a slightly higher incidence in men. Brain tumors rarely metastasize outside the central nervous system, but cause death by impairing vital functions. Brain tumors are classified as follows: (1) *dural meningiomas*, those arising from the coverings of the brain; (2) *acoustic neuromas*, those developing in or on the cranial nerves; (3) various *gliomas*, those originating in the brain tissue; and (4) *metastatic lesions* originating elsewhere in the body. Tumors of the pineal gland and pituitary and of cerebral blood vessels are also included in the types of brain tumors. Tumors may be benign or malignant. A benign tumor may occur in a vital area and have effects as serious as a malignant tumor.

Specific Tumors

- Gliomas, the most frequent brain neoplasm, cannot be totally removed because they spread by infiltrating into the surrounding neural tissue.
- Pituitary adenomas may cause symptoms as a result of mass (pressure) effects on adjacent structures or hormonal changes.
- Angiomas are found in or on the surface of the brain; they may never cause symptoms, or they may give rise to symptoms of brain tumor. The walls of the blood vessels in angiomas are thin, increasing the risk for cerebral vascular accident (stroke).
- Acoustic neuroma is a tumor of the eighth cranial nerve (hearing and balance). It may grow slowly and attain considerable size before it is correctly diagnosed.
- Meningiomas are common benign encapsulated tumors of arachnoid cells on the meninges. They are slow growing and occur most often in middle-aged women.

Clinical Manifestations
Increasing Intracranial Pressure Symptoms

- Headache, although not always present, is most common in the early morning and is made worse by coughing, straining, or sudden movement. Headaches are usually described as deep, expanding, or dull but unrelenting. Frontal tumors produce a bilateral frontal headache; pituitary gland tumors produce bitemporal pain; in cerebellar tumors, the headache may be located in the suboccipital region at the back of the head.
- Vomiting, seldom related to food intake, is usually due to irritation of the vagal centers in the medulla.
- Papilledema is associated with visual disturbances.
- Mental changes (eg, dullness and giddiness) are often general but can be localized.
- Pituitary adenomas may cause symptoms of hormone imbalance and Cushing's disease (eg, fat redistribution, hypertension, elevated serum glucose) in addition to general symptoms.

Localized Symptoms

The progression of the signs and symptoms is important because it indicates tumor growth and expansion.

- Tumor of the motor cortex: convulsive movements localized on one side of the body (jacksonian seizures)
- Occipital lobe tumors: visual manifestations, such as contralateral homonymous hemianopsia (visual loss in half of the visual field on the opposite side of tumor) and visual hallucinations
- Tumors of the cerebellum: dizziness, ataxic or staggering gait, with tendency to fall toward side of lesion; marked muscle incoordination; and nystagmus
- Tumors of the frontal lobe: personality disorders, changes in emotional state and behavior, and a disinterested mental attitude
- Tumors of the acoustic nerve may reveal loss of hearing, tinnitus, vertigo, staggering gait, painful sensations of

the face (numbness, tingling) and tongue, progressing to weakness and paralysis of the face

Diagnostic Evaluation
- History of the illness and manner in which the symptoms evolved
- Neurologic examination indicating areas involved
- CT, MRI, computer-assisted stereotactic (three-dimensional) biopsy, cerebral angiography, electroencephalogram, and cytologic studies of the cerebrospinal fluid

Medical Management
The objective is to remove or destroy all of the tumor or as much as possible without increasing the neurologic deficit (paralysis, blindness) or to achieve relief of symptoms by partial tumor removal (decompression), radiation therapy, chemotherapy, or a combination of these.

- Evaluation and treatment should be done as soon as possible before irreversible neurologic damage occurs.
- Most patients undergo a neurosurgical procedure, followed by radiation and possibly chemotherapy.

Other Therapies
- Corticosteroids to prevent postoperative swelling
- Intravenous autologous bone marrow transplantation for marrow toxicity associated with high dosages of drugs and radiation
- Radioisotopes (^{131}I) implanted directly into the brain tumor (brachytherapy)
- Gene-transfer therapy is an approach currently being tested

Nursing Management
- Evaluate gag reflex and ability to swallow preoperatively.
- Teach patient to direct food and fluids toward the unaffected side, assist the patient upright to eat, offering a

semisoft diet and having suction readily available, if diminished gag response.

- Reassess function postoperatively because changes can occur.
- Perform neurologic checks; monitor vital signs; maintain a neurologic flow record; space nursing interventions to prevent rapid increase in intracranial pressure (ICP).
- Reorient patient when necessary to person, time, and place.
- Use orienting devices (personal possessions, photographs, lists, clock); supervise and assist with self-care; monitor and intervene for prevention of injury.
- Carefully monitor patients with seizures.
- Check motor function at intervals; assess sensory disturbances.
- Evaluate speech; assess eye movement, pupil size, and reaction.

For more information, see Chapters 57 and 59 in Smeltzer and Bare: *Brunner and Suddarth's Textbook of Medical-Surgical Nursing,* 9th edition. Philadelphia: Lippincott Williams & Wilkins, 2000.

BRONCHIECTASIS

Bronchiectasis is a chronic, irreversible dilation and impaired mucociliary clearance of the bronchi and bronchioles. The result is retention of secretions, obstruction, and eventual alveolar collapse. Bronchiectasis may be caused by a variety of conditions, including pulmonary infections and obstruction of the bronchus; aspiration of foreign bodies, vomitus, or material from the respiratory tract; and pressure from tumors, dilated blood vessels, and enlarged lymph nodes. Bronchiectasis is usually localized in a lobe or segment of a lung (frequently the lower lobes). A person may be predisposed to bronchiectasis (history of recurrent respiratory infections, measles, influenza, tuberculosis, and immunodeficiency disorders). Patients with bronchiectasis almost always have bronchitis.

Clinical Manifestations
- Chronic cough and production of copious purulent sputum, which has a quality of "layering out" into three layers on standing: a frothy top layer, a middle clear layer, and a dense particulate bottom layer
- Hemoptysis, clubbing of the fingers, and repeated episodes of pulmonary infection

Diagnostic Evaluation
- Definite diagnostic clue is prolonged history of productive cough, with sputum consistently negative for tubercle bacilli.
- Diagnosis is established on the basis of computed tomography (CT) scan.
- Bronchogram is occasionally performed.

Medical Management
The objectives of treatment are to prevent and control infection and to promote bronchial drainage.

- Chest physiotherapy with percussion; postural drainage, expectorants, or bronchoscopy to remove bronchial secretions
- Antimicrobial therapy guided by sputum sensitivity studies
- Year-round regimen of antibiotics, alternating types of drugs at intervals
- Vaccination against influenza and pneumococcal pneumonia
- Bronchodilators; sympathomimetics (beta-adrenergic agonists)
- Increased oral fluid intake
- Smoking cessation
- Surgical intervention (segmental resection to lobe or lung removal), used infrequently

- In preparation for surgery: vigorous postural drainage, suction through bronchoscope, and antibacterial therapy

Nursing Management

See Nursing Management and Patient Education under Chronic Obstructive Pulmonary Disease and Preoperative and Postoperative Nursing Management for additional information.

For more information, see Chapter 21 in Smeltzer and Bare: *Brunner and Suddarth's Textbook of Medical-Surgical Nursing,* 9th edition. Philadelphia: Lippincott Williams & Wilkins, 2000.

BRONCHITIS, CHRONIC

Chronic bronchitis is defined as a productive cough that lasts 3 months a year for 2 consecutive years with other causes excluded. Chronic exposure to smoke or another pollutant irritates the airways resulting in hypersecretion of mucus and inflammation, thickened bronchial walls, and narrow bronchial lumen. Risk factors include cigarette smoking (major risk factor) or exposure to pollution or hazardous airborne substances. Patients have increased susceptibility to recurring infections of the lower respiratory tract.

Clinical Manifestations
- Chronic, productive cough in winter months, earliest sign; cough is exacerbated by cold weather, dampness, and pulmonary irritants
- History of cigarette smoking, frequent respiratory infections

Diagnostic Evaluation
- History, including family, exposure to irritants, including smoking habits
- Pulse oximetry, arterial blood gases, chest radiograph, pulmonary function studies, blood counts

Medical Management

Prevention

- Smoking cessation
- Minimized exposure to environmental irritants
- Prophylactic vaccination against influenza and pneumonia
- Antimicrobial therapy at the first sign of purulent sputum

Treatment

The main objectives of treatment are to keep the bronchials open and functioning, facilitate removal of secretions, and prevent disability.

- Note changes in the sputum pattern (nature, color, amount, thickness) and in the cough pattern.
- Treat recurrent bacterial infections with antibiotic therapy.
- Facilitate removal of secretions (bronchodilators).
- Provide for postural drainage and chest percussion.
- Give fluids orally or parenterally to liquefy secretions.
- Use steroid therapy when conservative measures fail.
- Patient must stop smoking (causes bronchoconstriction).
- Counsel patient to avoid respiratory irritants (eg, tobacco smoke).
- Immunize against common viral agents (influenza, pneumonia).
- Provide proper treatment for acute upper respiratory infections (antimicrobial therapy and sensitivity studies).

Nursing Management

See Preoperative and Postoperative Nursing Management and Patient Education under Chronic Obstructive Pulmonary Disease for additional information.

For more information, see Chapter 21 in Smeltzer and Bare: *Brunner and Suddarth's Textbook of Medical-Surgical Nursing,* 9th edition. Philadelphia: Lippincott Williams & Wilkins, 2000.

BUERGER'S DISEASE (THROMBOANGIITIS OBLITERANS)

Buerger's disease is a recurring inflammation of the intermediate and small arteries and veins of the lower and, rarely, upper extremities. It results in thrombus formation and occlusion of the vessels. It is believed to be an autoimmune vasculitis. It occurs most often in men between the ages of 20 and 35 years and has been reported in all races in many areas of the world. There is considerable evidence that heavy smoking or chewing of tobacco is either a causative or aggravating factor.

Clinical Manifestations
- Pain is the outstanding symptom; complaints of cramps in the feet (arches) after exercise (instep claudication); relieved by rest; involvement usually bilateral and symmetric
- Burning pain aggravated by emotional disturbances, nicotine, or chilling; digital rest pain (fingers or toes); a feeling of coldness or sensitivity to cold may be early symptoms
- Types of paresthesia may develop; pulses diminished or absent
- Color changes (rubor) of the feet progressing to cyanosis (in only one extremity or certain digits)
- Ulceration with gangrene eventually occurs

Diagnostic Evaluation
Segmental limb blood pressure, duplex ultrasound, and contrast angiography are used to identify occlusions.

Medical Management
See Medical Management under Peripheral Arterial Occlusive Disease for additional information.

The main objectives are to improve circulation to the extremities, prevent the progression of the disease, and protect the extremities from trauma and infection.

- Stop smoking completely.
- Vasodilators are rarely prescribed (cause dilation of healthy vessels only).
- Regional sympathetic block or ganglionectomy produce vasodilation and increase blood flow.
- Conservative débridement of necrotic tissue is used in treatment of ulceration and gangrene.
- If gangrene of a toe develops, usually a below-knee amputation, or occasionally an above-knee amputation, is necessary.
- Indications for amputation are worsening gangrene (especially if moist), severe rest pain, or sepsis secondary to gangrene.

Nursing Management

See Nursing Management under Peripheral Arterial Occlusive Disease for additional information.

 Gerontologic Considerations

In older patients, Buerger's disease may be followed by atherosclerosis of the larger vessels after involvement of the smaller vessels.

For more information, see Chapter 28 in Smeltzer and Bare: *Brunner and Suddarth's Textbook of Medical-Surgical Nursing,* 9th edition. Philadelphia: Lippincott Williams & Wilkins, 2000.

BURN INJURY

Burns are caused by a transfer of energy from a heat source to the body. The depth of the injury depends on the temperature of the burning agent and the duration of contact with the agent. Burns can be categorized as thermal, radiation, electrical, or chemical. Young children and elderly people are at particularly high risk for burn injury. Those younger than 5 years and older than 40 years are at risk for death after burn trauma.

Burn Depth

Burns are classified according to the depth of tissue destruction:

- Superficial partial-thickness (similar to first-degree), including sunburn; skin involvement includes the epidermis and may involve a portion of the dermis.
- Deep partial-thickness (similar to second-degree), including scald; skin involvement includes the epidermis and upper to deeper portions of the dermis.
- Full-thickness (third-degree), including flame, electric current; skin involvement includes the epidermis, entire dermis, and sometimes underlying tissue.

Extent of Surface Area Burned

Depth of burn is affected by the type of injury, causative agent, temperature of burning agent, duration of contact, and thickness of the burn patient's skin. Determination of how much surface area is affected is achieved by one of the following methods:

- Rule of nines: an estimation of the total body surface area (BSA) burned by dividing the body into multiples of nine
- Lund and Browder method: a more precise method of estimating extent of burned BSA that recognizes that the percentage of BSA surface of various anatomic parts (head and legs) changes with growth
- Palm method: a method to estimate percentage of scattered burns, using the size of the patient's palm (about 1% of BSA) for assessing extent of burn injury

Medical Management

Four major goals relating to burns are prevention; institution of life-saving measures for the severely burned person; prevention of disability and disfigurement; and rehabilitation.

Nursing Management: Burn Care During the Emergent and Resuscitative Phase

Assessment

- Review the initial assessment data obtained by prehospital providers. If needed, further assess the time of injury, mechanism of burn, whether the burn occurred in a closed space, the possibility of inhalation of noxious chemicals, and any related trauma.
- Focus on the major priorities of any trauma patient: A–airway, B–breathing, C–circulation (also cervical-spine immobilization and cardiac monitoring), D–disability, E–exposure, and F–fluid resuscitation. The burn wound is a secondary consideration, although aseptic management of burn wounds is continued.
- Monitor for respiratory status as first priority: airway patency and breathing adequacy.
- Note presence of increased hoarseness, stridor, abnormal respiratory rate and depth, or mental changes from hypoxia.
- Evaluate circulation: apical, carotid, and femoral pulses; start cardiac monitoring if indicated (eg, electrical injury, history of cardiac or respiratory problems or dysrhythmia).
- Check vital signs frequently using an ultrasound device if necessary.
- Check peripheral pulses on burned extremities hourly; use Doppler as needed.
- Monitor fluid intake (intravenous fluids) and output (urinary catheter) and measure hourly; assess urine-specific gravity, pH, protein, and hemoglobin; note amount of urine obtained when catheter inserted (indicates preburn renal function and fluid status).
- Arrange for patients with facial burns to be assessed for corneal injury.
- Assess body temperature, body weight, history of preburn weight, allergies, tetanus immunization, past medical-surgical problems, current illnesses, and use of medication.

- Assess depth of the wound, and identify areas of full- and partial-thickness injury.
- Assess neurologic status: consciousness; psychological status, pain and anxiety levels, and behavior.
- Assess patient's and family's understanding of injury and treatment; assess patient's support system and coping skills.

Major Nursing Diagnoses
- Impaired gas exchange related to carbon monoxide poisoning, smoke inhalation, and upper airway obstruction
- Ineffective airway clearance related to edema and effects of smoke inhalation
- Fluid volume deficit related to increased capillary permeability and evaporative fluid loss from the burn wound
- Hypothermia related to loss of skin microcirculation and open wounds
- Pain related to tissue and nerve injury and emotional impact of injury
- Anxiety related to fear and emotional impact of injury

Collaborative Problems/Potential Complications
- Acute respiratory failure
- Distributive shock
- Acute renal failure
- Compartment syndrome
- Paralytic ileus
- Curling's ulcer

Planning and Goals
The major goals for the emergent and resuscitative phase include maintenance of a patent airway and tissue oxygenation; restoration of optimal fluid and electrolyte balance and perfusion of vital organs; maintenance of adequate body temperature; minimal pain and anxiety; and absence of complications.

Nursing Interventions

PROMOTING GAS EXCHANGE AND
AIRWAY CLEARANCE

- Provide humidified oxygen, and monitor arterial blood gases (ABGs), pulse oximetry, and carboxyhemoglobin levels.
- Assess breath sounds, respiratory rate, rhythm, depth, and symmetry; monitor for hypoxia.
- Observe for signs of inhalation injury: blistering of lips or buccal mucosa, singed nostrils, burns of face, neck, or chest, increasing hoarseness, or soot in sputum or respiratory secretions.
- Report labored respirations, decreased depth of respirations, or signs of hypoxia to physician immediately; prepare to assist with intubation and escharotomies.
- Monitor mechanically ventilated patient closely.
- Institute aggressive pulmonary care measures: turning, coughing, deep breathing, periodic forceful inspiration using spirometry, and tracheal suctioning.
- Maintain proper positioning to promote removal of secretions and patent airway and to promote optimal chest expansion; use artificial airway as needed.
- Maintain asepsis to prevent contamination of the respiratory tract and infection that increases metabolic requirements.

RESTORING FLUID AND ELECTROLYTE BALANCE

- Insert large-bore intravenous catheters and an indwelling urinary catheter.
- Monitor vital signs and urinary output (hourly), central venous pressure, pulmonary artery pressure, and cardiac output. Note and report signs of hypovolemia or fluid overload.
- Provide intravenous fluids as prescribed, and titrate with urinary output; document intake and output and daily weight.
- Elevate head of patient's bed and burned extremities.

- Monitor serum electrolyte levels (eg, sodium, potassium, calcium, phosphorus, bicarbonate); recognize developing electrolyte imbalances.

MAINTAINING NORMAL BODY TEMPERATURE
- Provide warm environment through use of heat shield, space blanket, heat lights, or blankets.
- Assess core body temperature frequently.
- Work quickly when wounds must be exposed to minimize heat loss from the wound.

MINIMIZING PAIN AND ANXIETY
- Use a pain scale to assess pain level (ie, 1 to 10).
- Differentiate from hypoxia.
- Perform a respiratory assessment before giving analgesics to nonventilated patients.
- Administer intravenous analgesics as prescribed, and assess response to medication.
- Assess patient's and family's understanding of burn injury, coping strategies, family dynamics, and anxiety levels, and provide individualized responses to meet patient and family coping levels.
- Provide emotional support, reassurance, and simple explanations about procedures.
- Provide pain relief, and give antianxiety medications if patient remains highly anxious and agitated after psychological interventions.

MONITORING AND MANAGING
POTENTIAL COMPLICATIONS
- Acute respiratory failure: assess for increasing dyspnea, stridor, changes in respiratory patterns; monitor pulse oximetry, ABG values for decreasing pO_2 or oxygen saturation, and increasing CO_2; monitor chest radiographs; assess for cerebral hypoxia (eg, restlessness, confusion); report deteriorating respiratory status immediately to physician; and assist as needed with intubation or escharotomy.
- Distributive shock: monitor for early signs of shock (decreasing urine output, cardiac output, pulmonary

artery pressure (PAP), pulmonary capillary wedge pressure (PCWP), blood pressure, or increasing pulse) or progressive edema; manage by fluid resuscitation as ordered in response to physical findings; continue monitoring fluid status.

- Acute renal failure: monitor and report abnormal urine output and quality, blood urea nitrogen (BUN) and creatinine levels; assess for urine hemoglobin or myoglobin; administer fluids as prescribed.
- Compartment syndrome: assess neurovascular status of extremities hourly (warmth, capillary refill, sensation, and movement); report any extremity pain, loss of peripheral pulses or sensation; remove blood pressure cuff after each reading; elevate burned extremities; prepare to assist with escharotomies.
- Paralytic ileus: insert nasogastric tube and maintain on low intermittent suction until bowel sounds resume; assess abdomen regularly for distention and bowel sounds; begin oral feedings as soon as possible when ileus is resolved.
- Curling's ulcer: assess gastric aspirate for blood and pH; assess stools for occult blood; administer antacids and histamine blockers (eg, ranitidine [Zantac]) as prescribed.

Nursing Management: Burn Care During the Acute and Intermediate Phase

The acute or intermediate phase begins 42 to 72 hours after the burn injury. Burn wound care and pain control are priorities at this stage.

Assessment

- Focus on hemodynamic alterations, wound healing, pain and psychosocial responses, and early detection of complications.
- Measure vital signs frequently; respiratory and fluid status remain highest priority.
- Assess peripheral pulses frequently for first few days after the burn for restricted blood flow.

- Observe electrocardiogram for dysrhythmias resulting from potassium imbalance, preexisting cardiac disease, or the effects of electrical injury or burn shock.
- Assess residual gastric volumes and pH in patients with nasogastric tubes (for clues to early sepsis or need for antacid therapy).
- Note and report blood in gastric fluid or stool.
- Assess wound: size, color, odor, eschar, exudate, abscess formation under the eschar, epithelial buds, bleeding, granulation tissue appearance, progress of graphs and donor sites, and quality of surrounding skin. Report significant wound changes to physician.
- Focus on pain and psychosocial responses, daily body weight, caloric intake, general hydration, and serum electrolyte, hemoglobin, and hematocrit levels.
- Assess for excessive bleeding adjacent to areas of surgical exploration and débridement.

Major Nursing Diagnoses
- Fluid volume excess related to resumption of capillary integrity and fluid shift from interstitial to intravascular compartment
- Risk for infection related to loss of skin barrier and impaired immune response
- Altered nutrition: less than body requirements related to hypermetabolism and wound healing needs
- Impaired skin integrity related to open burn wounds
- Pain related to exposed nerves, wound healing, and treatments
- Impaired physical mobility related to burn wound edema, pain, and joint contractures
- Ineffective individual coping related to fear and anxiety, grieving, and forced dependence on health care providers
- Altered family processes related to burn injury
- Knowledge deficit about the course of burn treatment

Collaborative Problems/Potential Complications

- Congestive heart failure and pulmonary edema, sepsis, acute respiratory failure, acute respiratory distress syndrome, visceral damage (electrical burns)

Planning and Goals

The major goals may include restoration of normal fluid balance, absence of infection, attainment of anabolic state and normal weight, improved skin integrity, reduction of pain and discomfort, optimal physical mobility, adequate patient and family coping, adequate patient and family knowledge of burn treatment, and absence of complications.

Nursing Interventions

RESTORING NORMAL FLUID BALANCE

- Monitor intravenous and oral fluid intake; use intravenous infusion pumps or rate controllers.
- Measure intake and output and daily weight.
- Report changes in hemodynamics (pulmonary arterial, wedge, and central venous pressures, blood pressure, pulse rate) and urine output (less than 30 mL/h) to physician.
- Administer low-dose dopamine to increase renal perfusion and diuretics to promote increased urine output; monitor patient's response.

PREVENTING INFECTION

- Provide a clean and safe environment; protect patient from sources of cross-contamination (eg, visitors, other patients, staff, tubing, and lines).
- Caution patient to avoid touching wounds or dressings; bathe unburned areas and change linens regularly.
- Practice aseptic technique for wound care and invasive procedures.
- Closely scrutinize the burn wound to detect early signs of infection. Monitor culture results and white blood cell counts.

MAINTAINING ADEQUATE NUTRITION

- Initiate oral fluids slowly when bowel sounds resume.
- Collaborate with dietitian to plan a protein and calorie-rich diet acceptable to patient; encourage family to bring nutritious favorite foods; offer and provide nutritional and vitamin and mineral supplements.
- Document caloric intake; insert feeding tube if caloric goals cannot be met by oral feeding (for continuous or bolus feedings); note residual volumes. Total parenteral nutrition (TPN) may be required.
- Weigh patients daily and graph weights.
- Encourage and support the patient with anorexia to increase food intake; provide pleasant surroundings at mealtime; cater food preferences; and offer high-protein, high-vitamin snacks.

PROMOTING SKIN INTEGRITY

- Assess wound status; use creative approaches to wound dressing; support during emotionally distressing and painful wound care.
- Coordinate complex aspects of wound care and dressing changes.
- Assess and record any changes and progress in wound healing; inform all members of the health care team of changes in the wound or treatment.
- Assist patient and family by instruction, support, and encouragement to take an active part in dressing changes and wound care.
- Anticipate home care needs early; assess strengths of patient and family when preparing for discharge and home care.

RELIEVING PAIN AND DISCOMFORT

- Teach the patient relaxation techniques; give some control over wound care and analgesia; provide frequent reassurance.
- Provide guided imagery in altering patient perceptions and responses to pain; distraction, hypnosis, biofeedback, and behavioral modification are also useful.

- Administer minor antianxiety medications and analgesics before pain becomes too severe; assess and document the patient's response to medication; assess frequently for pain and discomfort.
- Work quickly to complete treatments and dressing changes; encourage to use analgesic medications before painful procedures.
- Promote comfort during healing phase by using oral antipruritic agents, a cool environment, lubrication of the skin, exercise and splinting to prevent skin contracture, and diversional activities.

PROMOTING PHYSICAL MOBILITY

- Prevent complications (atelectasis, pneumonia, edema, pressure ulcers, and contractures) resulting from immobility by deep breathing, turning, and proper repositioning.
- Modify interventions to meet the individual patient needs; encourage early sitting and ambulation; when legs are involved, apply elastic pressure bandages before the patient is placed in an upright position.
- Make aggressive efforts to prevent contractures and hypertrophic scarring of the wound area after wound closure for a year or more.
- Initiate passive and active range-of-motion (ROM) exercises from admission until after grafting within prescribed limitations.
- Apply splints or functional devices to extremities for contracture control; monitor for signs of vascular insufficiency and nerve compression.

STRENGTHENING COPING STRATEGIES

- Assist patient in developing effective coping strategies by setting specific expectations for behavior, promoting truthful communication to build trust, helping patient practice coping strategies, and giving positive reinforcement when appropriate.
- Demonstrate acceptance of the patient; enlist a noninvolved person for patient to vent feelings without fear of retaliation.

- Include patient in decisions regarding care; encourage patient to assert individuality and preferences; set realistic expectations for self-care.

SUPPORTING PATIENT AND FAMILY PROCESSES
- Support and address patient and family's verbal and nonverbal concerns.
- Instruct family in ways to support the patient; support the patient and family.
- Make psychological or social work referrals as needed.
- Provide thorough information about the patient's burn care and expected course of treatment.
- Initiate patient and family education at the time of burn management; assess and consider preferred learning styles; assess patient and family ability to grasp and cope with the information and barriers to learning when planning and executing teaching.

MONITORING AND MANAGING
POTENTIAL COMPLICATIONS
- Congestive heart failure: assess for decreased cardiac output, oliguria, jugular vein distention, edema, or onset of S_3 or S_4 heart sounds.
- Pulmonary edema: assess for increasing central venous pressure (CVP), pulmonary artery and wedge pressures, and crackles, and report promptly. Position comfortably with head elevated unless contraindicated; administer medications and oxygen as ordered, assess response.
- Sepsis: assess for increased temperature, increased pulse, widened pulse pressure, and flushed, dry skin in unburned areas (early signs), and note the trends in the date; perform wound and blood cultures as prescribed; give scheduled antibiotics on time.
- Acute respiratory failure and adult respiratory distress syndrome (ARDS): monitor respiratory status for dyspnea, change in respiratory pattern, and onset of adventitious sounds; assess for decrease in tidal volume and lung compliance in patients on mechanical ventilation.

The hallmark of onset of ARDS is hypoxemia on 100% oxygen, decreased lung compliance, and significant shunting; notify physician of deteriorating respiratory status.

- Visceral damage (from electrical burns): monitor ECG and report dysrhythmias; pay attention to pain related to deep muscle ischemia and report. Early detection may minimize severity of this complication; fasciotomies may be necessary to relieve swelling and ischemia in the muscles and fascia; monitor the patient for excessive blood loss and hypovolemia after fasciotomy.

🏠 Promoting Home and Community-Based Care

- Recognize that family roles are disrupted when patients are sent to burn centers; many centers are far from home, compounding role disruption.
- Give patient and family thorough information about the burn care and expected course of treatment.
- Assess patient's and family's abilities to process the educational content; do not provide information before they can cope with it.

Evaluation

EXPECTED OUTCOMES
- Achieves optimal fluid balance
- Experiences no localized or systemic infection
- Demonstrates anabolic nutritional status
- Demonstrates improved skin integrity
- Experiences minimal pain
- Demonstrates optimal physical mobility
- Uses appropriate coping strategies to deal with postburn problems
- Relates appropriately in patient and family processes
- Patient and family verbalize understanding of the treatment course
- Experiences no complications

Nursing Management: Burn Care for the Rehabilitation and Long-Term Phase

It is important that rehabilitation begin immediately after the burn has occurred. Wound healing, psychosocial support, and restoring maximum functional activity remain priorities. Maintaining fluid and electrolyte balance and improving nutrition status continue to be a focus.

Assessment

- In early assessment, obtain information about the patient's educational level, occupation, leisure activities, cultural background, religion, and family interactions.
- Assess self-concept, mental status, emotional response to injury and hospitalization, level of intellectual functioning, previous hospitalizations, response to pain and pain relief measures, and sleep pattern.
- Perform ongoing assessments relative to rehabilitation goals, including ROM of affected joints, functional abilities in activities of daily living (ADLs), early signs of skin breakdown from splints or positioning devices, evidence of neuropathies, activity tolerance, and condition of healing skin.
- Document participation and self-care abilities in wound care, ambulation, and feeding.
- Maintain comprehensive and continuous assessment for early detection of complications with specific assessments as needed for specific treatments, such as postoperative assessment of patient undergoing primary excision.

Major Nursing Diagnoses

- Activity intolerance related to pain on exercise, limited joint mobility, muscle wasting, and limited endurance.
- Body image disturbance related to altered physical appearance and self-concept.
- Knowledge deficit of postdischarge home care and follow-up needs.

Collaborative Problems/Potential Complications

- Contractures
- Inadequate psychological adaptation to burn injury

Planning and Goals

The goals include increased participation in ADLs; increased understanding of the injury, treatment, and planned follow-up care; adaptation and adjustment to alterations in body image, self-concept, and lifestyle; and absence of complications.

Nursing Interventions

PROMOTING ACTIVITY TOLERANCE

- Schedule care to allow periods of uninterrupted sleep.
- Communicate plan of care to family and other caregivers.
- Listen and reassure patient, and administer hypnotics, as prescribed, to promote sleep.
- Reduce metabolic stress by relieving pain, preventing chilling or fever, and promoting physical integrity of all body systems to help conserve energy; monitor fatigue, pain, and fever to determine amount of activity to be encouraged daily.
- Incorporate physical therapy exercises to prevent muscular atrophy and maintain mobility required for daily activities.
- Improve psychological outlook, and increase tolerance for activity by scheduling diversion activities in periods of increasing duration.

IMPROVING BODY IMAGE AND SELF-CONCEPT

- Refer patients to a support group to meet others with similar experiences and develop coping strategies to deal with losses.
- Assess patient's psychosocial reactions; provide support and develop a plan to help the patient handle these feelings.
- Promote a healthy body image and self-concept by helping patients practice responses to people who stare or ask about their injury.
- Recognize patient through small gestures such as providing a birthday cake, combing patient's hair before visi-

tors, and sharing information on cosmetic resources to enhance appearance.
- Teach patient to direct attention away from a disfigured body to the self within.
- Coordinate consultants, such as psychologists, social workers, vocational counselors, and teachers during rehabilitation.

MONITORING AND MANAGING POTENTIAL COMPLICATIONS
- Contractures: provide early and aggressive physical and occupational therapy; support patient if intervention with surgery is needed to achieve full range of motion.
- Impaired psychological adaptation to the burn injury: obtain psychological or psychiatric referral as soon as evidence of major coping problems appear.

Promoting Home and Community-Based Care

Teaching Patients Self-Care and Continuing Care
- Throughout the phases of burn care, make efforts to prepare patient and family for the care they will perform at home (instruct them about measures and procedures).
- Provide verbal and written instructions about wound care, prevention of complications, pain management, and nutrition.
- Include families in planning and carrying out care according to their interest, ability, and patient's needs.
- Encourage and support patients and families to handle follow-up wound care; coordinate all aspects of care.
- Refer patient for home care to provide assistance with wound care and exercises for patients with inadequate support systems.
- Inform and review with patient-specific exercises and use of elastic pressure garments and splints; provide written instruction.
- Evaluate patient status periodically by burn team for modification of home care instructions and planning for reconstructive surgery.

Gerontologic Considerations

Elderly people are at higher risk for burn injury because of reduced mobility, changes in vision, and decreased sensation in feet and hands. The morbidity and mortality associated with burns are often much greater than with younger patients. Thinning and loss of elasticity of the skin in elderly people predispose them to a deep injury from a thermal insult that might cause a less severe burn in a younger person.

Chronic illness decreases the aged person's ability to withstand the multisystem stressors of burn injury and requires close observation with even relatively small burns, during the emergent and acute phases. Acute oliguric renal failure is more common in elderly people than in those younger than 40 years of age. Suppressed immunologic response, high incidence of malnutrition, and inability to withstand metabolic stressors (cold environment) further compromise the patient's ability to heal. Eschar separation in full-thickness burns is delayed.

Nursing assessment should include particular attention to pulmonary function, response to fluid resuscitation, and signs of mental confusion or disorientation; careful history of preburn medications and preexisting illnesses is essential.

Contact social and community nursing services to provide for optimal care upon hospital discharge.

Evaluation

EXPECTED OUTCOMES
- Demonstrates activity tolerance required for desired daily activities
- Adapts to altered body image
- Demonstrates knowledge of required self-care and follow-up care
- Exhibits no complications

For more information, see Chapter 53 in Smeltzer and Bare: *Brunner and Suddarth's Textbook of Medical-Surgical Nursing,* 9th edition. Philadelphia: Lippincott Williams & Wilkins, 2000.

C

CANCER

Cancer is a disease process that begins when a normal cell is transformed by the genetic mutation of the cellular DNA. This mutated cell forms a clone and begins to proliferate abnormally, ignoring growth-regulating signals in the environment surrounding the cell. The cells acquire invasive characteristics, and changes occur in surrounding tissues. The cells infiltrate these tissues and gain access to lymph and blood vessels, which carry the cells to other areas of the body. This phenomenon is called *metastasis* (cancer spread to other parts of the body). Cancerous cells are described as malignant neoplasms. Cancer is second only to cardiovascular disease as a leading cause of death in the United States. Although cancer affects every age group, most cancers occur in people older than 65 years of age. Overall, the incidence of cancer is higher in men than in women and higher in industrialized sectors and nations. Certain categories of agents or factors implicated in carcinogenesis (malignant transformation) include viruses, physical agents, chemical agents, genetic or familial factors, dietary factors, and hormonal agents.

Clinical Manifestations
- Cancerous cells spread from one organ or body part to another by invasion and metastasis; therefore, manifestations related to system affected and degree of disruption. (See the specific type of cancer).
- Generally, cancer can cause anemia, weakness, weight loss (dysphagia, anorexia, blockage), and pain (often in late stages).

- Symptoms are often due to tissue destruction and replacement with nonfunctional cancer tissue or over-productive cancer tissue (eg, bone marrow disruption and anemia or excess adrenal steroid productions); pressure on surrounding structures, increased metabolic demands, and disruption of production of blood cells.

Diagnostic Evaluation
- Screening to detect early cancer usually focuses on cancers with the highest incidence or those that have improved survival rates if diagnosed early. Examples of these cancers include breast, colorectal, cervical, endometrial, testicular, skin, and oropharyngeal cancers.
- Patients with suspected cancer undergo extensive testing for the following reasons:
  - To determine the presence of tumor and its extent
  - To identify possible spread (metastasis) of disease or invasion of other body tissues
  - To evaluate the function of involved and uninvolved body systems and organs
  - To obtain tissue and cells for analysis, including tumor stage (tumor size, presence of metastasis, and grade classification, eg, TNM stage).
- Diagnostic tests may include imaging tests (magnetic resonance imaging [MRI], computed tomography [CT] scan, endoscopy, fluoroscopy, positron emission tomography [PET] scan, radioimmunoconjugates, ultrasonography; and biopsy.

TMN Classification System
Tumors are staged depending on size, lymph node involvement, and metastasis. Staging is also expressed in TNM symbols: T indicates primary tumor; N, lymph node involvement; and M, metastasis.

- *Stage I:* tumor less than 2 cm, negative lymph node involvement, no detectable metastases

- *Stage II:* tumor greater than 2 cm but less than 5 cm, negative or positive unfixed lymph node involvement, no detectable metastases
- *Stage III:* large tumor greater than 5 cm, or a tumor of any size with invasion of the skin or chest wall or positive fixed lymph node involvement in the clavicular area without evidence of metastases
- *Stage IV:* tumor of any size, positive or negative lymph node involvement, and distant metastases

Laboratory Values
- Tumor marker identification may be beneficial for some cancers.
- Complete blood count, electrolytes, hormone levels, liver enzyme studies, as well as other chemistry studies might be helpful in identifying secondary effects of tumor (eg, anemia, neutropenia).

Medical Management
The range of possible treatment goals may include complete eradication of malignant disease (*cure*), prolonged survival and containment of cancer cell growth (*control*), or relief of symptoms associated with the disease (*palliation*).

- A variety of therapies may be used, including surgery (eg, video-assisted endoscopic surgery, salvage surgery, electrosurgery, cryosurgery, chemosurgery, or laser surgery). Surgery could be for prophylactic, palliative, or reconstructive purposes.
- Radiation therapy and chemotherapy may be used individually or in combination.
- Biologic response modifier (BRM) therapy may be used at various times throughout treatment.

Nursing Management: The Patient With Cancer
Assessment
- Assess the patient for secondary problems, such as infection, reduced white blood cell (WBC) counts, bleeding, skin problems, nutritional problems, pain, fatigue, and psychological stress.

C

- Assess factors that can promote infection, such as impaired skin, chemotherapy, radiation and other therapy, malignancy, medications, age, chronic illness, intravenous line, urinary catheter, and other invasive procedures.
- Monitor laboratory studies (eg, WBC count for leukopenia or neutropenia).
- Frequently assess common sites of infection (eg, the pharynx, skin, perianal area, urinary tract, and respiratory tract) for signs of infection (fever, swelling, redness, drainage, and pain)
- Monitor the patient for sepsis, particularly if invasive catheters or infusion lines are in place.
- Assess patient for factors that may contribute to bleeding (eg, bone marrow suppression from radiation, chemotherapy, and other medications, such as aspirin, dipyridamole [Persantine], heparin, or warfarin [Coumadin]).
- Monitor common bleeding sites (eg, skin, mucous membranes; the intestinal, urinary, and respiratory tracts; and the brain).
- Monitor and report gross hemorrhage as well as blood in the stools, urine, sputum, or vomitus (melena, hematuria, hemoptysis, hematemesis), oozing at injection sites, bruising (ecchymosis), petechiae, and changes in mental status.
- Assess patient for risk factors for decreased skin integrity (eg, therapy effects, invasive diagnostic procedures, nutritional deficits, bowel and bladder incontinence, immobility, immunosuppression, and changes related to aging).
- Note skin lesions or ulcerations secondary to the tumor or therapy, particularly alterations throughout the gastrointestinal tract (eg, the oral mucous membranes), as well as their effects on the patient's nutritional status and comfort level.
- Note any alopecia (hair loss) and assesses the psychological impact of this side effect on the patient and the family.

- Assess the patient's nutritional status (weight, caloric intake and diet history, anorexia, changes in appetite, and cachexia (wasting, emaciation).
- Assess situations and foods that aggravate or relieve anorexia and the patient's medication history; determine difficulty in chewing or swallowing and occurrences of nausea, vomiting, or diarrhea.
- Assess clinical and laboratory data related to the patient's nutritional status (eg, anthropometric measurements (triceps skin fold and middle–upper arm circumference), serum protein levels (albumin and transferrin), lymphocyte count, skin response to intradermal injection of antigens, hemoglobin levels, hematocrit, urinary creatinine levels, and serum iron levels).
- Assess the level (pain assessment scale), source, and site of pain and factors that increase the patient's perception of pain (eg, fear and apprehension, fatigue, anger, and social isolation).
- Assess for feelings of weariness, weakness, lack of energy, inability to carry out necessary and valued daily functions, lack of motivation, and inability to concentrate.
- Assess physiologic and psychological stressors that can contribute to fatigue, including pain, nausea, dyspnea, fear, and anxiety or constipation.
- Assess the patient's mood and emotional reaction to the results of diagnostic testing and prognosis.
- Assess the patient's progress through the stages of grief and ability to talk about the diagnosis and prognosis with family.
- Identify potential threats to self-concept and body image, and assess the patient's ability to cope with these changes.

Major Nursing Diagnoses

Based on the assessment data, nursing diagnoses of the patient with cancer may include the following:

- Impaired tissue integrity related to the effects of treatment and the disease

- Altered nutrition: less than body requirements related to anorexia and gastrointestinal changes
- Pain and discomfort related to disease and treatment effects
- Fatigue related to physical and psychological stressors
- Grieving related to anticipated loss and altered role function
- Body image disturbance related to changes in appearance and role functions

Collaborative Problems/Potential Complications

Based on the assessment data, potential complications that may develop include the following:

- Infection and sepsis
- Hemorrhage
- Superior vena cava syndrome
- Spinal cord compression
- Hypercalcemia
- Pericardial effusion
- Disseminated intravascular coagulation
- Syndrome of inappropriate secretion of antidiuretic hormone
- Tumor lysis syndrome

Planning and Goals

The major goals for the patient may include maintenance of tissue integrity, maintenance of nutrition, relief of pain, relief of fatigue, effective progression through the grieving process, improved body image, and absence of complications.

Nursing Interventions

MAINTAINING TISSUE INTEGRITY

Some of the most frequently encountered disturbances include skin and tissue reactions to radiation therapy, stomatitis, alopecia, and metastatic skin lesions.

- Provide careful skin care to prevent further skin irritation, drying, and damage. Handle skin over the affected

area gently; avoid rubbing and use of hot or cold water, soaps, powders, lotions, and cosmetics.
- Instruct the patient to wear loose-fitting clothes and avoid clothes that constrict, irritate, or rub the affected area.
- Take care not to disrupt any blisters present to reduce the risk of introducing bacteria.
- Provide aseptic wound care (moisture, vapor-permeable dressing, and topical antibiotics, as ordered) on area of moist desquamation (painful, red, moist skin).

MANAGING STOMATITIS
- Instruct on, and assist patient with, good oral hygiene (brushing with soft-bristled toothbrush and nonabrasive toothpaste).
- Use oral swabs with spongelike applicators in place of a toothbrush for painful oral tissues, or oral rinses with saline solution or tap water.
- Assist patient with flossing, unless it causes pain or unless platelet levels are below 40,000 mm^3.
- Avoid products or foods that irritate or traumatize oral tissues or impair healing, such as alcohol-based mouth rinses and food that is difficult to chew or too hot or spicy.
- Lubricate the patient's lips to keep the tissues from becoming dry and cracked. Use a topical antiinflammatory agent and anesthetic agents if prescribed. Products that coat or protect oral mucosa are used to facilitate comfort and to promote healing and minimize discomfort. Give systemic analgesics as required.
- Encourage adequate fluid and food intake; administer parenteral hydration and nutrition as ordered.
- Administer topical or systemic antifungal and antibiotic drugs as prescribed to treat local or systemic infections.

ADDRESSING ALOPECIA
- Provide information about alopecia (include that hair usually begins to regrow after completing therapy, although the color and texture of the new hair may

change), and support the patient and family in coping with disturbing effects of therapy.

- Encourage the patient to acquire a wig or hairpiece before hair loss occurs so that the replacement matches the patient's own hair. Suggest that the use of attractive scarves and hats may make the patient feel less conspicuous.
- Refer patients to supportive programs, such as Look Good, Feel Better, offered by the American Cancer Society.

MANAGING MALIGNANT SKIN LESIONS

- Carefully assess and cleanse the skin, reducing superficial bacteria, controlling bleeding, reducing odor, and protecting the skin from pain and further trauma.
- Assist and guide the patient and family regarding care for these skin lesions at home; refer for home care as indicated.

PROMOTING NUTRITION

- Assist in selecting foods that the patient might eat despite altered sense of taste and smell and decreased appetite.
- Prepare foods in ways to make it look and taste appealing; avoiding unpleasant smells and unappetizing-looking food.
- Include family members in the plan of care to encourage adequate food intake.
- Consider the patient's preferences as well as physiologic and metabolic requirements in selecting foods.
- Provide and encourage the patient to eat small, frequent meals with additional supplements between meals.
- Offer oral hygiene and pain relief measures before mealtime to make meals more pleasant.
- Use additional strategies as indicated (eg, changing the feeding schedule, using simple diets, and relieving diarrhea).
- Administer enzyme and vitamin replacement if ordered for malabsorption; administer total parenteral nutrition (TPN) if ordered for severe malabsorption.

- Teach the patient and family how to care for venous access devices and how to administer TPN; refer for home care nurses to assist with or supervise TPN in the home, as needed.
- Before invasive nutritional strategies are instituted, assess the patient carefully and discuss the options with the patient and family (creative dietary therapies, enteral [tube] feedings, or TPN).
- Direct nursing care toward preventing trauma, infection and other complications that increase metabolic demands.

RELIEVING PAIN
- Use a multidisciplinary team approach to determine optimal management of the patient's pain.
- Help patients and families play an active role in managing pain.
- Provide education and support to correct fears and misconceptions about opioid use.

DECREASING FATIGUE
- Help the patient and family to understand that fatigue is usually an expected and temporary side effect of the cancer process and the treatments employed.
- Help the patient to identify sources of fatigue.
- Develop ways to conserve energy to help the patient plan daily activities, alternating periods of rest and activity.
- Encourage regular, light exercise, which may decrease fatigue and facilitate coping.
- Encourage the patient to maintain as normal a lifestyle as possible by continuing with those activities valued and enjoyed by the patient.
- Encourage both patients and families to plan to reallocate responsibilities, such as attending to child care, cleaning, and preparing meals. A patient who is employed full-time may need to reduce the number of hours worked each week.
- Assist the patient and family in coping with these changing roles and responsibilities.

- Address factors that contribute to fatigue and implement pharmacologic and nonpharmacologic strategies to manage pain.
- Provide nutrition counseling to patients who are not eating enough calories or protein; small, frequent meals require less energy for digestion.
- Monitor serum hemoglobin and hematocrit levels for deficiencies, and administer blood products as prescribed.
- Monitor patients for alterations in oxygenation and electrolyte balances.
- Arrange for physical therapy and assistive devices are for patients with impaired mobility.

IMPROVING BODY IMAGE AND SELF-ESTEEM

A positive approach is essential when caring for the patient with an altered body image. To help the patient retain control and a sense of self-worth, it is important to encourage independence and continued participation in self-care and decision making.

- Assist patient to assume those tasks and participate in those activities that are personally of most value.
- Encourage the patient to express any negative feelings or threats to body image.
- Serve as a listener and counselor to the patient and family.
- Refer the patient and family to a support group for additional assistance in coping with the changes resulting from cancer or its treatment.
- Consult with a cosmetologist who might provide ideas about hair or wig styling, make-up, and the use of scarves and turbans to help with body image concerns.
- Encourage patients who are experiencing alterations in sexuality and sexual function to share and discuss concerns openly with their partner. Explore alternative forms of sexual expression with the patient and partner to promote positive self-worth and acceptance.
- Assist the patient and partner in seeking further counseling if serious physiologic, psychological, or communica-

tion difficulties related to sexuality or sexual function are identified.

ASSISTING IN THE GRIEVING PROCESS

- Answer any questions the patient and family may have, and clarify information provided by the physician.
- Assess the response of the patient and family to the diagnosis and planned treatment, and assist them in framing their questions and concerns.
- Identify resources and support people (eg, clergy, counselor, and other support available through hospitals and various community organizations).
- Assist patient and family with communicating and sharing their concerns with each other.
- Encourage the patient and family to verbalize their feelings in an atmosphere of trust and support.
- If the patient enters the terminal phase of disease, assist the patient and family to come to grips with their reactions and feelings (physical support, such as holding the patient's hand or just being with the patient at home or at the bedside).
- Maintain contact with the surviving family members after death of the cancer patient, which may help them to work through their feelings of loss and grief.

MONITORING AND MANAGING
POTENTIAL COMPLICATIONS

- Use strict asepsis when handling intravenous lines, catheters, and other invasive equipment.
- Avoid exposure of the patient to others with an active infection and to crowds.
- Place patients with profound immunosuppression, such as recipients of bone marrow transplants, in a protective environment whereby the room and its contents are sterilized and the air filtered.
- Provide immunosuppressed patients with low-bacterial diets, avoiding fresh fruits and vegetables.
- Avoid invasive procedures, such as injections, vaginal or rectal examinations, rectal temperatures, and surgery.

- Encourage the patient to do coughing and deep-breathing exercises frequently to prevent potential respiratory problems.
- Teach the patient and family to recognize signs and symptoms of infection to report, perform effective hand washing, use antipyretics, maintain skin integrity, and self-administer hematopoietic growth factors when indicated.

TREATING SEPTIC SHOCK
- Assess frequently for infection and inflammation throughout the course of the disease.
- Prevent septicemia and septic shock, or detect and report for prompt treatment. Monitor for signs and symptoms of septic shock (altered mental status, either subnormal or elevated temperature, cool and clammy skin, decreased urine output, hypotension, dysrhythmias, electrolyte imbalances, and abnormal arterial blood gas values).
- Instruct patient and family members about signs of septicemia, methods for preventing infection, and actions to take if infection or septicemia occurs (See Septic Shock).

MANAGING BLEEDING AND HEMORRHAGE
- Monitor laboratory values, and continue to assess the patient for bleeding.
- Take steps to prevent trauma and minimize the risk of bleeding by encouraging the patient to use a soft, not stiff, toothbrush and an electric, not straight-edged, razor.
- Avoid unnecessary invasive procedures (eg, rectal temperatures, intramuscular injections, and catheterization).
- Assist the patient and family to identify and remove environmental hazards that may lead to falls or other trauma.
- Provide soft foods, increased fluid intake, and stool softeners, if prescribed, to reduce trauma to the gastrointestinal tract.

- Handle and move the joints and extremities gently to minimize the risk of spontaneous bleeding.
- Monitor serum hemoglobin and hematocrit carefully for changes indicating blood loss.
- Test all urine, stool, and emesis for occult blood.
- Perform neurologic assessments to detect changes in orientation and behavior.
- Administer fluids and blood products as prescribed to replace any losses and vasopressor drugs and supplemental oxygen as prescribed to maintain blood pressure and ensure tissue oxygenation.

🏠 Promoting Home and Community-Based Care

Teaching Patients Self-Care
- Provide information needed by the patient and family to address the most immediate care needs likely to be encountered at home.
- Verbally review, and reinforce with written information, the side effects of treatments and changes in the patient's status that should be reported.
- Discuss strategies to deal with side effects of treatment with patients and their families.
- Identify learning needs based on the priorities identified by the patient and family as well as on the complexity of home-provided care.
- Instruct the patient and family and provide ongoing support that allows them to feel comfortable and proficient in managing treatments at home.
- Refer the patient for home care nursing to provide care and support for patients receiving advanced technical care.
- Provide follow-up visits and phone calls to patient and family, and evaluate patient progress and ongoing needs.

Continuing Care
- Refer patient for home care (assessment of the home environment, suggestions for modifications to assist the patient and family in addressing the patient's physical

C

needs, physical care, and ongoing assessment of the psychological and emotional effects of the illness on the patient and the family).
- Assess the adequacy of pain management and the effectiveness of other strategies to prevent or manage the side effects of treatment modalities.
- Facilitate the coordination of patient care by maintaining close communication with all health care providers involved in each patient's care.
- Make referrals and coordinate available community resources (eg, local office of the American Cancer Society, home aides, church groups, and support groups) to assist patients and caregivers.

Evaluation
EXPECTED OUTCOMES
- Maintains adequate tissue (skin and mucous membrane) integrity
- Maintains adequate nutritional status
- Achieves relief of pain and discomfort
- Demonstrates increased activity tolerance and decreased fatigue
- Progresses through the grieving process
- Exhibits improved body image and self-esteem
- Experiences no complications, such as inflammation, infection, or sepsis, and no episodes of bleeding or hemorrhage

Nursing Management: The Patient Undergoing Surgery for Cancer
- Complete a thorough preoperative assessment for all factors that may affect patients undergoing surgical procedures.
- Provide time and assist the patient and family in dealing with the possible changes and outcomes resulting from the surgery; provide education and emotional support by assessing patient and family needs and exploring with them their fears and coping mechanisms, encouraging

them to take an active role in decision making when possible.

- Explain and clarify information the physician has provided to the patient or family about the results of diagnostic testing and surgical procedures, if asked.
- Communicate frequently with the physician and other health care team members to ensure that information provided is consistent.
- After surgery, assess the patient's responses to the surgery, and monitor for possible complications, such as infection, bleeding, thrombophlebitis, wound dehiscence, fluid and electrolyte imbalance, and organ dysfunction.
- Provide for patient comfort.
- Provide postoperative teaching that addresses wound care, activity, nutrition, and medication information.
- Initiate plans for discharge, follow-up care, and treatment as early as possible to ensure continuity of care.
- Encourage the patient and families to use community resources, such as the American Cancer Society or Make Today Count, for support and information.

Nursing Management: The Patient Undergoing Radiation Therapy

- Answer questions and allay fears of the patient and family about the effects of radiation on others, on the tumor, and on the patient's normal tissues and organs.
- Explain the procedure for delivering radiation, and describe the equipment, the duration of the procedure (often minutes only), the possible need for immobilizing the patient during the procedure, and the absence of new sensations, including pain during the procedure.
- If a radioactive implant is used, inform the patient about the restrictions placed on visitors and health care personnel and other radiation precautions as well as the patient's own role before, during, and after the procedure.

- Maintain a patient with an intracavitary delivery device on bed rest and log-roll to prevent displacement; provide a low-residue diet and antidiarrheal agents to prevent bowel movement during therapy to prevent the radioisotopes from being displaced. Maintain an indwelling urinary catheter to ensure that the bladder empties.
- For safety in brachytherapy, assign the patient to a private room, posting appropriate notices about radiation safety precautions; have staff members wear dosimeter badges, making sure that pregnant staff members are not assigned to this patient's care; prohibit visits by children or pregnant women; limit visits from others to 30 minutes daily, and instruct and monitor visitors to ensure they maintain a 6-foot distance from the radiation source.
- Assess the patient's skin, nutritional status, and general feeling of well-being.
- Assess the skin and oral mucosa frequently for changes (particularly if radiation therapy is directed to these areas). Protect the skin from irritation, and instruct the patient to avoid using ointments, lotions, or powders on the area.
- Assist the weak or fatigued patient with activities of daily living and personal hygiene, including gentle oral hygiene to remove debris, prevent irritation, and promote healing.
- Reassure the patient by explaining that these symptoms are a result of the treatment and do not represent deterioration or progression of the disease.
- Follow the instructions provided by the radiation safety officer from the radiology department which identify the maximum time a health care provider can spend safely in the patient's room, the shielding equipment to be used, and special precautions and actions to be taken if the implant is dislodged. Explain the rationale for these precautions to the patient.

Nursing Management: The Patient Undergoing Chemotherapy

- Assess the patient's nutritional and fluid and electrolyte status frequently, and use creative ways to encourage an adequate fluid and dietary intake.
- Due to increased risk of anemia, infection, and bleeding disorders, focus nursing assessment and care on identifying and modifying factors that further increase the patient's risk.
- Use aseptic technique and gentle handling to prevent infection and trauma; closely monitor laboratory test results (blood cell counts), and promptly report untoward changes and signs of infection or bleeding.
- Carefully select peripheral veins and perform venipuncture, and carefully administer drugs. Monitor for indications of extravasation during drug administration (eg, absence of blood return from the intravenous catheter, resistance to flow of intravenous fluid, or swelling, pain, or redness at the site).
- If extravasation is suspected, stop the drug administration immediately, and apply ice to the site (unless the extravasated vesicant is a vinca alkaloid).
- Assist patient with delayed nausea and vomiting (occurring later than 48 to 72 hours after chemotherapy) by teaching the patient to take antiemetic medications as necessary for the first week at home after chemotherapy and by teaching relaxation techniques and imagery, which can help to decrease stimuli contributing to symptoms.
- Alter the patient's diet to include small, frequent meals, bland foods, and comfort foods, which may reduce the frequency or severity of these symptoms.
- Monitor blood cell counts frequently, note and report neutropenia, and protect the patient from infection and injury, particularly while the blood cell counts are depressed.
- Monitor blood urea nitrogen (BUN), serum creatinine, creatinine clearance, and serum electrolyte levels, and report any findings that indicate decreasing renal func-

tion. Provide adequate hydration and alkalinization of
the urine to prevent formation of uric acid crystals, and
administer allopurinol as ordered to prevent renal
damage.

- Monitor closely for signs of congestive heart failure and
for pulmonary fibrosis (eg, pulmonary function test
results).
- Inform patients and their partners about potential
changes in reproduction resulting from chemotherapy
and possible options. (Banking of sperm is recommended for men before treatments.) Advise patients and
their partners to use reliable birth control while receiving chemotherapy because sterility is not certain.
- Inform patients that the taxanes and plant alkaloids,
especially vincristine, can cause peripheral neuropathies,
loss of deep tendon reflexes, and paralytic ileus, but that
these side effects are usually reversible and disappear
after completion of chemotherapy.
- Help patient and family members plan strategies to
combat fatigue.
- Use precautions developed by the Occupational Safety
and Health Administration (OSHA), Oncology Nursing
Society (ONS), hospitals, and other health care agencies
to protect the health care personnel who have handled
chemotherapeutic agents.

Nursing Management: The Patient
Undergoing Bone Marrow Transplantation

- Before bone marrow transplantation (BMT), perform
nutritional assessments and extensive physical examinations and ensure that organ function tests, as well as psychological evaluations, are completed as ordered.
- Assure that the patient's social support systems and
financial and insurance resources are also evaluated.
- Reinforce information for informed consent.
- Provide patient teaching about the procedure and pre-
transplantation and posttransplantation care.
- During the treatment phase, closely monitor for signs of
acute toxicities (eg, nausea, diarrhea, mucositis, and

hemorrhagic cystitis), and give constant attention to the patient.

- During the bone marrow or stem cell infusions, monitor vital signs and blood oxygen saturation; assess for adverse effects (eg, fever, chills, shortness of breath, chest pain, cutaneous reactions, nausea, vomiting, hypotension or hypertension, tachycardia, anxiety, and taste changes); and provide ongoing support and patient teaching.
- Because patients are at high risk for dying from sepsis and bleeding, support the patient with blood products and hemopoietic growth factors and protection from infection.
- Assess for early graft-versus-host disease (GVHD) effects to the skin, liver, and gastrointestinal tract as well as gastrointestinal complications (eg, fluid retention, jaundice, abdominal pain, ascites, tender and enlarged liver, and encephalopathy).
- Monitor for pulmonary complications, such as pulmonary edema, and interstitial and other pneumonias, which often complicate the recovery after BMT.
- Provide for ongoing nursing assessments in follow-up visits to detect late effects (100 days or later) after BMT, such as infections (eg, varicella zoster), restrictive pulmonary abnormalities, and recurrent pneumonias, as well as chronic GVHD involving the skin, liver, intestine, esophagus, eye, lungs, joints, and vaginal mucosa. Cataracts may develop after total-body irradiation.
- Provide ongoing psychosocial patient assessments, including the stressors affecting patients at each phase of the transplantation experience.
- Assess and address the psychosocial needs of the marrow donors and family members. Educate and support donor and family members to reduce anxiety and promote coping. Family members must also be assisted to maintain realistic expectations of themselves as well as of the patient.

Nursing Management: The Patient With Hyperthermia

- Explain to patient and family about the procedure, its goals, and its effects.
- Assess the patient for adverse effects, and make efforts to reduce their occurrence and severity.
- Provide local skin care at the site of the implanted hyperthermic probes.

Nursing Management: The Patient Undergoing Biologic Response Modifier Therapy

- Assess the need for education, support, and guidance for both the patient and family (often the same needs as patients having other treatment approaches, but may be perceived as a last chance effort by patients who have not responded to standard treatments).
- Monitor the therapeutic and adverse effects (eg, fever, myalgia, nausea, and vomiting, as seen with interferon therapy), and life-threatening side effects (eg, capillary leak syndrome, pulmonary edema, and hypotension).
- Assess the impact of adverse and side effects on the patient's quality of life.
- Work closely with physicians in assessing and managing potential toxicities of BRM therapy.
- Use accurate observations and careful documentation with administration of investigational agents for data collection.

Promoting Home and Community-Based Care

- Teach patients and families, as needed, how to administer BRM agents through subcutaneous injections.
- Arrange for home care nurses to monitor the patient's responses to treatment, and provide teaching and continued care.

Nursing Management: The Patient Undergoing Photodynamic Therapy

- Teach the patient that the major side effect of therapy is photosensitivity for 4 to 6 weeks after treatment.
- Instruct patients to protect themselves from direct and indirect sunlight to prevent skin burns.
- Observe and teach patients to observe local reactions in the area treated.
- Monitor liver and renal function for transient abnormalities.
- Educate, assist, and provide emotional support to the patient and family.

For more information, see Chapter 15 in Smeltzer and Bare: *Brunner and Suddarth's Textbook of Medical-Surgical Nursing,* 9th edition. Philadelphia: Lippincott Williams & Wilkins, 2000.

CANCER OF THE BLADDER

Cancer of the urinary bladder is seen more frequently in people aged 50 to 70 years and affects men more than women (3:1). There are two forms of bladder cancer: superficial (which tends to recur) and invasive. Tumors usually arise at the base of the bladder and involve the ureteral orifices and bladder neck. The predominate cause is cigarette smoking. Chronic schistosomiasis (parasitic infection that irritates the bladder) is also a risk factor. Cancers arising from the prostate, colon, and rectum in men and from the lower gynecologic tract in women may metastasize to the bladder.

Clinical Manifestations

- Gross painless hematuria is the most common symptom.
- Infection of the urinary tract is common and produces frequency, urgency, and dysuria.
- Any alteration in voiding or change in the urine is indicative.
- Pelvic or back pain may occur with metastasis.

Diagnostic Evaluation

Biopsies of the tumor and adjacent mucosa are definitive, but the following procedures are also used:

- Cystoscopy, biopsy of tumor and adjacent mucosa
- Excretory urography
- Computed tomography (CT) scan
- Ultrasonography
- Bimanual examination under anesthesia
- Cytologic examination of fresh urine and saline bladder washings

Medical Management

Treatment of bladder cancer depends on the grade of tumor, the stage of tumor growth, and the multicentricity of the tumor. Age and physical, mental, and emotional status are considered in determining treatment modalities.

- Transurethral resection (TUR) or fulguration for simple papillomas with intravesical bacille Calmette Guérin (BCG)
- Monitoring of benign papillomas with cytology and cystoscopy periodically for the rest of patient's life
- Simple cystectomy or radical cystectomy for invasive or multifocal bladder cancer
- Chemotherapy with a combination of methotrexate, 5-fluorouracil (5-FU), vinblastine, doxorubicin (Adriamycin), and cisplatin (M-VAC), possibly by topical chemotherapy applied directly to the bladder wall
- Radiation of tumor preoperatively to reduce microextension and viability
- Radiation therapy in combination with surgery to control inoperable tumors
- Cytotoxic agent infusions through the arterial supply of the involved organ
- Hydrostatic therapy: for advanced bladder cancer or patients with intractable hematuria (after radiation therapy)
- Formalin, phenol, or silver nitrate instillations to achieve relief of hematuria and strangury (slow and painful discharge of urine) in some patients

Nursing Management

See Nursing Management for the patient undergoing cancer surgery, radiation, and chemotherapy under Cancer for additional information.

For more information, see Chapter 41 in Smeltzer and Bare: *Brunner and Suddarth's Textbook of Medical-Surgical Nursing,* 9th edition. Philadelphia: Lippincott Williams & Wilkins, 2000.

CANCER OF THE BREAST

Carcinoma of the breast is a pathologic entity that starts with a genetic alteration in a single cell and may take 2 years to become palpable. The most common type of breast cancer is infiltrating ductal carcinoma (75% of cases), which has a poorer prognosis than other types of breast cancer. Infiltrating lobular carcinoma accounts for 5% to 10% of cases. These tumors occur in an area of ill-defined thickening and are multicentric tumors. Infiltrating ductal and lobular carcinomas usually spread to bone, lung, liver, adrenals, pleura, skin, or brain. Several less common invasive cancers, such as medullary carcinoma (6% of cases), mucinous cancer (3% of cases), tubular ductal cancer (2% of cases) have very favorable prognoses. There is no one specific cause; rather, a combination of genetic, hormonal, and possibly environmental events may contribute to its development. If lymph nodes are unaffected, prognosis is better. The key to improved cure rates is early diagnosis before metastasis.

Risk Factors

- Previous breast cancer: the risk of developing cancer in the other breast increases 1% each year.
- Genetic alterations (BRCA1 or BRCA2), which may be inherited or acquired, indicate risk.
- Prolonged exposure to hormonal stimulation, that is, early menarche before 12 years of age, nulliparity, first birth after 30 years of age, and late menopause after 55

years of age, oral contraceptives, hormone replacement therapy, cigarette smoking, and high-fat diet have been weakly associated factors.

Protective Factors
Protective factors may include regular vigorous exercise, pregnancy before 30 years of age, and breastfeeding.

Clinical Manifestations
- Symptoms are insidious; generally, the lesions are non-tender, fixed, and hard with irregular borders; most occur in the upper outer quadrant, more often on the left breast.
- Pain is usually absent except in later stages; some women have no symptoms and no palpable lump but have an abnormal mammogram.
- Without detection and treatment, the following may occur: dimpling or peau d'orange (orange-peel skin), asymmetry and an elevation of the affected breast, nipple retraction, lesions fixed to the chest wall, ulceration, and metastasis.

Diagnostic Evaluation
- Fine-needle aspiration
- Biopsy (eg, excisional, core, stereotactic)
- Needle localization

Staging of Breast Cancer
See Staging of Cancer under Cancer.

Medical Management
- Modified radical mastectomy: entire breast tissue removed along with axillary lymph nodes
- Breast-conserving surgery: lumpectomy, segmental mastectomy, or quadrantectomy, and axillary node dissection followed by radiation therapy to residual microscopic disease
- Lymphatic mapping and sentinel node biopsy, possibly sparing the patient unnecessary node dissection

- A course of external-beam radiation therapy to the tumor mass to decrease chance of recurrence and eradicate residual cancer
- Chemotherapy to eradicate micrometastatic spread of the disease: cyclophosphamide (cytoxan) (C), methotrexate (M), fluorouracil (F), doxorubicin (Adriamycin) (A). and paclitaxel (Taxol) (T).
- CMF or CAF regimen common; or ACT may be used
- Autologous bone marrow transplant (ABMT) is increasingly being used; current use of growth factors to stimulate the bone marrow have led to an overall decline in mortality.
- Hormonal therapy based on the index of estrogen and progesterone receptors; tamoxifen is the primary hormonal agent used to suppress hormonal-dependent tumors; others are anastrozole (Arimidex), megestrol (Megace), diethylstilbestrol (DES), fluoxymesterone (Halotestin), and aminoglutethimide (Cytadren)
- Elective reconstructive surgery provides considerable psychological benefit but is contraindicated if cancer is locally advanced, metastatic, or inflammatory

Nursing Management

See Nursing Management: The Patient With Cancer under Cancer for additional information.

Assessment

PREOPERATIVE

- Assess the reaction of the patient to the diagnosis and ability to cope with it.
- Take a complete health and gynecologic history.
- Ask pertinent questions about coping skills, support systems, knowledge deficit, and presence of discomfort.
- Perform a complete physical assessment, with particular attention to breasts and related mass signs and symptoms.

POSTOPERATIVE

- Monitor pulse and blood pressure for signs of shock and hemorrhage.

- Avoid blood pressure readings, injections, intravenous lines, and venipunctures on the operative side to prevent infection and compromised circulation.
- Inspect dressings for bleeding on a regular basis; monitor drainage; turn and encourage deep breathing; assess graft areas for unusual redness, pain, swelling, or drainage.

Major Nursing Diagnoses

PREOPERATIVE
- Anxiety related to cancer diagnosis
- Risk for ineffective coping (individual or family) related to the diagnosis of breast cancer and related treatment options

POSTOPERATIVE
- Pain related to surgical procedure
- Impaired skin integrity due to surgical incision
- Risk for infection related to surgical incision and presence of surgical drains
- Knowledge deficit about breast cancer and treatment options
- Risk for sexual dysfunction related to loss of body part, change in self-image, and fear of partner's responses
- Self-care deficit related to partial immobility of upper extremity on operative side

Collaborative Problems/Potential Complications
- Lymphedema
- Infection
- Hematoma formation

Planning and Goals
The major goals of the patient may include increased knowledge about the disease and its treatment; reduction of preoperative and postoperative fear, emotional stress, and anxiety; improvement of decision-making ability; pain management; maintenance of skin integrity; improved self-concept; active participation in self-care activities; improved sexual function; and the absence of complications.

Nursing Interventions

REDUCING STRESS AND IMPROVING COPING SKILLS

- Preoperatively, give patient time to absorb significance of diagnosis, and give information to help evaluate available treatment options.
- Promote the best preoperative physical, psychological, and nutritional conditions possible.
- Arrange for patient to discuss concerns with those who will be administering care and, if desired, a breast cancer survivor. Use careful guidance and supportive counseling to assist the patient who cannot make a decision about treatment.
- Avoid forcing patient to look at incision site if not ready.
- Elicit assistance from supportive family or friends to promote acceptance of body alteration.
- Recognize that spouse or partner is often in need of guidance, support, and education to cope with the crisis.

CORRECTING KNOWLEDGE DEFICIT

- With consideration for timing and amount of information, discuss uses of medications, goals, extent and duration of treatment, side-effect management, and possible reactions after treatment, as well as issues, such as prostheses and plastic surgery, chosen by the patient.
- Be aware of and reinforce information given by doctor (eg, diagnosis and treatment options)

MAINTAINING SKIN INTEGRITY

- Maintain patency of surgical drain to prevent fluid accumulation under the chest wall incision; monitor dressing and drains frequently.
- Inform of decreased sensation in the operative area because of nerve disruption; teach signs of infection or irritation.
- Patient usually may shower on second day and wash incision, and dressing is applied for 7 days. After incision is healed, lotions or creams may be applied to area to increase skin elasticity.

C

- Use dressing changes as an opportunity to discuss incision with patient.

RELIEVING PAIN AND DISCOMFORT
- Encourage patient to use analgesics before exercise or bedtime and to take a warm shower to relieve referred muscle pain.
- Elevate the involved extremity moderately.

PROMOTING SELF-CARE
- Provide information about development of postoperative surgical edema and strategies to prevent it; cuts, bruises, and infections on the operative side are dangerous precursors to problems.
- Encourage ambulation when patient is free of postanesthesia nausea and is tolerating fluids; initiate full range-of-motion exercises and hand exercises (3 times/day for 20 minutes) to promote circulation and muscle strength and to prevent stiffness. If skin graft or tight surgical incision is present, see prescribed exercises.
- Promote self-care, exercise of both arms, and maintenance of good posture.
- Encourage normal household and work-related arm activities, avoiding heavy lifting (eg, arm movements when walking, cleanliness of operative site).
- Avoid injury to operative side; check with physician before introducing strenuous activity.

IMPROVING SEXUAL FUNCTION
- Discuss how patient sees self and possible decreased libido related to fatigue, nausea, or anxiety.
- Clarify misconceptions (eg, that cancer can be transmitted sexually).
- Encourage couple to discuss fears, needs, and desires.
- Suggest variations in time of day for sexual activity (when least tired) or positions that are most comfortable, and alternative options (eg, hugging, kissing, manual stimulation).

- Refer to psychosocial resources (eg, psychologist, psychiatric clinical nurse specialist, social worker, or sex therapist) if indicated or desired.

MANAGING POTENTIAL COMPLICATIONS
- Facilitate development of collateral or auxiliary lymph drainage by promoting movement and exercise (eg, hand pumps) through postoperative education.
- Elevate arm on pillow so that the hand and elbow are higher than shoulder.
- Obtain referral for patient to therapist for custom-made elastic sleeves, exercises, manual lymph drainage, or special pump to decrease swelling.
- Teach patient proper incision care and signs and symptoms of infection and when to contact surgeon or nurse.
- Monitor the surgical site for gross swelling or drainage output, and notify surgeon promptly; maintain a calm demeanor with the patient.
- If ordered, apply an elastic bandage wrap and ice pack to the surgical site.

🏠 Promoting Home and Community-Based Care

Teaching Patients Self-Care
- Assess patient's readiness to assume self-care, and focus on teaching incision care, signs to report, pain management, arm exercises, hand and arm care, and drainage management; include family member.
- Follow patient with telephone calls for concerns about incision, pain management, and patient and family adjustment;
- Teach how to empty reservoir and measure drainage if discharged with a drain in place.

Continuing Care
- Reinforce and repeat earlier teaching postoperatively, as needed; teach or reinforce breast self-examination, and encourage patient to perform monthly.

- Refer patient for home care as indicated or desired by patient.
- Reinforce need for follow-up visits to the physician.

Evaluation

EXPECTED OUTCOMES

Preoperative

- Exhibits knowledge about diagnosis and treatment options
- Verbalizes willingness to deal with anxiety and fears
- Demonstrates ability to cope with diagnosis and treatment
- Demonstrates ability to make decisions regarding treatment options in a timely manner

Postoperative

- Exhibits clean dry and intact surgical incision without signs of inflammation or infection
- Reports pain has decreased and states pain management strategies
- Lists signs and symptoms of infection to be reported
- Verbalizes feelings regarding change of body image
- Participates actively in self-care activities

For more information, see Chapter 44 in Smeltzer and Bare: *Brunner and Suddarth's Textbook of Medical-Surgical Nursing,* 9th edition. Philadelphia: Lippincott Williams and Wilkins, 2000.

CANCER OF THE CERVIX

Cancer of the cervix is predominantly (90%) squamous cell cancer and also includes adenocarcinomas. It is less common than it once was because of early detection by Papinacolaou's (Pap) test but remains the third most common reproductive cancer in women. It occurs most commonly between the ages of 30 and 45 years but can occur in women as young as 18 years of age. Risk factors vary from multiple sex partners to smoking to chronic cervical infection.

Clinical Manifestations

- Cervical cancer is most often asymptomatic. When discharge, irregular bleeding, or bleeding after sexual intercourse occurs, the disease may be advanced.
- Vaginal discharge gradually increases in amount, becomes watery, and finally is dark and foul smelling because of necrosis and infection of the tumor mass.
- Bleeding occurs at irregular intervals between periods or after menopause, may be slight (enough to spot undergarments), and is usually noted after mild trauma (intercourse, douching, or defecation).
- As disease continues, bleeding may persist and increase.
- Nerve involvement, producing excruciating pain in the back and legs, occurs as cancer advances and tissues outside the cervix are invaded, including lymph glands anterior to the sacrum.
- Extreme emaciation and anemia, often with fever due to secondary infection and abscesses in the ulcerating mass, and fistula formation may occur in the final stage.

Diagnostic Evaluation

- Abnormal Pap test followed by biopsy, dilation and curettage (D & C), computed tomography (CT), magnetic resonance imaging (MRI), intravenous urography (IVU), cytogram, and barium radiographs.
- Clinical staging of the disease with the International Classification staging system or TNM classification.

Medical Management

- Conservative treatments include cryotherapy (freezing with nitrous oxide), laser therapy, loop electrosurgical excision procedure (LEEP), or conization (removing a cone-shaped portion of cervix).
- Simple hysterectomy if invasion is less than 3 mm.
- For invasive cancer, radical hysterectomy, radiation (external-beam or brachytherapy), or chemotherapy (cisplatin, carboplatin, and paclitaxel [Taxol]) or a combination of these approaches.
- For recurrent cancer, pelvic exenteration is considered.

Nursing Management: The Patient Undergoing Hysterectomy

See Nursing Management: The Patient With Cancer under Cancer for additional care measures and nursing care of patients with varied treatment regimens.

Assessment

Assess the health history; perform a physical and pelvic examination and laboratory studies; gather data on the patient's psychosocial supports and responses.

Major Nursing Diagnoses

- Anxiety related to the diagnosis of cancer, fear of pain, perceived loss of femininity, and disfigurement.
- Body image disturbance related to altered fertility, fears about sexuality, and relationships with partner and family.
- Pain related to surgery and other adjuvant therapy.
- Knowledge deficit of the perioperative aspects of hysterectomy and self-care.

Collaborative Problems/Potential Complications

- Hemorrhage
- Deep vein thrombosis
- Bladder dysfunction

Planning and Goals

The major goals of the patient may include relief of anxiety, self-acceptance after loss of the uterus, absence of pain or discomfort, increased knowledge of self-care requirements, and prevention of complications.

Nursing Interventions

RELIEVING ANXIETY

- Determine how this experience affects the patient.
- Allow the patient to verbalize feelings and identify strengths.

IMPROVING BODY IMAGE
- Assess how the patient feels about having a hysterectomy related to the nature of diagnosis, significant others, religious beliefs, and prognosis.
- Acknowledge the patient's concerns: ability to have children, loss of femininity, impact on sexual relations.
- Educate the patient about sexual relations: sexual satisfaction, orgasm arises from clitoral stimulation, sexual feeling or comfort related to shortened vagina.
- Explain that depression and heightened emotional sensitivity are expected because of upset hormonal balances.
- Exhibit interest, concern, and willingness to listen to fears.

RELIEVING PAIN
- Administer analgesics to relieve pain and promote movement and ambulation.
- Observe nasogastric tube patency (if tube is present).
- Resume food and fluids gradually when peristalsis is auscultated.
- Apply heat to abdomen, or insert a rectal tube, if prescribed.

MONITORING AND MANAGING COMPLICATIONS
- Hemorrhage: count perineal pads used, and assess extent of saturation; monitor vital signs; check abdominal dressings for drainage; give guidelines for restricting activity to promote healing and prevent bleeding.
- Deep vein thrombosis: apply elastic antiembolism stockings; encourage and assist in changing positions frequently; assist with early ambulation; monitor leg pain and positive Homans' sign; instruct patient to avoid prolonged pressure at the knees and immobility.
- Bladder dysfunction: monitor urinary output and assess for abdominal distention after catheter is removed; initiate measures to encourage voiding.

Promoting Home and Community-Based Care

C

Teaching Patients Self-Care
- Tailor information according to needs: no menstrual cycles, need for hormones.
- Instruct patient to resume activities gradually; no sitting for long periods.
- Teach that showers are preferable to tub baths to reduce risk of infection and injury getting in and out of tub.
- Avoid lifting, straining, sexual intercourse, or driving until advised by physician.
- Report vaginal discharge, foul odor, excessive bleeding, leg redness or pain, or elevated temperature to health care professional promptly.

Continuing Care
- Initiate follow-up telephone contact with patient to address concerns and determine progress.
- Remind patient to discuss hormonal replacement therapy with primary physician, if ovaries were removed.
- Reinforce information regarding resumption of sexual intercourse.
- Reinforce with patient importance of follow-up appointments.

Evaluation

EXPECTED OUTCOMES
- Experiences decreased anxiety
- Accepts changes related to surgery
- Experiences minimal pain and discomfort
- Verbalizes knowledge and understanding of self-care
- Experiences no complications

For more information, see Chapter 43 in Smeltzer and Bare: *Brunner and Suddarth's Textbook of Medical-Surgical Nursing,* 9th edition. Philadelphia: Lippincott Williams & Wilkins, 2000.

CANCER OF THE COLON AND RECTUM (COLORECTAL CANCER)

Colorectal cancer is predominantly (95%) adenocarcinoma, with colon cancer affecting more than twice as many people as rectal cancer. It may start as a benign polyp and become malignant and spread (most often to the liver). Risk factors include age greater than 85 years, family history of colon cancer or polyps, history of inflammatory bowel disease, and a diet high in fat, protein, and beef and low in fiber. Almost three out of four patients could be saved by early diagnosis and prompt treatment; the low 5-year survival rate of 40% to 50% is due primarily to late diagnosis.

Clinical Manifestations
- Changes in bowel habits (most common presenting symptom), passage of blood in the stools (second most common symptom)
- Many asymptomatic for long periods, seeking medical help only when the above is noted
- Unexplained anemia, anorexia, weight loss, and fatigue
- Right-sided lesions, possibly accompanied by dull abdominal pain and melena
- Left-sided lesions, associated with obstruction (abdominal pain and cramping, narrowing stools, constipation, and distention); and bright red blood in stool
- Rectal lesions, associated with tenesmus (ineffective painful straining at stool), rectal pain, the feeling of incomplete evacuation after a bowel movement, alternating constipation and diarrhea, and bloody stool
- Signs of complications: partial or complete bowel obstruction, perforation, abscess formation, peritonitis, sepsis, or shock

Diagnostic Evaluation
- Abdominal and rectal examination, fecal occult blood testing, barium enema, proctosigmoidoscopy, and colonoscopy, biopsy, or cytology smears
- Carcinoembryonic antigen (CEA) studies (reliable in predicting prognosis and recurrence)

Medical Management
- Treatment of cancer depends on stage of disease and related complications.
- Obstruction is treated with intravenous fluids and nasogastric suction and with blood therapy if bleeding is significant.
- Supportive therapy and adjuvant therapy (eg, chemotherapy, radiation therapy, immunotherapy) are included.
- Surgery is the primary treatment for most colon and rectal cancers; type of surgery depends on location and size of tumor; it may be curative or palliative.
- Cancers limited to one site are removable through a colonoscope.
- Laparoscopic colotomy with polypectomy; the neodymium yttrium aluminum garnet (Nd:YAG) laser is effective in some lesions.
- Bowel resection with anastomosis and possible temporary or permanent colostomy or ileostomy (less than one third of patients).

Nursing Management
Assessment
- Obtain a health history, noting symptoms as stated previously (eg, fatigue, elimination pattern, diet, history of weight loss).
- Note presence and character of abdominal or rectal pain; current drug therapy; past medical history; description of color, odor, consistency of stool and presence of blood or mucus; weight loss.

- Auscultate abdomen for bowel sounds; palpate for areas of tenderness, distention, solid masses; inspect stool for blood.

Major Nursing Diagnoses

- Altered nutrition: less than body requirements related to nausea and anorexia
- Risk for fluid volume deficit related to vomiting and dehydration
- Anxiety related to impending surgery and diagnosis of cancer
- Risk for ineffective management of therapeutic regimen related to knowledge deficit concerning the diagnosis, surgical procedure, and self-care after discharge.
- Impaired skin integrity related to surgical incisions and stoma
- Body image disturbance related to colostomy

Collaborative Problems/Potential Complications

- Intraperitoneal infection
- Complete large bowel obstruction
- Gastrointestinal bleeding and hemorrhage
- Bowel perforation
- Peritonitis, abscess, sepsis

Planning and Goals

The major goals of the patient may include attaining optimal level of nutrition and maintaining fluid and electrolyte balance; reducing anxiety; adequate elimination of body waste products; adequate protection of peristomal skin; acquiring knowledge of diagnosis, treatment, and surgical procedure and self-care after discharge; maintaining optimal tissue healing and skin (ostomy) integrity; exploring and verbalizing feelings and concerns about colostomy and impact on self; and preventing complications.

Nursing Interventions

PREPARING THE PATIENT FOR SURGERY

- Physically prepare patient for surgery (diet high in calories, protein, and carbohydrates and low in residue; full liquid diet 24 to 48 hours before surgery, or total parenteral nutrition [TPN], if prescribed).
- Administer antibiotics, laxatives, enemas, or irrigations as ordered.
- Perform intake and output measurement of hospitalized patient; nasogastric tube and intravenous fluid management
- Monitor hydration status (eg, skin turgor, mucous membranes).
- Monitor for signs of obstruction or perforation (increased abdominal distention, loss of bowel sounds, pain, or rigidity).
- Reinforce and supplement patient's knowledge about diagnosis, prognosis, surgical procedure, and expected level of function postoperatively. Include information about postoperative wound and ostomy care, dietary restrictions, pain control, and medical management.

See Nursing Management under Cancer for additional information.

MAINTAINING OPTIMAL NUTRITION

- Provide a diet high in calories, protein, and carbohydrates and low in residue.
- Provide a full liquid diet 24 to 48 hours before surgery, if prescribed.
- Administer TPN for hospitalized patient.
- Monitor intake and output; administer and monitor intravenous fluids and electrolytes as ordered.
- Insert and monitor nasogastric tube, and note drainage.

MAINTAINING FLUID AND ELECTROLYTE BALANCE

- Administer antiemetics, and restrict fluids and food to prevent vomiting; monitor abdomen for distention, loss of bowel sounds, or pain or rigidity (signs of obstruction or perforation).

- Record intake and output, and restrict fluids and oral food to prevent vomiting.
- Monitor serum electrolytes to detect hypokalemia and hyponatremia.
- Assess vital signs to detect signs of hypovolemia: tachycardia, hypotension, and decreased pulse volume.
- Assess hydration status, and report decreased skin turgor, dry mucous membranes, concentrated urine, and increased urine specific gravity.

PROVIDING EMOTIONAL SUPPORT
- Assess the patient's level of anxiety and coping mechanisms used to deal with stress.
- Provide privacy, if desired; suggest and instruct in relaxation exercises and visualization; listen to patient who wishes to express feelings.
- Arrange meetings with a member of the clergy, if desired.
- Provide meetings for patient and family with physicians and nurses to discuss the treatment and prognosis; a meeting with an enterostomal therapist may be useful.
- Promote patient comfort by a relaxed and empathetic attitude.
- Explain all tests and procedures in language the patient understands; repeat as needed.

SUPPORTING A POSITIVE BODY IMAGE
- Encourage the patient to verbalize feelings and concerns.
- Provide a supportive environment and attitude to promote the patient's adaptation to lifestyle changes related to stoma care.

MONITORING AND MANAGING COMPLICATIONS
- Before and after surgery, observe for symptoms of complications; report; and institute necessary care.
- Administer antibiotics as ordered to reduce intestinal bacteria in preparation for bowel surgery.
- Postoperatively, examine wound dressing frequently during first 24 hours, checking for infection, dehiscence, hemorrhage, and excessive edema.

Promoting Home and Community-Based Care

Teaching Patients Self-Care

- Assess patient's needs and desires for information, and provide information to patient and family (see Providing Emotional Support earlier under Nursing Interventions).
- Provide patients being discharged with specific information, individualized to their needs.
- If patient has an ostomy, include information about ostomy care and complications to observe for symptoms, including obstruction, infection, stoma stenosis, retraction or prolapse, and periostomal skin irritation.
- Provide dietary instructions to help patients identify and eliminate irritating foods that can cause diarrhea or constipation.
- Provide patients with a list of medications prescribed for them, with information on action, purpose, and possible side effects.
- Demonstrate and review treatments and dressing changes, and encourage the family to participate.
- Provide patient with specific directions about when to call the physician and what complications require prompt attention (eg, bleeding, abdominal distention and rigidity, diarrhea, and the dumping syndrome).
- Review side effects of radiation therapy (anorexia, vomiting, diarrhea, and exhaustion) if necessary.
- Refer patient for home nursing care as indicated.

Gerontologic Considerations

Colon and rectal cancers are considered the most common malignancies in old age except for prostatic cancer in men. Symptoms are often insidious; fatigue is almost always present, due primarily to iron-deficiency anemia. Other commonly reported symptoms are abdominal pain, obstruction, tenesmus, and rectal bleeding.

Colon cancer in the elderly has been closely associated with dietary carcinogens, lack of fiber, and excess fat. After surgery, the elderly may experience decreased vision and hearing as well as difficulty with skills that require fine motor coordination, which may require the patient to have help in handling ostomy equipment and periostomal care. Most elderly patients require 6 months before they feel comfortable with their ostomy care.

Arteriosclerosis causes decreased blood flow to the wound and stoma site. As a result, healing time may be prolonged. Some patients experience delayed elimination after irrigation because of decreased peristalsis and mucus production.

Evaluation

EXPECTED OUTCOMES
- Experiences reduced anxiety
- Acquires information about diagnosis, surgical procedure, preoperative preparation, and self-care after discharge
- Maintains clean incision, stoma, and perineal wound
- Verbalizes feelings and concerns about self
- Recovers without complications

For more information, see Chapter 35 in Smeltzer and Bare: *Brunner and Suddarth's Textbook of Medical-Surgical Nursing,* 9th edition. Philadelphia: Lippincott Williams & Wilkins, 2000.

CANCER OF THE ENDOMETRIUM

Cancer of the uterine endometrium (fundus or corpus) is most often adenocarcinoma originating in the lining of the uterus. This cancer is the fourth most common in women and the most common pelvic neoplasm. Risk factors include age (advanced), and weight (obesity). Women receiving hormone replacement therapy (HRT) without progesterone are at particular risk. Other risk factors include nulliparity and late menopause.

Clinical Manifestations
Postmenopausal bleeding raises suspicion of endometrial cancer.

Diagnostic Evaluation
- Annual checkups, including gynecologic examination
- Regular endometrial aspiration or biopsy (primary diagnostic)
- Ultrasonography

Medical Management
Treatment is based on the stage of the disease.
- Treatment consists of total hysterectomy and bilateral salpingo-oophorectomy.
- Intercavitary irradiation or external pelvic irradiation may be part of the preoperative and postoperative treatments.
- Hormonal therapy or chemotherapy may be used to treat recurrent lesions beyond the vagina.

Nursing Management
See Nursing Management under Cancer of the Cervix for additional information.

For more information, see Chapter 43 in Smeltzer and Bare: *Brunner and Suddarth's Textbook of Medical-Surgical Nursing,* 9th edition. Philadelphia: Lippincott Williams & Wilkins, 2000.

CANCER OF THE ESOPHAGUS

Carcinoma of the esophagus is usually of the squamous cell epidermoid type; the incidence of adenocarcinoma of the esophagus is increasing in the United States. Tumor cells may involve the esophageal mucosa and muscle layers and can spread to the lymphatics; in latter stages, they may obstruct the esophagus, perforate the mediastinum, or erode into the great vessels. Risk factors include gender (male), race (African American), age (greater risk in fifth decade of life), and locale (much higher incidence in China and northern Iran). Risk factors also include chronic irritation, use of alcohol and tobacco. In other parts of the world, there has been association with use of opium pipes; ingestion of exceptionally hot beverages, and nutritional deficiencies, mainly lack of fruits and vegetables.

Clinical Manifestations

The patient usually presents with advanced ulcerated lesion of the esophagus.

- Dysphagia, first with solid foods and eventually liquids
- Feeling of a lump in the throat and painful swallowing
- Substernal pain or fullness; regurgitation of undigested food with foul breath and hiccoughs later
- Hemorrhage; progressive loss of weight and strength due to starvation.

Diagnostic Evaluation

- Esophagogastroduodenoscopy with biopsy and brushings confirms the diagnosis in 95% of cases.
- Other studies include bronchoscopy and mediastinoscopy.

Medical Management

Treatment goals of esophageal cancer may be directed toward cure if found in an early stage; in late stages, palliation is the goal of therapy. Each patient is approached in a way that appears best for that individual.

- Surgery, radiation, chemotherapy, or a combination of these modalities, depending on extent of disease
- Palliative treatment done to maintain esophageal patency: dilation of the esophagus, laser therapy, radiation, and chemotherapy
- Esophagectomy through thorax or abdomen or free jejunal graft transfer

Nursing Management
See Nursing Management of the Patient With Cancer under Cancer for additional information.

Assessment
- Obtain a complete health history (appetite, discomfort in swallowing, food associated with pain)
- Question past or present causative factors of esophageal discomfort (eg, alcohol or tobacco use).

Major Nursing Diagnoses
- Altered nutrition: less than body requirement related to difficulty swallowing
- Risk for aspiration due to difficulty swallowing and/or tube feeding
- Pain related to difficulty swallowing
- Knowledge deficit about esophageal cancer, diagnostic studies, management, and rehabilitation

Planning and Goals
Goals of care include improved nutritional and physical condition in preparation for surgery, radiation therapy, or chemotherapy; absence of respiratory compromise; relief of pain; increased knowledge level; and absence of postoperative complications.

Nursing Interventions
- Observe carefully for regurgitation, dyspnea, and aspiration postoperatively.
- Monitor for signs of infection or leakage through the anastomosis; monitor temperature.

PREPARING THE PATIENT FOR SURGERY
- Educate the patient about the nature of the postoperative equipment that will be used (eg, chest drainage, nasogastric suction, parenteral fluid therapy, and gastric intubation).

DECREASING THE RISK FOR ASPIRATION

- Place the patient in semi-Fowler's, and later Fowler's, position after waking from anesthesia to prevent reflux of gastric secretions.
- Instruct patient in the use of oral suction.

PROMOTING WOUND HEALING

- If grafting was done, check for graft viability hourly for the first 12 hours.
- Assess graft for color and presence of pulse (with Doppler).
- If an endoprosthesis has been inserted or anastomosis performed, *do not manipulate nasogastric tube,* mark tube for position immediately postoperative, and notify physician if displacement occurs.

PROMOTING ADEQUATE NUTRITION

- Guide patient through a weight gain program based on a high-calorie and high-protein diet in liquid or soft form, with small, frequent feedings.
- Initiate and monitor total parenteral nutrition, if needed.
- Monitor nutrition status continually.
- Encourage small sips of water, later puréed, small feedings after feeding begins; involve family, home-cooked food may be preferred.
- Administer antacids for gastric distress; liquid supplements may be more easily tolerated.
- Discontinue parenteral fluids when food intake is sufficient; instruct patient to chew sufficiently.
- Keep patient upright for at least 2 hours after each meal to assist in movement of food.
- If patient drools, place a wick-type piece of gauze at corner of the mouth to direct secretions to dressing or emesis basin. Provide oral suction as needed.
- Assess for aspiration of saliva into the tracheobronchial tree (danger of pneumonia).

Promoting Home and Community-Based Care

Teaching Patients Self-Care
- Help patient plan for needed physical and psychological adjustment and for follow-up care, if an ongoing condition exists.
- Provide special equipment, if required, and teach patient and family how to use the equipment.
- Help patient in planning meals, using medications as prescribed, and resuming activity.
- Educate patient about nutritional requirements and how to measure the adequacy of nutrition.
- Educate and assist elderly and debilitated patients, in particular, in ways to adjust their limitations and resume important activities.

Continuing Care
- Instruct patient and family in ways to promote nutrition, such as food preparation, six small meals.
- Teach patient and family what to observe and how to handle signs of complications.
- Assist patient to adjust the medication schedule to daily activities as much as possible.
- Instruct patient about management of equipment and treatments.
- Teach patient how to keep comfortable and how to obtain needed physical and emotional support.
- Refer for home health care as indicated.

Evaluation
EXPECTED OUTCOMES
- Achieves an adequate nutritional intake
- Does not aspirate or develop pneumonia
- Is free of pain or able to control pain within a tolerable level

• Increases knowledge level of esophageal condition, treatment, and prognosis

For more information, see Chapter 32 in Smeltzer and Bare: *Brunner and Suddarth's Textbook of Medical-Surgical Nursing,* 9th edition. Philadelphia: Lippincott Williams & Wilkins, 2000.

CANCER OF THE KIDNEYS (RENAL TUMORS)

The most common type of renal tumor (85%) is renal cell or renal adenocarcinoma. Risk factors include gender (male), tobacco use, occupational exposure to industrial chemicals, obesity, and dialysis. These tumors may metastasize early to the lungs, bones, liver, brain, and contralateral kidney. One third of patients have metastatic disease at the time of diagnosis.

Clinical Manifestations
• Many tumors are without symptoms and are discovered as a palpable abdominal mass on routine examination.
• The classic triad, occurring in only 10% of patients, is hematuria, pain, and a mass in the flank.
• The usual sign that first calls attention to the tumor is painless hematuria, either intermittent and microscopic or continuous and gross.
• Dull pain occurs in the back from pressure from compression of the ureter, extension of the tumor, or hemorrhage into the kidney tissue.
• Colicky pains occur if a clot or mass of tumor cells passes down the ureter.
• Symptoms from metastasis may be the first manifestation of renal tumor, including unexplained weight loss, increasing weakness, and anemia.

Diagnostic Evaluation
• Intravenous urography
• Cystoscopic examination

- Nephrotomograms, renal angiograms
- Ultrasonography
- Computed tomography (CT) scan

Medical Management

The goal of management is to eradicate the tumor before metastasis occurs.

- Radical nephrectomy is the preferred treatment, including removal of the kidney, adrenal gland, and surrounding fat, fascia, and lymph nodes; partial nephrectomy may be used for some patients.
- Radiation therapy, hormonal therapy, or chemotherapy may be used with surgery; immunotherapy may be helpful.
- Renal artery embolization may be used in metastasis to occlude the blood supply to the tumor and kill the tumor cells. Treat a postinfarction syndrome of flank and abdominal pain, elevated temperature, and gastrointestinal complaints with parenteral analgesics, antiemetics, restricted oral intake, and intravenous fluids.
- Biologic therapy includes interleukin-2 (IL-2), lymphokine-activated killer (LAK) cells, or possibly interferon.

Nursing Management

See Nursing Management: The Patient With Cancer under Cancer for additional information.

Nursing Interventions

- Assist patient physiologically and psychologically in preparation for extensive diagnostic and therapeutic procedures; monitor carefully for signs of dehydration and exhaustion.
- After surgery, give frequent analgesia for pain and muscle soreness.
- Provide assistance with turning; encourage to turn, cough, and take deep breaths to prevent atelectasis and other pulmonary complications.

- Support patient and family in coping with diagnosis and uncertainties about outcome and prognosis.

🏠 Promoting Home and Community-Based Care

Teaching Patients Self-Care
- Teach patient to inspect and care for the incision and perform other general postoperative care.
- Teach patient activity and lifting restrictions, driving, and use of pain medications.
- Provide instructions about follow-up care and need to notify physician about fever, breathing difficulty, wound drainage, blood in urine, pain, or swelling of the legs.
- Instruct patient and family in need for follow-up care to detect signs of metastases; evaluate all subsequent symptoms with possible metastases in mind.
- Emphasize that a yearly physical examination and chest radiograph throughout life is required for patients who have had surgery for renal carcinoma.

Continuing Care
- With follow-up chemotherapy, inform the patient and family thoroughly, including treatment plan or chemotherapy protocol, what to expect with visits, and how to notify the physician; explain the need for periodic evaluation of renal function (creatinine clearance, blood urea nitrogen [BUN], and creatinine).
- Reassure the patient and family about the patient's well-being.
- Refer to home care nurse as needed to monitor and support patient and coordinate services and resources needed by the patient.

For more information, see Chapter 41 in Smeltzer and Bare: *Brunner and Suddarth's Textbook of Medical-Surgical Nursing*, 9th edition. Philadelphia: Lippincott Williams & Wilkins, 2000.

CANCER OF THE LARYNX

Cancer of the larynx is most often squamous cell and may occur in the glottic area—vocal cords (two thirds of cases), supraglottic area, and subglottis. This cancer is potentially curable if detected early. Risk factors include gender (male), age (50 to 70 years), tobacco (smoke, smokeless), and alcohol use and their combined effects; vocal straining; chronic laryngitis; industrial exposure to carcinogens; nutritional deficiencies (riboflavin); and family predisposition.

Clinical Manifestations
- Hoarseness, noted early with cancer in glottic area; harsh, low-pitched voice
- Pain and burning in the throat when drinking hot liquids and citrus juices
- Lump felt in the neck
- Late symptoms: dysphagia, dyspnea, unilateral nasal obstruction or discharge, persistent hoarseness or ulceration, and foul breath
- Enlarged cervical nodes, weight loss, general debility, and pain radiating to the ear suggestive of metastasis

Diagnostic Evaluation
- Indirect laryngoscopy
- Direct laryngoscopic examination under general anesthesia
- Biopsy of suspicious tissue with staging using the TNM classification developed by the American Joint Committee on Cancer
- Other tests: computerized tomography (CT) scan; magnetic resonance imaging (MRI) to assess adenopathy; positron emission tomography (PET) to detect recurrence of tumor after treatment

Medical Management
Treatment varies with the extent of malignancy; options include radiation therapy, chemotherapy, and surgery, or combinations.

- Complete dental examination to rule out oral disease
- Dental problems resolved before scheduling surgery if possible
- Radiation therapy achieves excellent results in early-stage glottic tumors, when only one cord is affected and mobile; may be used preoperatively to reduce tumor size or as a palliative measure
- Partial laryngectomy recommended in early stages of glottic cancer with only one vocal cord involved; high cure rate
- Supraglottic (horizontal) laryngectomy used in early supraglottic tumors; true cords and trachea remain intact; radical neck dissection performed on involved side; voice preserved
- Hemilaryngectomy (vertical partial laryngectomy) performed when the tumor extends beyond the vocal cord but is less than 1 cm and is only in the subglottic area
- Total laryngectomy with permanent tracheal stoma for cancer that extends beyond the vocal cords or for recurrent or persistent cancer; radical neck dissection recommended; loss of voice but normal swallowing
- Speech therapy when indicated: esophageal speech, electrolarynx, or tracheoesophageal puncture

Nursing Management: The Patient Undergoing Laryngectomy

See Nursing Management: The Patient With Cancer under Cancer for additional nursing care related to other treatment regimens.

Assessment

- Assess for hoarseness, sore throat, dyspnea, dysphagia, or pain and burning in the throat.
- Palpate the neck for swelling.
- Assess patient's ability to hear, see, read, and write; evaluation by speech therapist if indicated.
- Determine the nature of the surgery; assess the psychological status of the patient; evaluate patient's and fam-

ily's coping methods preoperatively and postoperatively; give effective support.

Planning and Goals

The major goals of the patient may include attainment of an adequate level of knowledge related to treatment, reduction in anxiety, maintenance of a patent airway, improvement in communication, attainment of optimal levels of nutrition and hydration, maintenance of a positive body image and self-esteem, management of self-care, adherence to rehabilitative program, home maintenance management, and prevention of complications.

Major Nursing Diagnoses

Based on all the assessment data, major nursing diagnoses may include the following:

- Knowledge deficit about the surgical procedure and postoperative course
- Anxiety related to the diagnosis of cancer and impending surgery
- Ineffective airway clearance related to surgical alterations in the airway
- Impaired verbal communication related to removal of the larynx and to edema
- Altered nutrition: less than body requirements related to swallowing difficulties
- Disturbance in body image, self-concept, and self-esteem related to major neck surgery
- Self-care deficit related to postoperative care
- Potential for noncompliance with rehabilitative program and home maintenance management

Collaborative Problems/Potential Complications

Based on assessment data, potential complications that may develop include the following:
- Respiratory distress (hypoxia, airway obstruction, tracheal edema)
- Hemorrhage

- Infection
- Wound breakdown

Nursing Interventions

PROVIDING PATIENT EDUCATION

- Clarify any misconceptions, and give patient and family educational materials about surgery (written and audio-visual) for review and reinforcement.
- Explain to patient that natural voice will be lost if complete laryngectomy is planned.
- Assure patient that much can be done through training in a rehabilitation program.
- Review equipment and treatments that will be part of the postoperative care.
- Teach coughing and deep-breathing exercises; provide for return demonstration.

REDUCING ANXIETY AND DEPRESSION

- Assess patient's psychological preparation, and give patient opportunity to verbalize feelings and share perceptions; give patient and family complete, concise answers to questions.
- Arrange a visit from a postlaryngectomy patient to help patient cope with situation and know successful rehabilitation is possible.

MAINTAINING A PATENT AIRWAY

- Position in semi-Fowler's or Fowler's position after recovery from anesthesia.
- Encourage to turn and deep breathe; suction if necessary; early ambulation.
- Observe for signs and symptoms of respiratory distress and hypoxia: restlessness, irritation, agitation, confusion, tachypnea, tachycardia, use of accessory muscles, and decreased oxygen saturation.
- Rule out obstruction immediately by suctioning and having patient cough and take deep breaths.
- Contact physician immediately if nursing measures do not improve respiratory status.

- Use medications that depress respirations with caution; monitor for respiratory depression.
- Care for the laryngectomy tube the same way as a tracheostomy tube; maintain humidification.
- Keep stoma clean by daily cleansing as prescribed, and wipe opening clean as needed after coughing.

PROMOTING COMMUNICATION
AND SPEECH REHABILITATION

- Implement a system of communication, such as "magic slate" or hand signals.
- Use nonwriting arm for intravenous infusions.
- If patient cannot write, use alternate systems, such as hand signals or a picture-word-phrase board.
- Work with patient, speech therapist, and family to find least frustrating system of communication.
- Inform patient of alternative communication methods; most common are esophageal speech, the electrolarynx, and tracheal esophageal puncture.

PROMOTING ADEQUATE NUTRITION

- Maintain patient NPO for 10 to 14 days, and provide alternative sources of nutrition as ordered: intravenous fluids, enteral feedings, and total parenteral nutrition (TPN); explain nutritional plan to patient and family.
- Start oral feedings with thick fluids for easy swallowing; instruct to avoid sweet foods, which increase salivation and suppress appetite; introduce solid foods as tolerated.
- Instruct to rinse mouth with warm water or mouthwash and brush teeth frequently.
- Observe patient for difficulty swallowing (particularly with eating); report occurrence to physician.

PROMOTING A POSITIVE BODY IMAGE AND
INCREASING SELF-ESTEEM

- Encourage patient to express feelings about changes from surgery (fear, anger, depression, and isolation); be a good listener and a support to the patient and family; explain tubes, dressings, and drains.

- Use a positive approach; promote participation in self-care activities as soon as possible.
- Refer to a support group, such as A Lost Chord or A New Voice clubs, and I Can Cope.

MONITORING AND MANAGING POTENTIAL POSTOPERATIVE COMPLICATIONS

Complications after laryngectomy include respiratory distress (hypoxia, airway obstruction, tracheal edema), bleeding, infection, and wound breakdown.

- See Maintaining a Patent Airway, earlier, for respiratory distress.
- Note pale, cold, clammy skin, which may indicate active bleeding.
- Observe wound drainage; measure and record.
- Contact physician immediately if any active bleeding occurs.
- Monitor vital signs for changes: increase in pulse, decrease in blood pressure, or rapid, deep respirations.
- Observe for early signs and symptoms of infection: change in type of wound drainage, increased areas of redness or tenderness at surgical site, purulent drainage, odor, and increase in wound drainage.
- Observe the stoma area for wound breakdown, hematoma, and bleeding, and report significant changes to the surgeon.
- Monitor patient carefully, particularly for carotic hemorrhage (see Nursing Alert, later).

Promoting Home and Community-Based Care

Teaching Patients Self-Care

- Provide discharge instructions as soon as patient able to participate; assess readiness to learn.
- Assess knowledge about self-care management; reassure patient and family that strategies can be mastered.
- Give specific information about tracheostomy and stomal care, wound care, and oral hygiene, including suctioning and emergency measures.

C

- Keep orifice clean and clear of mucus; wash skin around stoma at least twice daily; if crusting occurs, lubricate stoma with a non–oil-based ointment.
- Instruct patient to provide adequate humidification of the environment; minimize air-conditioning.
- Inform patient to expect a diminished sense of taste and smell after surgery.
- Teach patient to take precautions when showering to prevent getting water into the stoma.
- Discourage swimming because the patient with a laryngectomy can drown.
- Recommend avoidance of hairsprays, loose hair, and powders getting into stoma.
- Stress that activity should be undertaken in moderation; when tired, the patient has more difficulty speaking with new voice.

Continuing Care
- Encourage patient to visit physician regularly for physical examinations and advice.
- Recommend carrying proper identification to alert first-aid giver to special requirements of cardiopulmonary resuscitation.
- Teach family mouth-to-stoma ventilation and to keep prerecorded emergency messages for police, fire department, and other rescue services for patient to use at home.
- Refer to home care agency for patient and family assistance, follow-up assessment, and teaching.

⚡ NURSING ALERT
Postoperatively, the nurse must be alert for the possible serious complications of rupture of the carotid artery. Should this occur, apply direct pressure over the artery, summon assistance, and provide psychological support until the vessel can be ligated.

Evaluation

EXPECTED OUTCOMES

- Acquires an adequate level of knowledge, verbalizing an understanding of the surgical procedure and performing self-care adequately
- Demonstrates less anxiety and depression
- Maintains a clear airway
- Acquires effective communication techniques
- Maintains balanced nutrition and adequate fluid intake
- Exhibits improved body image, self-esteem, and self-concept
- Exhibits no complications
- Adheres to rehabilitation and home care program

For more information, see Chapter 20 in Smeltzer and Bare: *Brunner and Suddarth's Textbook of Medical-Surgical Nursing,* 9th edition. Philadelphia: Lippincott Williams & Wilkins, 2000.

CANCER OF THE LIVER

Few cancers originate in the liver. Primary tumors ordinarily occur in patients with chronic liver disease (cirrhosis). Hepatocellular carcinoma (HCC) is the most common type of primary liver tumor. It is usually nonresectable because of rapid growth and metastasis elsewhere. Other types include cholangiocellular carcinoma (CCC) and combined HCC and CCC. If found early, resection may be possible; however, early detection is rare.

Cirrhosis, hepatitis B and C, and exposure to certain chemical toxins have been implicated in the etiology of HCC. Cigarette smoking, especially when combined with alcohol use, has also been identified as a risk factor. Other substances that have been implicated include alfatoxins and other similar toxic molds. Half of all advanced liver cancer cases are metastases from other primary sites.

Clinical Manifestations
- Early manifestations include pain (dull ache in upper right quadrant, epigastrium, or back), recent loss of weight, loss of strength, anorexia, and anemia.
- Liver enlargement and irregular surface may be noted on palpation.
- Jaundice is present only if larger bile ducts are occluded.
- Ascites occurs if portal veins are obstructed or tumor tissue is seeded in the peritoneal cavity.

Diagnostic Evaluation
Diagnosis is made on the basis of clinical signs and symptoms, history and physical examination, and results of laboratory and radiographic studies, liver scans, computed tomography (CT) scans, ultrasounds, magnetic resonance imaging (MRI), arteriography, laparoscopy, or biopsy.

Medical Management
Radiation Therapy
- Intravenous injection of antibodies that specifically attack tumor-associated antigens.
- Percutaneous placement of a high-intensity source for interstitial radiation therapy.

Chemotherapy
- Systemic chemotherapy and regional infusion are used to administer antineoplastic agents.
- An implantable pump is used to deliver a high-concentration chemotherapy to the liver through the hepatic artery.

Percutaneous Biliary Drainage
- Percutaneous biliary drainage is used to bypass biliary ducts obstructed by the liver, pancreatic, or bile ducts in patients with inoperable tumors or those who are poor surgical risks.
- Complications include sepsis, leakage of bile, hemorrhage, and reobstruction of the biliary system.

- Observe patients for fever and chills, bile drainage around the catheter, changes in vital signs, and evidence of biliary obstruction, including increased pain or pressure, pruritus, and recurrence of jaundice.

Other Nonsurgical Treatment Modalities

- Hyperthermia: heat is directed to tumors to cause necrosis of the tumors while sparing normal tissue.
- Cryosurgery is a newer treatment modality.
- Embolization of the arterial blood flow to the tumor; effective in small tumors; alcohol injection may be used to cause tumor necrosis.
- Immunotherapy: lymphocytes with antitumor reactivity are administered to the patient.

Surgical Management

Hepatic lobectomy can be performed when the primary hepatic tumor is localized or when the primary site can be completely excised and the metastasis is limited. Capitalizing on the regenerative capacity of the liver cells, 90% of the liver has been successfully removed. The presence of cirrhosis limits the ability of the liver to regenerate.

PREOPERATIVE EVALUATION AND PREPARATION

- Evaluate and address patient's nutritional, fluid, psychological, and physical needs before surgery.
- Prepare the intestinal tract with cathartics, colonic irrigation, and intestinal antibiotics.

ANATOMIC (SURGICAL) DIVISION OF THE LOBES
WITH RESECTION

LIVER TRANSPLANTATION TO TREAT LIVER TUMORS

- Removal of the liver and its replacement by a healthy donor organ has been successful.
- Recurrence rate of primary liver malignancy after transplantation is 70% to 85%.

Nursing Management

See Nursing Management under Cancer for additional information.

Nursing Interventions

POSTOPERATIVE

- Assess for potential problems related to cardiopulmonary involvement, vascular complications, and respiratory and liver dysfunction.
- Give careful attention to metabolic abnormalities (glucose, protein, and lipids).
- Give constant close monitoring and care for the first 2 or 3 days.
- Encourage early ambulation, and initiate other postoperative care measures.
- Closely monitor the patient undergoing cryosurgery for hypothermia, hemorrhage, bile leak, and myoglobinuria.

Promoting Home and Community-Based Care

Teaching Patients Self-Care

- Instruct family to assess and report complications and side effects of the chemotherapy.
- Instruct about the importance of follow-up visits to permit frequent checks on the response of the patient and the tumor to chemotherapy, condition of the site of the pump insertion, and occurrence of toxic effects.
- Encourage patient to resume activities as soon as possible, but caution to avoid activities that may damage the pump.

Continuing Care

- Instruct regarding signs of complications, and encourage the patient to notify nurse or physician if problems or questions occur.
- Teach irrigation technique to avoid introducing bacteria (eg, not aspirating or drawing back into syringe).

- Refer the patient for home care; the nurse serves a vital role in assisting the patient and family to cope with the symptoms that may occur and with the prognosis in the following ways:
  - Collaborate with the health care team, patient, and family to identify and implement pain management strategies and approaches to management of other problems: weakness, pruritus, inadequate dietary intake, jaundice, and symptoms associated with metastasis to other sites.
  - Assist patient and family in decision making about hospice care and initiation of referrals.
- Encourage patient to discuss end-of-life care.
- Provide reassurance and instructions to patient and family to reduce fear that the percutaneous biliary drainage catheter will fall out.
- Provide verbal and written instruction as well as demonstration of biliary catheter care to patient and family; instruct in techniques to keep catheter site clean and dry and to assess the catheter and its insertion site.

For more information, see Chapter 36 in Smeltzer and Bare: *Brunner and Suddarth's Textbook of Medical-Surgical Nursing,* 9th edition. Philadelphia: Lippincott Williams & Wilkins, 2000.

CANCER OF THE LUNG (BRONCHOGENIC CARCINOMA)

Lung cancers arise from a transformed epithelial cell in tracheobronchial airways. A carcinogen (cigarette smoke, radon gas, other occupational and environmental agents) damages the cell, causing abnormal growth and development into a malignant tumor. The survival rate is low because of spread to regional lymphatics (in 70% of patients) by the time of diagnosis. There are four major cell types of lung cancer. Epidermoid or squamous cell carcinoma (25% to 40% of patients) is more centrally located, adenocarcinoma (25% to 45%) presents as peripheral masses and often metastasizes, large cell carcinoma (10% to 15%) is a fast-growing tumor that often arises peripherally. Small cell (oat cell) carcinoma (15% to 20% of cases) usually arises in the major bronchi.

Risk factors include tobacco smoke, secondhand smoke, environmental (air) pollution, occupational exposure, and radon. Other risk factors may include dietary factors (vitamin A and beta-carotene deficiency from low fruit and vegetable intake), genetic predisposition, and other underlying respiratory diseases, such as chronic obstructive pulmonary disease and tuberculosis.

Clinical Manifestations
- Lung cancer begins insidiously over several decades and is often asymptomatic until late in its course.
- Signs and symptoms depend on location, tumor size, degree of obstruction, and existence of metastases.
- Most common symptom is a persistent and nonproductive cough, which later progresses to producing thick, purulent sputum. *A cough that changes in character should arouse suspicion of lung cancer.*
- Wheezing occurs when the bronchus becomes partially obstructed; expectoration of blood-tinged sputum occurs.
- A recurring fever may exist in some patients.
- Chest pain or shoulder pain may indicate chest wall or pleural involvement. Pain is a late symptom and may be related to bone metastasis.
- Chest pain, tightness, hoarseness, dysphagia, head and neck edema, and symptoms of pleural or pericardial infusion exist if the tumor spreads to adjacent structures and lymph nodes.
- Common sites of metastases are lymph nodes, bone, brain, contralateral lung, adrenal glands, and liver.
- Weakness, anorexia, and weight loss appear late.

Diagnostic Evaluation

- Chest films, sputum examinations, endoscopy or bronchoscopy, mediastinoscopy, fine-needle aspiration (FNA), biopsy
- Various computed tomography (CT) and magnetic resonance imaging (MRI) scans
- Pulmonary function tests, arterial blood gas analysis, ventilation-perfusion scans, and exercise testing
- Staging of the tumor refers to the anatomic extent of the tumor, spread to the regional lymph nodes, and metastatic spread.

See Diagnostic Evaluation and Staging of Cancer under Cancer for additional information.

Medical Management

See Medical Management under Cancer for additional information.

The objective of management is to provide the maximum likelihood of cure. Treatment depends on cell type, stage of the disease, and physiologic status.

- Treatment may involve surgery (preferred unless contraindicated); lung resection is beneficial.
- Radiation therapy, chemotherapy, and immunotherapy may be used separately or in combination and with surgery.
- Immunotherapy (minimal success in the past) is still investigational.
- Newer therapies (gene, tumor antigens) are under study.

Nursing Management

See Nursing Management under Cancer for additional information.

Nursing Interventions

MANAGING SYMPTOMS

- Instruct the patient and family about the side effects of specific treatments and strategies to manage them.

RELIEVING BREATHING PROBLEMS
- Maintain airway patency; remove secretions.
- Encourage deep breathing, aerosol therapy, oxygen therapy; mechanical ventilation may be necessary.
- Encourage patient to assume positions that promote lung expansion.
- Teach breathing exercises, relaxation techniques, and energy conservation.
- Refer for pulmonary rehabilitation as indicated.

REDUCING FATIGUE
- Assess level of fatigue; identify potentially treatable causes.
- Educate patient in energy conservation techniques.
- Refer to physical or occupational therapist as indicated.

PROVIDING PSYCHOLOGICAL SUPPORT
- Help patient and family deal with poor prognosis and progression of the disease (when indicated).
- Assess psychological aspects and assist patient to cope.
- Assist patient and family with informed decision-making regarding treatment options.
- Support patient and family in end-of-life decisions and treatment options.

For more information, see Chapter 21 in Smeltzer and Bare: *Brunner and Suddarth's Textbook of Medical-Surgical Nursing,* 9th edition. Philadelphia: Lippincott Williams & Wilkins, 2000.

CANCER OF THE ORAL CAVITY

Cancer of the oral cavity may occur in any part of the mouth (lips, lateral tongue, floor of mouth most common) or throat and is highly curable if discovered early. It is associated with use of alcohol and tobacco. Risk factors also include age (older than 60 years, but seen increasingly under age 30 years), gender (male), smokeless tobacco use (buccal mucosa and gingiva), dietary deficiency, and smoked meats as well as chronic irritation by a warm pipe stem or prolonged exposure to sun and wind (lip cancer).

Clinical Manifestations
- Most common complaint: painless sore or mass that will not heal.
- Typical lesion is a painful indurated ulcer with raised edges.
- As the cancer progresses, patient may complain of tenderness; difficulty in chewing, swallowing, and speaking; coughing of blood-tinged sputum; or enlarged cervical lymph nodes.

Diagnostic Evaluation
Oral examination, assessment of lymph nodes, and biopsies on suspicious lesions (not healed within 2 weeks).

Medical Management
Management varies with the nature of the lesion, preference of the physician, and patient choice. Resectional surgery, radiation therapy, chemotherapy, or a combination may be effective.

- Lip cancer: small lesions are excised liberally; larger lesions may be treated by radiation therapy.
- Tongue cancer: treated aggressively, recurrence rate is high. Radiation and surgery (resection or hemiglossectomy) are performed.
- Radical neck dissection for metastases of oral cancer to lymphatic channel in the neck region with reconstructive surgery.

Nursing Management
See Nursing Management under Cancer for additional information.

Assessment
- Assess patient's history to determine teaching and learning needs and symptoms requiring medical evaluation. Include questions related to oral cavity: oral and dental hygiene; dentures or partial plate; alcohol and tobacco use, also smokeless chewing tobacco; lesions or irritated areas in the mouth, tongue, or throat; recent history of sore throat or bloody sputum; discomfort caused by certain foods.
- Perform physical examination: inspect and palpate internal and external structures of the mouth and throat; examine for moisture, color, texture, symmetry, and presence of lesions; examine neck for enlarged lymph nodes. Use gloves to examine the patient's oral cavity.

Major Nursing Diagnoses
- Altered oral mucous membrane related to pathologic condition, infection, or chemical or mechanical trauma (eg, medications, ill-fitting dentures).
- Altered nutrition: less than body requirements related to inability to ingest adequate nutrients secondary to oral or dental conditions.
- Body image disturbance related to a physical change in appearance resulting from a disease condition or its treatment
- Pain related to oral lesion or treatment
- Impaired verbal communication related to treatment
- Risk for infection related to disease or treatment
- Knowledge deficit about disease process and treatment plan

Planning and Goals
The major goals of the patient may include improved condition of the oral cavity and mucous membrane, improved nutritional intake, attainment and maintenance of positive self-image, attainment of comfort, alternative communication methods, remaining free of infection, demonstrating understanding of the disease and treatment.

Nursing Interventions

PROMOTING MOUTH CARE

- Identify patients at risk for oral complications, and assist with methods to decrease complications.
- Instruct the patient in importance and techniques of preventive mouth care: soft toothbrush, floss, or irrigating solution such as baking soda in water, double-strength hydrogen peroxide, or normal saline.

COMBATING XEROSTOMIA (DRYNESS OF MOUTH)

- Advise patient to avoid dry, bulky, and irritating foods and fluids, alcohol, and tobacco.
- Encourage patient to increase fluids and to use a humidifier during sleep.
- Provide synthetic saliva, moisturizing gel, or saliva production stimulant for patient, if needed.

RELIEVING STOMATITIS OR MUCOSITIS

- Start prophylactic mouth care as soon as chemotherapy or radiation therapy begins; if poor dentition, tooth extraction, or fluoride treatment may be needed.

ENSURING ADEQUATE FOOD AND FLUID INTAKE

- Perform dietary assessment with calorie count, and recommend changes in consistency of foods and frequency of eating based on disease condition and patient preferences; dietitian consult may be beneficial.
- Help attain and maintain desirable body weight and level of energy; promote the healing of tissue.

SUPPORTING A POSITIVE SELF-IMAGE

- Encourage patient to verbalize perceived change in body appearance; realistically discuss actual changes or losses.
- Offer support while patient verbalizes fears and negative feelings (withdrawal, depression, anger).
- Reinforce strengths, achievements, and positive attributes; support from groups, clergy, or other may be helpful.
- Note signs of grieving, and record emotional changes and progress toward positive self-esteem.

C

MINIMIZING DISCOMFORT AND PAIN
- Provide patient with an analgesic, such as viscous lidocaine (Xylocaine viscous 2%).
- Avoid foods that are spicy, hot, or hard.
- Instruct patient about mouth care.

PROMOTING EFFECTIVE COMMUNICATION
- Assess patient's ability to communicate in writing preoperatively.
- Provide a "magic slate" or pen and paper to communicate postoperatively.
- Provide a communication board if unable to write; involve a speech therapist postoperatively.

PROMOTING INFECTION CONTROL
- Evaluate laboratory results frequently; check temperature every 6 to 8 hours for elevation that may indicate infection, monitor for signs of infection such as redness, swelling, drainage, or tenderness.
- Prohibit visitors who may transmit microorganisms.
- Avoid trauma to sensitive skin tissues; use strict aseptic technique when changing dressings.
- Provide instruction about antibiotics.

Promoting Home and Community-Based Care

Teaching Patients Self-Care
- Assess patient needs, and instruct patient regarding mouth care, nutrition, infection prevention, and signs and symptoms of complications; refer to home care nurse for physical care, assessment, and further teaching.
- Prepare an individualized plan of care; if prostheses are used, teach patient in the use and care of these and the importance of clean dressings and strict oral hygiene.
- Determine what equipment is needed (eg, suction or tracheostomy tube) and where items can be obtained.
- Give consideration to humidification and aeration of patient's room and measures to control odors.
- Instruct patient and family in use of enteral or parenteral feedings (if unable to take foods orally).

- Provide information regarding signs of obstruction, hemorrhage, infection, depression, and withdrawal to caregivers.
- Instruct in the importance of follow-up visits to monitor patient's condition and to receive directions about modifications in treatment or general care; reinforce instructions to promote patient self-care and comfort.

Evaluation

EXPECTED OUTCOMES
- Acquires information about course of treatment
- Demonstrates good respiratory exchange
- Is free of infection
- Has graft that is pink and warm to touch
- Maintains adequate intake of foods and fluids
- Demonstrates ability to cope
- Verbalizes comfort
- Attains maximal mobility

For more information, see Chapter 32 in Smeltzer and Bare: *Brunner and Suddarth's Textbook of Medical-Surgical Nursing,* 9th edition. Philadelphia: Lippincott Williams & Wilkins, 2000.

CANCER OF THE OVARY

Ovarian cancer is most distressing because it is usually (75% of cases) diagnosed in advanced stage. Peak incidence is in the fifth decade of life. No definitive causative factors have been determined, but oral contraceptives appear to provide a protective effect. Serous adenocarcinoma is the most common type of tumor. Risk factors include high-fat diet; smoking; alcohol; use of talcum powder on perineal area; history of breast, colon, or endometrial cancer; and family history of breast or ovarian cancer. Nulliparity, infertility, and anovulation are additional risks.

Clinical Manifestations

- Irregular menses, increasing premenstrual tension, menorrhagia with breast tenderness, early menopause, abdominal discomfort, dyspepsia, pelvic pressure, and urinary frequency
- Flatulence, fullness after a light meal, and increasing abdominal girth significant
- A combination of a long history of ovarian dysfunction and vague gastrointestinal symptoms or a palpable ovary in a postmenopausal woman significant

Diagnostic Evaluation

- No screening mechanism exists; tumor markers are being explored.
- Any enlarged ovary must be investigated; pelvic examination does not detect early ovarian cancer.

Medical Management

- Surgical removal is the treatment of choice.
- Preoperative workup can include barium enema, proctosigmoidoscopy, upper gastrointestinal series, chest radiograph, intravenous pyelogram (IVP), and intravenous urography.
- Staging of the tumor is done to direct treatment.
- Total abdominal hysterectomy with bilateral salpingo-oophorectomy and omentectomy for early disease.
- Radiation therapy and intraperitoneal isotopes are sometimes used.
- Gene therapy is a future possibility.
- Chemotherapy, including liposomal and intraperitoneal delivery, is the most common form of treatment for advanced disease (eg, cisplatin, paclitaxel [Taxol]).
- Bone marrow transplantation and peripheral blood stem cell support may be used with chemotherapy.

Nursing Management

Assessment

- Be alert for manifestations and report to physician.

- Monitor for complications of therapy and abdominal surgery.
- Determine emotional needs, including desire for child-bearing.

Nursing Interventions

Nursing measures include treatment related to surgery, radiation, chemotherapy, and palliation. Emotional support is provided by giving comfort measures, showing attentiveness and caring. Allow patients to express feelings about condition and death. See Nursing Interventions under Cancer and under Preoperative and Postoperative Nursing Management.

For more information, see Chapter 43 in Smeltzer and Bare: *Brunner and Suddarth's Textbook of Medical-Surgical Nursing,* 9th edition. Philadelphia: Lippincott Williams & Wilkins, 2000.

CANCER OF THE PANCREAS

Cancer of the pancreas may arise in any portion of the pancreas, producing symptoms that vary, depending on the location of the lesion and whether functioning insulin-secreting pancreatic islet cells are involved. It occurs most frequently in the fifth to seventh decades of life. Risk factors include exposure to industrial chemicals or toxins in the environment; a diet high in fat, meat, or both; and cigarette smoking. Pancreatic cancer is also associated with hereditary pancreatitis, diabetes mellitus, and chronic pancreatitis. Tumors that originate in the head of the pancreas are the most common and obstruct the common bile duct; functioning islet cell tumors are responsible for the syndrome of hyperinsulinism, particularly in islet cell tumors. Zollinger-Ellison tumors of the islets of Langerhans are associated with hypersecretion of gastric acid. The pancreas can also be the site of metastasis from other tumors. Pancreatic carcinoma has a 3% survival rate at 5 years regardless of stage of disease at diagnosis.

Clinical Manifestations

- Abdominal pain, jaundice, or both present in 90% of patients, and weight loss is considered a classic sign and may appear only when the disease is far advanced.
- Rapid, profound, and progressive weight loss occur.
- Malabsorption of nutrients and fat-soluble vitamins, anorexia and malaise, and clay-colored stools and dark urine are common with tumors in the head of the pancreas.
- Vague upper or mid-abdominal pain or discomfort unrelated to any gastrointestinal function; radiates as a boring pain in the midback, and is more severe at night and when lying supine; pain is often progressive and severe; the formation of ascites is common.
- Onset of symptoms of insulin deficiency (diabetes): glucosuria, hyperglycemia, and abnormal glucose tolerance may be an early sign of carcinoma; meals often aggravate epigastric pain.
- Zollinger-Ellison tumors may cause hypersecretion of gastric acid, resulting in ulcers in the stomach, duodenum, and jejunum.

Diagnostic Evaluation

- Ultrasound and computed tomograph (CT) scan, endoscopic retrograde cholangiopancreatography (ERCP) with cell analysis, percutaneous fine-needle biopsy, percutaneous transhepatic cholangiography (PTC), angiography, laparoscopy or duodenography
- Glucose tolerance test used to diagnose a pancreatic islet tumor

Medical Management

- Surgical procedure is extensive to remove resectable localized tumors (eg, pancreatectomy, Whipple resection). If tumor is Zollinger-Ellison and is not removable, a total gastrectomy may be necessary.
- Diet high in protein with pancreatic enzymes, adequate hydration, vitamin K, and treatment of anemia with blood components and total parenteral nutrition (TPN)

administration may be instituted before surgery when indicated.
- Treatment is often limited to palliative measures owing to the widespread metastases, especially to the liver, lungs, and bones.
- Radiation and chemotherapy may be used; intraoperative radiation therapy (IORT) or interstitial implantation of radioactive sources may be used for relief of pain.
- A biliary stent may be used to relieve jaundice.

Nursing Management

See Preoperative and Postoperative Nursing Management for additional information.

- Provide pain management and attention to nutrition, be alert for hypoglycemia with the patients with pancreatic islet tumor.
- Provide skin care and measures to relieve pain and discomfort associated with jaundice, anorexia, and profound weight loss.
- Monitor patient postoperatively: vital signs, arterial blood gases and pressures, pulse oximetry, laboratory values, and urine output.
- Provide emotional support to the patient and family before, during, and after treatment.
- Consider patient-controlled analgesia (PCA) for severe, escalating pain.

🏠 Promoting Home and Community-Based Care

Teaching Patients Self-Care
- If chemotherapy is elected, focus teaching on prevention of side effects and complications of agents used.
- If surgery was performed, teaching addresses management of the drainage system and monitoring for complications.
- Teach the patient and family strategies to prevent skin breakdown, relieve pain, pruritus, and anorexia, including instruction about PCA, TPN, and diet modification

with pancreatic enzymes if indicated because of malabsorption and hyperglycemia; monitor serum glucose levels if patient had a pancreatic islet tumor.

- Discuss and arrange for palliative care with the patient and family in an effort to relieve patient discomfort, assist with care, and comply with end-of-life decisions.
- Instruct the family about changes in the patient's status that should be reported to the physician.
- Refer patient for home care for help dealing with problems, discomforts, and the psychological effects; discharge to a long-term care setting with communication to staff about prior teaching.

For more information, see Chapter 38 in Smeltzer and Bare: *Brunner and Suddarth's Textbook of Medical-Surgical Nursing,* 9th edition. Philadelphia: Lippincott Williams & Wilkins, 2000.

CANCER OF THE PROSTATE

Cancer of the prostate is the most common cancer in men, the second most common cause of cancer deaths in American men older than 55, and the most prevalent cancer overall in African American men. About 1 in 15 men in the United States develop prostate cancer. Risk factors include increasing age and possibly a high-fat diet.

Clinical Manifestations
- Usually asymptomatic in early stage
- Nodule felt within the substance of the gland or extensive hardening in the posterior lobe

Advanced Stage
- Lesion is stony hard and fixed.
- Obstructive symptoms occur late in the disease: difficulty and frequency of urination, urinary retention, decreased size and force of the urinary stream.
- Cancer metastasizes to bone, lymph nodes, brain, and lungs.

- Symptoms of metastases include backache, hip pain, perineal and rectal discomfort, anemia, weight loss, weakness, nausea, and oliguria; hematuria may result from urethral or bladder invasion.
- Sexual dysfunction occurs.

Diagnostic Evaluation

- To promote early detection, every man older than 50 years of age should have a digital rectal examination (DRE) as part of his regular health checkup—key to a higher cure rate.
- Diagnosis is confirmed by histologic examination of tissue, transurethral resection open prostatectomy, and fine-needle aspiration.
- Prostate-specific antigen (PSA) level, transrectal ultrasound, bone scan, radiographs, excretory urography, renal function tests, computed tomography (CT) scans on lymphangiography, or monoclonal antibody-based imaging may also be used.

Medical Management

Treatment is based on the stage of the disease and on the patient's age and symptoms. PSA concentration is used to monitor patient response to cancer therapy and to detect local progression and early recurrence.

Radical Prostatectomy

- Removal of the prostate and seminal vesicles through suprapubic (greater blood loss), perineal (easily contaminated, incontinence, impotence, and rectal injury common), or retropubic (infection can readily start) surgery.
- This procedure is performed in patients who have potentially curable disease and life expectancy of 10 years of more.
- Sexual impotency and various degrees of urinary incontinence follow radical prostatectomy.

Radiation Therapy
- If cancer is in the early stage, treatment may be curative radiation therapy.
- For locally advanced cancer, hormonal treatments are given before and after radiation.
- Side effects, usually transitory, include inflammation of the rectum, bowel, and bladder.
- There is better preservation of sexual potency, and young patients may prefer this treatment modality.

Hormonal Therapy
- Method of control rather than cure
- Accomplished by either orchiectomy or administration of estrogens
- Diethylstilbestrol (DES) is the most widely used estrogen
- Luteinizing hormone–releasing hormone (LHRH) agonists and antiandrogen drugs such as flutamide also used

Other Therapies
- Transurethral resection of the prostate (TUR or TURP) or transurethral incision of the prostate (TUIP) for benign condition
- Cryosurgery for those who cannot physically tolerate surgery or for recurrence.
- Chemotherapy (doxorubicin, cisplatin, and cyclophosphamide)
- Repeated TUR to keep urethra patent; suprapubic or transurethral catheter drainage when repeat TUR is impractical
- Opioid or nonopioid medications (antiandrogen, prednisone, and mitoxantrone) to control pain with metastasis to the bone
- Blood transfusions to maintain adequate hemoglobin levels
- Prosthetic penile implants or other options to create penile erection, for the patient with impotence

Nursing Management: The Patient Undergoing Prostatectomy

Assessment

- Take complete history with emphasis on urinary function and the effect of the underlying disorder on patient's lifestyle.
- Note reports of urgency, frequency, nocturia, dysuria, urinary retention, hematuria, or decreased ability to initiate voiding.
- Note family history of cancer, heart disease, or kidney disease, including hypertension.

Major Nursing Diagnoses

PREOPERATIVE

- Anxiety related to the inability to void
- Pain related to bladder distention
- Knowledge deficit about factors related to the problem and the treatment protocol

POSTOPERATIVE

- Pain related to the surgical incision, catheter placement, and bladder spasms
- Knowledge deficit about postoperative and convalescent management

Collaborative Problems/Potential Complications

- Hemorrhage and shock
- Infection
- Thrombosis
- Catheter obstruction

Planning and Goals

The major preoperative goals of the patient may include reduced anxiety and increased knowledge about prostate problem and the perioperative experience. The major postoperative goals may include correction of fluid volume disturbances, relief of pain and discomfort, ability to perform self-care activities, and absence of complications.

Nursing Interventions

PREOPERATIVE

Reducing Anxiety
- Provide privacy, and establish a trusting and professional relationship.
- Encourage verbalization of feelings and concerns.
- Clarify the nature of the surgery and expected postoperative outcomes.

Relieving Discomfort
- Place on bed rest; administer analgesics; initiate measures to relieve anxiety.
- Monitor voiding patterns; watch for bladder distention.
- Insert indwelling catheter if urinary retention is present or if laboratory test results indicate azotemia.
- Prepare patient for a cystostomy, if urinary catheter is not tolerated.

  See Preoperative and Postoperative Nursing Management for additional information.

Preparing Patient for Treatment
- Explain diagnostic tests, surgery procedure, and drainage system.
- Answer questions and provide patient support.
- Establish a private time for patient to review the anatomy and function of affected parts.
- Explain rationale for preoperative antiembolism stockings.
- Administer enema, if ordered.

POSTOPERATIVE

Relieving Pain
- Distinguish cause and location of pain, including bladder spasms.
- Give analgesics for incisional pain and smooth muscle relaxants for bladder spasm.
- Monitor drainage tubing, and irrigate drainage system to correct any obstruction.
- Secure the catheter to the leg or abdomen.

- Monitor dressings, and adjust to ensure they are not too snug, too saturated, or improperly placed.
- Provide stool softener, prune juice, or an enema, if prescribed.

Monitoring and Managing Complications
- Hemorrhage: observe catheter drainage, note bright red bleeding with increased viscosity and clots; monitor intake and output and vital signs; administer medication, intravenous fluids, and blood as prescribed. Provide explanations and reassurance to patient and family.
- Infection: assess for urinary tract infection and epididymitis; administer antibiotics as prescribed. Provide sitz bath and heat lamps to promote healing after sutures are removed. Use aseptic technique with dressing changes; avoid rectal thermometers, tubes, and enemas.
- Thrombosis: assess for deep vein thrombosis and pulmonary embolism; apply antiembolism stockings. Assist patient to progress from dangling the day of surgery to ambulating the next morning; encourage patient to walk but not sit for long periods of time. Monitor the patient receiving heparin for excessive bleeding.
- Obstructed catheter: Observe the lower abdomen for bladder distention. Provide for patent drainage system; perform gentle irrigation as prescribed to remove blood clots.

Promoting Home and Community-Based Care

Teaching Patients Self-Care
- Teach patient and family how to manage drainage system, monitor urinary output, perform wound care, and use strategies to prevent complications.
- Inform patient about signs and symptoms that should be reported to the physician (eg, blood in the urine, decreased urine output, fever, change in wound drainage, or calf tenderness).
- Teach perineal exercises to help regain urinary control.

- Teach patient not to engage in any Valsalva effort, which increases venous pressure and may produce hematuria.
- Avoid long motor trips and strenuous exercise, which increases tendency to bleed.
- Inform patient that spicy foods, alcohol, and coffee can cause bladder discomfort.
- Encourage fluids to avoid dehydration and clot formation.

Continuing Care
- Refer for home care if indicated.
- Remind patient that return of bladder control may take time.

Evaluation
EXPECTED OUTCOMES
Preoperative
- Demonstrates reduced anxiety and decreased pain
- Relates understanding of the surgical procedure and postoperative care

Postoperative
- Relates relief of discomfort
- Responds positively to self-care measures
- Remains free of complications

For more information, see Chapter 45 in Smeltzer and Bare: *Brunner and Suddarth's Textbook of Medical-Surgical Nursing,* 9th edition. Philadelphia: Lippincott Williams & Wilkins, 2000.

CANCER OF THE SKIN

Skin cancer is the most common and most successfully treated form of cancer in the United States. Exposure to the sun is the leading cause; incidence is related to the cumulative amount of exposure to the sun. Those at greatest risk are people with light complexions. Others at risk are outdoor workers, elderly people with sun-damaged skin, workers exposed to chemical agents (eg, arsenic, coal, tar); conditions causing scarring or chronic irritation may also lead to cancer. The two types of skin cancer are basal cell carcinoma (BCC), which arises from the basal cell layer of the epidermis or hair follicles (most common and rarely metastasizes; recurrence is common) and squamous cell carcinomas (SCC), a malignant proliferation arising from the epidermis (an invasive carcinoma).

Clinical Manifestations

- BCC generally appears on sun-exposed areas of the body; presents as a small, waxy nodule with rolled translucent pearly borders; telangiectatic vessels may present. Other variants may appear as shiny, flat, gray, or yellowish plaques.
- SCC usually appears on sun-damaged skin; may arise from normal skin or preexisting lesions; appears as a rough, thickened, scaly tumor; and may be asymptomatic or may involve bleeding.

Diagnostic Evaluation

- Biopsy and histologic evaluation of lesion and regional lymph nodes

Medical Management

The goal of treatment is to eradicate or completely destroy all the tumor.

- The method of treatment depends on tumor location, cell type, cosmetic desires, history of previous treatment, whether the tumor is invasive, and presence of metastatic nodes.
- Excision, Mohs' micrographic surgery, electrosurgery, cryosurgery, and radiation therapy are possible treatment methods.

Nursing Management: The Patient With Skin Cancer, Including Malignant Melanoma

Assessment
- Ask patient specifically about pruritus, tenderness, and pain.
- Question patient about changes in preexisting moles or the development of new pigmented lesions; assess people at risk carefully.
- Assess patient and family knowledge regarding prevention of skin cancer and treatment regimen.
- Inspect skin under good lighting with a magnifying lens; note skin irregularity and changes in mole: the abcd's—asymmetry, border irregularity, color, diameter exceeding 6 mm.
- In dark-complexioned people, melanomas are noted in less pigmented sites (eg, palms, soles).

Major Nursing Diagnoses
- Pain related to surgical excision and grafting
- Anxiety and depression related to possible life-threatening consequences of cancer and possible disfigurement (melanomas)
- Knowledge deficit about prevention, early signs of skin cancer, and treatment regimen

Collaborative Problems/Potential Complications
- Metastasis
- Infection of the surgical site

Planning and Goals
The major goals of the patient may include relief of pain and discomfort, reduction of anxiety, knowledge of early signs of melanoma, and absence of complications.

Nursing Interventions
RELIEVING PAIN AND DISCOMFORT
- Anticipate need for pain medication
- Administer analgesic medication before pain is severe

REDUCING ANXIETY
- Allow patient to express feelings about the seriousness of the neoplasm; convey understanding of patient's anger and depression.
- Reinforce diagnosis, answer questions, clarify information, and help clarify misconceptions (in BCC and SCC, emphasize that these are the most successfully treated cancers).
- Emphasize patient's resources, coping mechanisms, and social support systems.

MONITORING AND MANAGING
POTENTIAL COMPLICATIONS
- Monitor and document symptoms that may indicate metastasis: lung (dyspnea, shortness of breath, cough), bone (pain, decreased mobility), liver (change in enzyme levels, pain, jaundice).
- Plan nursing care according to the patient's symptoms.
- Provide time for the patient to express fears and concerns regarding the future.
- Deliver supportive care, provide and clarify information about therapy, and teach side effects and ways to manage them; instruct the patient and family about expected outcomes of treatment.

Promoting Home and Community-Based Care

Teaching Patients Self-Care
- Teach patient early signs of skin cancer and melanoma; encourage monthly examination of skin and scalp.
- Emphasize the relationship of cancer to sunlight and encourage the use of precautions.
- Postoperatively, teach patient to protect the wound from physical trauma, external irritants, and contamination.
- Advise regarding dressing protocols; watch for excessive bleeding.
- Instruct to drink liquids through a straw if lesion is in the oral area; limit excessive talking and facial movement.

Continuing Care

- Educate regarding unnecessary exposure to the sun, use of sunscreens, and protective clothing if patient must be in sun.
- Educate to have a follow-up evaluation throughout lifetime; watch for development of new lesions.

For more information, see Chapter 52 in Smeltzer and Bare: *Brunner and Suddarth's Textbook of Medical-Surgical Nursing,* 9th edition. Philadelphia: Lippincott Williams & Wilkins, 2000.

CANCER OF THE STOMACH

Cancer of the stomach is usually adenocarcinoma and typically occurs in people older than 40 years of age and occasionally in younger people. Most stomach cancers occur in the lesser curvature or antrum of the stomach and infiltrate surrounding mucosa, stomach wall, adjacent organs, and structures. The incidence of gastric cancer is much greater in Japan. Diet appears to be a significant factor (ie, high in smoked foods and lacking in fruits and vegetables). Other factors related to the incidence include chronic inflammation of the stomach, pernicious anemia, achlorhydria, gastric ulcers, *Helicobacter pylori* bacteria, and heredity. Prognosis is poor because most patients have metastases (liver, pancreas, and esophagus or duodenum) at the time of diagnosis.

Clinical Manifestations

- Early stages: symptoms may be absent or may resemble those of patients with benign ulcers (ie, pain relieved with antacids).
- Progressive disease: symptoms include indigestion (more than 4 weeks' duration indicates need for complete gastrointestinal tract radiographic examination), anorexia, dyspepsia, weight loss, abdominal pain (usually a late symptom), constipation, anemia, nausea and vomiting, and ascites (with metastasis of liver).

Diagnostic Evaluation
- Radiograph of upper gastrointestinal system with barium
- Endoscopy for biopsy and cytologic washings
- Computed tomography (CT) scan, bone scan, and liver scan to determine extent of metastasis
- Complete radiographic examination of the gastrointestinal tract if dyspepsia of more than 4 weeks' duration in any person older than 40 years of age.

Medical Management
- Removal of gastric carcinoma; cure if tumor can be removed while still localized to the stomach
- Effective palliation (to prevent symptoms such as obstruction) by resection of the tumor; radical subtotal gastrectomy; total gastrectomy with anastomosis of esophagus and jejunum
- Chemotherapy for further disease control or for palliation (5-fluorouracil, doxorubicin [Adriamycin], mitomycin C)
- Radiation for palliation
- Tumor marker assessment to determine treatment effectiveness

Nursing Management
Assessment
- Elicit history of dietary intake (intake of smoked or cured foods and of fruits and vegetables).
- Identify weight loss and amount; assess appetite and eating habits, include pain assessment.
- Obtain cigarette smoking history: how many a day, how long has patient been smoking, any stomach discomfort during or after smoking?
- History of alcohol intake: how much?
- Obtain family history of cancer (first- or second-degree relatives).
- Assess psychosocial support (marital status, coping skills, emotional and financial resources).
- Perform complete physical examination (palpate abdomen for tenderness, masses, or ascites).

Major Nursing Diagnoses
- Anxiety related to the disease and anticipated treatment
- Altered nutrition: less than body requirements related to anorexia
- Pain related to the presence of abnormal epithelial cells
- Anticipatory grieving related to the diagnosis of cancer
- Knowledge deficit regarding self-care activities

Planning and Goals
The major goals of the patient include reduction of anxiety, attainment of optimum nutrition, relief of pain, and adjustment to the diagnosis and to anticipated lifestyle changes.

Nursing Interventions
REDUCING ANXIETY
- Provide a relaxed, nonthreatening atmosphere (helps patient express fears, concerns, and anger).
- Encourage family in efforts to support the patient, offering assurance and supporting positive coping measures.
- Advise about any procedures and treatments.
- Suggest that patient discuss feelings with support person (eg, clergy), if desired.

PROMOTING OPTIMAL NUTRITION
- Encourage small, frequent feedings of nonirritating foods to decrease gastric irritation.
- Facilitate tissue repair by ensuring food supplements are high in calories and vitamins A, C, and iron.
- Administer parenteral vitamin B_{12} indefinitely if a total gastrectomy is performed.
- Monitor the rate and frequency of intravenous therapy.
- Record intake, output, and daily weights (patient is attaining or gaining weight).
- Assess signs of dehydration (thirst, dry mucous membranes, poor skin turgor, tachycardia, decreased urine output).
- Review results of daily laboratory studies to note any metabolic abnormalities (sodium, potassium, glucose, blood urea nitrogen).
- Administer antiemetics as prescribed.

RELIEVING PAIN
• Administer analgesics as prescribed (continuous infusion of a narcotic).
• Assess frequency, intensity, and duration of pain to determine effectiveness of analgesic.
• Work with patient to help manage pain (eg, position changes, decreased environmental stimuli, restricted visiting).
• Suggest nonpharmacologic methods for pain relief (eg, imagery, distraction, relaxation tapes, back rubs, and massage).
• Encourage periods of rest and relaxation.

PROVIDING PSYCHOSOCIAL SUPPORT
• Help patient express fears and concerns about the diagnosis.
• Allow patient freedom to grieve; answer patient's questions honestly.
• Encourage patient to participate in treatment decisions.
• Support patient's disbelief and time needed to accept diagnosis.
• Offer emotional support, and involve family members and significant others whenever possible; reassure that emotional responses are normal and expected.
• Be aware of mood swings and defense mechanisms (denial, rationalization, displacement, regression).
• Provide professional services as necessary (eg, clergy, psychiatric clinical nurse specialists, psychologists, social workers, and psychiatrists).

🏠 Promoting Home and Community-Based Care

Teaching Patients Self-Care
See Nursing Management under Cancer for additional information.
• Teach self-care activities specific to treatment regimen.
• Include information about diet and nutrition, treatment regimens, activity and lifestyle changes, pain management, and complications for which to observe.

- Explain that the possibility of dumping syndrome exists with any enteral feeding, and teach ways to manage it.
- Explain to the patient the necessity of daily rest periods and frequent visits to physician after discharge.
- Refer for home care; nurse can supervise any enteral or parenteral feeding and teach patient and family members how to use equipment and formulas as well as how to detect complications.
- Teach patient to record daily intake, output, and weight.
- Teach patient how to cope with pain, nausea, vomiting, and bloating.
- Teach patient to recognize and report those complications that require medical attention, such as bleeding (overt or covert hematemesis, melena), obstruction, perforation, or any symptoms that become consistently worse.
- Teach patient how to care for the incision and how to examine the wound for signs of infection.
- Explain chemotherapy or radiation regimen and the care needed during and after treatment.

For more information, see Chapter 34 in Smeltzer and Bare: *Brunner and Suddarth's Textbook of Medical-Surgical Nursing,* 9th edition. Philadelphia: Lippincott Williams & Wilkins, 2000.

CANCER OF THE TESTIS

Testicular cancer is the most common cancer in men 15 to 35 years of age and the second most common cancer in men aged 35 to 39 years. Testicular cancer is classified as germinal or nongerminal. Most neoplasms are germinal, arising from the germinal cells of the testes (seminomas, teratocarcinomas, choriocarcinomas, yolk sac carcinomas, and embryonal carcinomas). Nongerminal tumors arise from the epithelium. The cause of testicular tumors is unknown, but cryptorchidism, infections, and genetic and endocrine factors appear to play a part in their development. Testicular tumors are usually malignant and tend to metastasize early, spreading from the testicles to the lymph nodes in the retroperitoneum and to the lungs.

Clinical Manifestations
- Symptoms appear gradually, with a mass or lump on the testicle.
- Painless enlargement of the testis occurs; the patient may complain of heaviness in the scrotum, inguinal area, or lower abdomen.
- Backache, pain in the abdomen, loss of weight, and general weakness may result from metastasis.

Diagnostic Evaluation
- Testicular self-examination is an effective early detection method.
- Elevated alpha-fetoprotein and human chorionic gonadotropin are used as tumor markers.
- Tumor marker levels are used for diagnosis, staging, and monitoring the response to treatment.

Medical Management
The goals of management are to eradicate the disease and achieve a cure. Treatment selection is based on cell type and anatomic extent of the disease.

- Orchiectomy and retroperitoneal lymph node dissection (RPLND)
- Sperm banking
- Postoperative radiation of the lymph nodes from the iliac region to the diaphragm to treat seminomas
- Multiple chemotherapy agent; good results may be obtained by combining different types of treatments, including surgery, radiation therapy, and chemotherapy

Nursing Management
See Nursing Management under Cancer for additional information.

🏠 **Promoting Home and Community-Based Care**

Teaching Patients Self-Care
- Address issues related to body image and sexuality.
- Encourage patient to maintain a positive attitude during course of therapy.
- Inform patient that radiation therapy will not necessarily cause infertility, nor does unilateral excision of a tumor necessarily decrease virility.
- Encourage follow-up evaluation studies because a patient with a history of one tumor of the testis has a greater chance of developing subsequent tumors.

For more information, see Chapter 45 in Smeltzer and Bare: *Brunner and Suddarth's Textbook of Medical-Surgical Nursing,* 9th edition. Philadelphia: Lippincott Williams & Wilkins, 2000.

CANCER OF THE THYROID

Cancer of the thyroid is less prevalent than other forms of cancer. The most common type, papillary adenocarcinoma, accounts for more than half of thyroid malignancies; it starts in childhood or early adult life, remains localized, and eventually metastasizes. When papillary adenocarcinoma occurs in an elderly patient, it is more aggressive. Risks include gender (female) and external irradiation of the head, neck, or chest in infancy and childhood. Follicular adenocarcinoma usually appears in patient older than 40 years of age.

Clinical Manifestations
- Lesions that are single, hard, and fixed on palpation suggest malignancy.

Diagnostic Evaluation
- Needle biopsy or aspiration biopsy of the thyroid gland

- Ultrasound, magnetic resonance imaging (MRI), computed tomography (CT), thyroid scans, radioactive iodine uptake studies, and thyroid suppression tests

Medical Management

- The treatment of choice is surgical removal (total or near-total thyroidectomy).
- Modified or extensive radical neck dissection is done if lymph node involvement is present.
- Radioactive iodine (^{131}I) is used to eradicate residual thyroid tissue.
- Thyroid hormone is administered in suppressive doses after surgery to lower the levels of thyroid-stimulating hormone (TSH) to a euthyroid state.
- Lifelong thyroxine (T_4) is required if remaining thyroid tissue is inadequate to produce sufficient hormone.
- Radiation therapy is administered by several routes.
- Chemotherapy is used only occasionally.

Nursing Management

See Nursing Management under Cancer for additional information.

 Promoting Home and Community-Based Care

Teaching Patients Self-Care

- Encourage follow-up for recurrence of cancer: total-body scans are done 2 to 4 months and 1 year after surgery. If measurements are stable, a final scan is obtained in 3 to 5 years.
- Before planned total body scans, stop thyroid hormones for 6 weeks.
- Monitor T_4, TSH, serum calcium, and phosphorus levels to determine if thyroid supplementation is adequate, and maintain calcium balance.

Continuing Care

- Emphasize the importance and provide instructions about the need to take exogenous thyroid hormone.

- Reinforce that surgery combined with radioiodine produces a higher survival rate than surgery alone.
- Instruct in assessment and management of side effects of radiation therapy.

For more information, see Chapter 38 in Smeltzer and Bare: *Brunner and Suddarth's Textbook of Medical-Surgical Nursing,* 9th edition. Philadelphia: Lippincott Williams & Wilkins, 2000.

CANCER OF THE VAGINA

Cancer of the vagina usually results from metastasized choriocarcinoma or from cancer of the cervix or adjacent organs, such as the uterus, vulva, bladder, or rectum. Primary cancer of the vagina is uncommon. Risk factors include cervical cancer, in utero exposure to diethylstilbestrol (DES), previous vaginal or vulvar cancer, previous radiation therapy, history of human papillomavirus (HPV), or of pessary use.

Clinical Manifestations
- Often asymptomatic, but slight bleeding after intercourse may be reported.
- Spontaneous bleeding, vaginal discharge, pain, urinary or rectal symptoms

Diagnostic Evaluation
- Colposcopy for women exposed to DES in utero
- Papanicolaou's (Pap) smear of the vagina

Medical Management
- Laser treatment, chemotherapeutic cream, and radiation therapy, depending on the extent of the disease.
- Surgery: radical node dissection (local excision)

Nursing Management
Nursing Interventions
- Encourage close follow-up by health care providers.

- Provide emotional support.
- Teach specific vaginal dilating procedures for those who have had vaginal reconstructive surgery.
- Inform patient that water-soluble lubricants are helpful in reducing dyspareunia.
- Assist patient to explore all aspects and effects of radiation therapy, chemotherapy, or surgery on an individual basis.

For more information, see Chapter 43 in Smeltzer and Bare: *Brunner and Suddarth's Textbook of Medical-Surgical Nursing*, 9th edition. Philadelphia: Lippincott Williams & Wilkins, 2000.

CANCER OF THE VULVA

Primary cancer of the vulva is seen mostly in postmenopausal women; its incidence in younger women is rising. More whites than nonwhites are affected. Squamous cell carcinoma accounts for most primary vulvar tumors. The median age for cancer limited to the vulva is 44 years; median age for invasive vulvar cancer is 61 years. Little is known about what causes this disease; however, risk factors are hypertension, obesity, and diabetes.

Clinical Manifestations
- Long-standing pruritus and soreness are the most common symptoms; itching occurs in half of all patients.
- Bleeding, foul-smelling discharge, and pain are signs of advanced disease.
- Early lesions appear as chronic dermatitis; later, a lump that continues to grow and becomes a hard, ulcerated, cauliflower-like growth.

Diagnostic Evaluation
- Vulvar examination
- Biopsy

Medical Management

- Preinvasive (vulvar carcinoma in situ): local excision, laser vaporization, chemotherapeutic creams (fluorouracil), or cryosurgery
- Invasive: wide excision or vulvectomy (primary treatment), radiation (unresectable tumors), radical vulvectomy with bilateral groin dissection

Nursing Management: The Patient Undergoing a Vulvectomy

Assessment

- Develop a rapport between patient and nurse; ascertain health habits and receptivity for learning.
- Give preoperative preparation and psychological encouragement.

Major Nursing Diagnoses

- Anxiety related to the diagnosis and surgery.
- Alteration in skin integrity related to wound drainage.
- Pain related to surgical incision and subsequent wound care.
- Sexual dysfunction related to change in body part.
- Self-care deficit related to lack of understanding of perineal care and general health status.

Collaborative Problems/Potential Complications

- Wound infection and sepsis
- Deep vein thrombosis
- Hemorrhage

Planning and Goals

The major goals for the patient may include acceptance of and preparation for surgical intervention, recovery of optimal sexual function, ability to perform adequate and appropriate self-care, and prevention of complications.

Nursing Interventions

PREOPERATIVE
Relieving Anxiety
- Allow patient time to talk and ask questions.
- Advise patient that the possibility of having sexual relations is good and that pregnancy is possible after a simple vulvectomy.
- Reinforce information about the surgery, and address the patient's questions and concerns.

POSTOPERATIVE
Relieving Pain and Discomfort
- Administer analgesics preventively.
- Position patient to relieve tension on incision, and give soothing back rubs.

Improving Skin Integrity
- Provide pressure-reducing mattress.
- Install over-bed trapeze.
- Protect intact skin from drainage and moisture.
- Monitor for accumulation of purulent material (suppuration) under the graft.
- Assist the patient to keep the perineal area clean and dry.
- Assess and document surgical site characteristics and drainage.

Supporting Positive Sexuality and Sexual Function
- Establish a trusting nurse–patient relationship.
- Encourage patient to share and discuss concerns with sexual partner.
- Consult with surgeon to clarify expected changes.
- Refer the patient and partner to a sex counselor, as indicated.

Monitoring and Managing Potential Complications
- Monitor closely for local and systemic signs and symptoms of infection: purulent drainage, redness, increased pain, fever, increased white blood cell count.
- Assist in obtaining tissue specimens for culture.
- Administer antibiotics as prescribed.

- Avoid cross-contamination; carefully handle catheters, drains, and dressings.
- Provide a low-residue diet to prevent straining on defecation and wound contamination.
- Discourage sitz bath because of risk for infection.
- Assess for signs and symptoms of deep vein thrombosis and pulmonary embolism; apply elastic antiembolism stockings; encourage ankle exercises.
- Encourage and assist in frequent position changes, avoiding pressure behind the knees.
- Monitor closely for signs of hemorrhage and hypovolemic shock.

Promoting Home and Community-Based Care

Teaching Patients Self-Care
- Encourage patient to share concerns as patient recovers.
- Encourage participation in dressing changes and self-care.
- Give complete instructions to family member or other who will provide posthospital care regarding wound care, urinary catheterization, and possible complications.

Continuing Care
- Encourage communication with home care nurse to ensure continuity of care.
- Reinforce teaching with follow-up call between home visits.

Evaluation
EXPECTED OUTCOMES
- Adjusts to the trauma of the surgical experience
- Obtains pain relief
- Maintains skin integrity
- Performs adequate and appropriate self-care and prevention of complications

---

For more information, see Chapter 43 in Smeltzer and Bare: *Brunner and Suddarth's Textbook of Medical-Surgical Nursing,* 9th edition. Philadelphia: Lippincott Williams & Wilkins, 2000.

CARDIAC ARREST

Cardiac arrest occurs when the heart suddenly ceases to produce an effective pulse and blood circulation. All heart action may stop, or asynchronized muscular twitchings (ventricular fibrillation) may occur. There is an immediate loss of consciousness and absence of pulses and audible heart sounds. Dilation of the pupils begins within 45 seconds. Seizures may or may not occur. Cardiac arrest may be due to a cardiac electrical event (ventricular fibrillation or tachycardia, bradycardia, atrioventricular [AV] block, pulseless electrical activity [PEA], or asystole).

Clinical Manifestations

There is an interval of about 4 minutes between cessation of circulation and development of irreversible brain damage. Interval varies with age of the patient. During this period, the diagnosis of cardiac arrest must be made and circulation restored. The most reliable sign of arrest is the absence of a carotid pulsation.

Medical and Nursing Management

- Initiate immediate cardiopulmonary resuscitation (CPR).
- Institute follow-up monitoring once the patient is successfully resuscitated.

For more information, see Chapter 27 in Smeltzer and Bare: *Brunner and Suddarth's Textbook of Medical-Surgical Nursing,* 9th edition. Philadelphia: Lippincott Williams & Wilkins, 2000.

CARDIAC FAILURE

Cardiac failure (congestive heart failure) is the inability of the heart to pump sufficient blood to meet the needs of the tissues for oxygen and nutrients. The term *congestive heart failure* is most commonly used when referring to left-sided and right-sided failure. The underlying mechanism of cardiac failure involves impairment of the contractile properties of the heart, which leads to a lower-than-normal cardiac output. Common underlying conditions include myocardial dysfunction (coronary atherosclerosis, cardiomyopathy, and inflammatory or degenerative muscle disease) and arterial hypertension.

A number of systemic factors can contribute to the development and severity of cardiac failure. Increased metabolic rate (fever, thyrotoxicosis), hypoxia, and anemia require an increased cardiac output to satisfy systemic oxygen demand. Dysrhythmia decreases the efficiency of myocardial function.

Clinical Manifestations
- Inadequate tissue perfusion
- Diminished cardiac output with accompanying dizziness, confusion, fatigue, exercise or heat intolerance, cool extremities, and oliguria
- Congestion of tissues
- Increased pulmonary venous pressure (pulmonary edema) manifested by cough and shortness of breath
- Increased systemic venous pressure as evidenced in generalized peripheral edema and weight gain

Left-Sided Cardiac Failure
- Most often precedes right-sided cardiac failure
- Pulmonary congestion; dyspnea, cough, fatigability; tachycardia with an S_3 heart sound, anxiety, restlessness
- Orthopnea, proximal nocturnal dyspnea (PND)
- Cough may be dry and nonproductive but is most often moist
- Bibasilar crackles advancing to crackles in all lung fields
- Large quantities of frothy sputum, which is sometimes pink (blood-tinged)

Right-Sided Cardiac Failure
- Congestion of the viscera and peripheral tissues
- Edema of the lower extremities (dependent edema), usually pitting edema, weight gain, hepatomegaly

- Distended neck veins, ascites, anorexia, and nausea
- Nocturia and weakness

Diagnostic Evaluation
- Evaluation of the clinical manifestations
- Hemodynamic monitoring
- Echocardiogram (ejection fraction)

Medical Management
The goals of treatment are to reduce the workload on the heart, increase the force and efficiency of myocardial contractions with pharmacologic agents, and eliminate the excessive accumulation of body water.

- Smoking, alcohol, and excess fluid intake prohibited
- Medication and oxygen, as indicated
- Coronary bypass surgery, innovative therapies as indicated (eg, mechanical assist devices, transplantation)
- Pharmacologic therapy (used alone or in combination)
  - Vasodilator therapy (angiotensin-converting enzyme [ACE] inhibitors), diuretic therapy, and cardiac glycosides
  - Dobutamine, milrinone, anticoagulants, beta-blockers, as indicated
  - Possibly antihypertensives or antianginal medications
- Nutritional therapy
  - Sodium restriction, avoidance of excess fluid intake to prevent, control, or eliminate edema

---

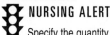 **NURSING ALERT**
Specify the quantity of sodium in milligrams (there are 393 mg of sodium in 1000 mg of salt).

Nursing Management
Assessment
The focus of the nursing assessment for the patient with cardiac failure is directed toward observing for signs and

symptoms of pulmonary and systemic fluid overload. All untoward signs are recorded and reported.

- Note report of sleep disturbance due to shortness of breath, and number of pillows used for sleep.
- Note activities reported to cause shortness of breath.
- Respiratory: auscultate lungs at frequent intervals to determine presence or absence of crackles and wheezes. Note rate and depth of respirations.
- Cardiac: auscultate for the presence of an S_3 heart sound, which may mean pump is beginning to fail; signs of fluid overload (orthopnea, paroxysmal nocturnal dyspnea, and dyspnea on exertion).
- Assess sensorium and level of consciousness.
- Periphery: assess dependent parts of the patient's body for perfusion and edema and the liver for hepatojugular reflux and jugular vein distention
- Intake and output and weight: measure carefully; weigh patient daily.

Major Nursing Diagnoses
- Activity intolerance related to imbalance between oxygen supply and demand secondary to decreased cardiac output
- Fatigue secondary to cardiac failure
- Excess fluid volume related to excess fluid or sodium intake or retention secondary to congestive heart failure and its medical therapy
- Anxiety related to breathlessness and restlessness secondary to inadequate oxygenation
- Powerlessness related to inability to perform role responsibilities secondary to chronic illness and hospitalizations
- Noncompliance related to lack of knowledge
- Knowledge deficit of self-care program related to nonacceptance of necessary lifestyle changes

Collaborative Problems/Potential Complications
- Cardiogenic shock
- Thromboembolism
- Pericardial effusion and pericardial tamponade
- Dysrhythmias

Planning and Goals

The major goals of the patient may include promotion of activity while maintaining vital signs within identified range; reduction of fatigue; relief of fluid overload symptoms; decreased anxiety or increased ability to manage anxiety; knowledge of self-care program; and verbalization of ability to make decisions and influence outcomes.

Nursing Interventions

PROMOTING ACTIVITY TOLERANCE

- Monitor the patient's response to activities; instruct patient to avoid prolonged bed rest; the patient should rest if symptoms are severe, otherwise, assume regular activity.
- Encourage the patient to perform an activity more slowly than usual, for a shorter duration, or with assistance initially.
- Identify barriers that could limit abilities to perform an activity, and discuss methods of adjusting an activity to ensure pacing but still accomplish the task (eg, patient may chop or peel vegetables while sitting at the kitchen table rather than standing at a kitchen counter).
- Take vital signs, especially pulse, before, during, and immediately after an activity to identify whether within the predetermined range; the heart rate should return to baseline within 3 minutes. If the patient tolerates the activity, develop short-term and long-term goals to increase gradually the intensity, duration, or frequency of activity.
- Refer to a cardiac rehabilitation program as needed, especially for those patients with a recent myocardial infarction (MI), recent open heart surgery, or increased anxiety.

REDUCING FATIGUE

- Collaborate with the patient on developing a schedule that promotes pacing and prioritization of activities; alternate activities with periods of rest; avoid having two significant energy-consuming activities occur on the same day or in immediate succession.

- Encourage family members to stagger visits to allow for rest between visits or calls; identify a spokesperson to relay messages from and to other friends and family members.
- Identify the patient's peak and low periods of energy, and plan energy-consuming activities accordingly.
- Explain that small, frequent meals tend to decrease the amount of energy needed for digestion while providing adequate nutrition.
- Help the patient develop a positive outlook focused on the patient's strengths, abilities, and interests.

MANAGING FLUID VOLUME
- Administer diuretics early in the morning so that diuresis does not disturb patient's nighttime rest.
- Monitor the patient's fluid status closely: auscultate the lungs, compare daily body weights, monitor intake and output.
- Teach the patient to adhere to a low-sodium diet by reading food labels and avoiding commercially prepared convenience foods.
- Assist the patient to adhere to any fluid restriction by planning the distribution throughout the day while maintaining the patient's dietary preferences.
- Monitor intravenous fluids closely; contact the physician or pharmacist about the possibility of double-concentrating any medications.
- Position the patient, or teach the patient how to assume a position, that shifts fluid away from the heart (increase the number of pillows, elevate the head of the bed, place the bed legs on 20- to 30-cm [8- to 10-inch] blocks, or patient may prefer to sit in a comfortable armchair to sleep).
- Assess for skin breakdown, and institute preventive measures (frequent changes of position, positioning to avoid pressure, elastic pressure stockings, and leg exercises).

CONTROLLING ANXIETY

- Decrease anxiety so that the patient's cardiac work is also decreased.
- Administer oxygen during the acute stage to diminish the work of breathing and to increase the comfort of the patient.
- When the patient exhibits anxiety, takes steps to promote physical comfort and psychological support; a family member's presence provides reassurance.
- Speak in a slow, calm, and confident manner; state specific, brief directions for an activity, when necessary.
- When the patient is comfortable, teach the patient ways to control anxiety and avoid anxiety-provoking situations (relaxation techniques).
- Assist in identifying factors that contribute to anxiety (lack of sleep, lack of information, misinformation, or poor nutritional status).
- Promote physical comfort, provide accurate information, and teach the patient to avoid situations that tend to promote anxiety and agitation.

✸ NURSING ALERT

Cerebral hypoxia with superimposed carbon dioxide retention, if present in cardiac failure, may cause the patient to react to sedative-hypnotic medications with confusion and increased anxiety. Administer sedative-hypnotic medications with caution because hepatic congestion may result in a decreased ability of the liver to metabolize the medication within a normal time frame to prevent toxicity. Avoid use of restraints with cases of confusion and anxiety reactions. The patient who insists on getting out of bed at night can be seated comfortably in an armchair.

MINIMIZING POWERLESSNESS

- Assess for factors contributing to a perception of powerlessness, and intervene accordingly.
- Take time to listen actively to patients often; encourage them to express their concerns and questions.

- If indicated, review hospital policies and standards that tend to promote powerlessness, and advocate for their elimination or change.
- Provide the patient with decision-making opportunities with increasing frequency and significance; provide encouragement and praise while identifying the patient's progress; assist the patient to differentiate between those factors that can be controlled and those that cannot.

Promoting Home and Community-Based Care

Teaching Patients Self-Care
- Provide patient education, and involve the patient in implementing the therapeutic regimen to promote understanding and compliance.
- Support the patient and family, and encourage them to ask questions so that information can be clarified and understanding enhanced.
- Adapt the teaching plan according to cultural factors.
- Teach patients and their families how the progression of the disease is influenced by compliance with the treatment plan.
- Convey that monitoring symptoms and daily weights, restricting sodium intake, avoiding excess fluids, preventing infection, avoiding noxious agents such as alcohol and tobacco, and participating in regular exercise all aid in preventing the exacerbation of cardiac failure.

Continuing Care
- Reinforce and clarify information about diet and fluid restrictions, monitor symptoms and daily body weight, and reinforce follow-up health care expectations.
- Provide assistance in scheduling and keeping appointments.
- Encourage the patient to increase gradually self-care and responsibility for accomplishing the daily requirements of the therapeutic regimen.

- Refer the patient for home care if indicated (elderly patients or patients who have long standing heart disease and whose physical stamina is compromised).
- The home care nurse should assess the physical environment of the home and the family or friend support system and suggest adaptions in the home environment that best meet the patient's activity limitations.

Evaluation

EXPECTED OUTCOMES

- Demonstrates tolerance for increased activity
- Experiences less fatigue and dyspnea
- Maintains fluid balance
- Experiences less anxiety
- Adheres to self-care regimen
- Makes decisions regarding care and treatment

For more information, see Chapter 27 in Smeltzer and Bare: *Brunner and Suddarth's Textbook of Medical-Surgical Nursing,* 9th edition. Philadelphia: Lippincott Williams & Wilkins, 2000.

CARDIOMYOPATHIES

The cardiomyopathies are a group of diseases that affect the structure and function of the myocardium. The three types of cardiomyopathies are classified according to the structural and functional abnormalities of the heart muscle: (1) dilated or congestive cardiomyopathy (most common); (2) hypertrophic cardiomyopathy (obstructive or nonobstructive); and (3) restrictive cardiomyopathy (rarest). These diseases lead to severe heart failure, significant dysrhythmias, and often death. Cardiomyopathy is a series of progressive events that culminate in impaired pumping of the left ventricle, which enlarges to accommodate the demands of increased systemic vascular resistance and eventually fails. Failure of the right ventricle usually accompanies this process.

Clinical Manifestations
- May occur at any age and affects both men and women
- Present initially with signs and symptoms of heart failure
- Early: shortness of breath on exertion, proximal nocturnal dyspnea (PND), cough, chest pain, palpitations, fatigue, dizziness, and syncope
- Systemic venous congestion, jugular vein distention, pitting edema of dependent body parts, hepatic engorgement, and tachycardia with physical examination

Diagnostic Evaluation
- Patient history; rule out other causes of failure
- Electrocardiogram (ECG), chest radiograph, echocardiogram, cardiac catheterization, and possibly an endomyocardial biopsy

Medical Management
- Medical management is directed toward determining and managing possible underlying or precipitating causes, correcting the heart failure, and controlling dysrhythmias.
- Surgical intervention, including a myectomy, or a heart transplantation is considered when heart failure has progressed beyond being medically responsive.
- In some cases, ventricular assist devices are necessary to support the failing heart until a suitable donor becomes available.

Nursing Management
Assessment
- Take detailed history of presenting signs and symptoms and possible etiologic factors.
- Careful psychosocial history: identify family support system and involve family in patient management.
- Physical assessment directed toward signs and symptoms of congestive heart failure. Evaluate fluid volume status, vital signs (pulse pressure), auscultation for a systolic murmur, and palpation for a shift to the left of the point of maximum impulse.

- Use cardiac monitor if dysrhythmia is a significant problem.

Major Nursing Diagnoses
- Decreased cardiac output related to structural disorders secondary to cardiomyopathy or dysrhythmia.
- Altered tissue perfusion related to decreased peripheral blood flow.
- Impaired gas exchange related to pulmonary congestion secondary to myocardial failure.
- Activity intolerance related to excessive fluid volume.
- Anxiety related to the disease process.
- Powerlessness related to disease process.
- Noncompliance with the self-care program.

Collaborative Problems/Potential Complications
- Cardiac failure
- Ventricular and atrial dysrhythmias

Planning and Goals
The major goals of the patient include improved or maintained cardiac output, increased activity tolerance, reduction of anxiety, compliance with self-care program, and absence of complications.

Nursing Interventions
IMPROVING CARDIAC OUTPUT AND RELIEVING RESPIRATORY DIFFICULTIES
- Assist the patient into a resting position during a symptomatic episode.
- Administer oxygen if indicated.
- Note and document patient's response (daily weight, oxygen saturation); correlate interventions with patient's response.
- Administer prescribed medications on time.
- Assist patient to rest at the bedside in a chair for most comfort. Keep patient warm and change position frequently.

- Keep patient warm, and change positions frequently to stimulate circulation and reduce skin breakdown.

INCREASING ACTIVITY TOLERANCE
- Plan nursing care so that activities occur in cycles, alternating rest with activity.
- Help patient learn to conserve energy.

REDUCING ANXIETY
- Provide the patient with appropriate information about signs and symptoms.
- Provide an atmosphere in which the patient feels free to verbalize fears.
- Assist patient to accomplish a goal, no matter how small, to enhance a sense of well-being.
- Provide time for the patient to discuss concerns if facing death or awaiting transplantation.
- Give spiritual, psychological, and emotional support.
- Establish trust with patient, and provide realistic hope to reduce anxiety while awaiting a donor heart.

🏠 Promoting Home and Community-Based Care

Teaching Patients Self-Care
- Teach patient what self-care activities are necessary and how to perform them at home.
- Maintain attention to a medication program and dietary restrictions to prevent cardiac failure.
- Allow patient and significant others the freedom to begin the grieving process when they can no longer be helped by any therapeutic technique.

Continuing Care
- Refer patient for home care and support.
- Teach patients about medication regimen and dietary and fluid restrictions.
- Assist in review of lifestyle, and suggest strategies to incorporate therapeutic activities to balance lifestyle and work.

- Teach patient and family the symptoms that should be reported to the physician.
- Establish trust with patient, and provide support during the process of end-of-life decision making.

Evaluation

EXPECTED OUTCOMES
- Demonstrates improved cardiac function
- Increases activity tolerance
- Experiences reduction of anxiety
- Complies with the self-care program

For more information, see Chapter 26 in Smeltzer and Bare: *Brunner and Suddarth's Textbook of Medical-Surgical Nursing,* 9th edition. Philadelphia: Lippincott Williams & Wilkins, 2000.

CATARACTS

A cataract is an opacity of the normally clear, transparent crystalline lens. It is community associated with aging but can develop at any age. It may also be associated with blunt or penetrating trauma, long-term corticosteroid use, systemic disease such as diabetes mellitus, hypoparathyroidism, radiation exposure, exposure to long hours or bright sunlight (ultraviolet light), or other eye disorders. Vision impairment depends on the size, density, and location in the lens.

Clinical Manifestations
- Diminished visual acuity, disabling glare, dimmed or blurred vision with distortion of images, poor night vision
- Yellowish, gray, or white pupil
- Develops gradually over a period of years, and as the cataract worsens, stronger glasses no longer improve sight
- May develop in both eyes, although one is more compromised than the other

Diagnostic Evaluation

- Degree of visual acuity directly proportionate to density of the cataract
- Snellen visual acuity test
- Ophthalmoscopy
- Slit-lamp biomicroscopic examination
- A-scan ultrasound

Medical Management

- There is no medical treatment for cataracts, although use of vitamins C and E and beta-carotene is being investigated; glasses or contact, bifocal, or magnifying lenses may improve vision. Mydriatics can be used short-term, but glare is increased.
- Two surgical techniques are available: intracapsular cataract extraction (ICCE) and extracapsular cataract extraction (ECCE). Less than 15% of people with cataracts require surgery.
- Indications for surgery are loss of vision that interferes with normal activities or a cataract that is causing glaucoma.
- Cataracts are removed under local anesthesia on an out-patient basis.
- Lens replacement may involve aphakic eyeglasses, contact lens, and intraocular lens (IOL) implants.
- When both eyes have cataracts, one eye is surgically treated at a time.

Nursing Management

 ## Promoting Home and Community-Based Care

Teaching Patients Self-Care

- Provide postoperative discharge teaching concerning eye medications, cleansing and protection, activity level and restrictions, diet, pain control, positioning, office appointments, expected postoperative course, and symptoms to report immediately to the surgeon.

- Instruct patient to make arrangements for transportation home, care during that evening, and a follow-up visit to the surgeon the next day.
- Instruct patient to restrict bending and lifting heavy objects.
- Instruct patient to wear eye shield at night and eye-glasses (sunglasses in bright light) during the day for 2 weeks.

Continuing Care
- Caution patient that vision may blur for several days to weeks.
- Inform patient that vision gradually improves as the eye heals; IOL implants improve vision faster than glasses or contact lenses.
- Reinforce that vision correction is needed for remaining visual acuity deficit.

For more information, see Chapter 54 in Smeltzer and Bare: *Brunner and Suddarth's Textbook of Medical-Surgical Nursing,* 9th edition. Philadelphia: Lippincott Williams & Wilkins, 2000.

CEREBRAL VASCULAR ACCIDENT (STROKE)

A stroke, or "brain attack," is a sudden loss of brain function resulting from a disruption of the blood supply to a part of the brain. It is usually the result of long-standing cerebrovascular disease. Stroke is the primary neurologic problem in the United States and in the world. Strokes are usually hemorrhagic (15%) or nonhemorrhagic (85%). Nonhemorrhagic strokes usually result from one of three events: (1) thrombosis, (2) cerebral embolism, or (3) ischemia. The result is an interruption in the blood supply to the brain, causing temporary or permanent loss of movement, thought, memory, speech, or sensation.

Risk Factors
- Hemorrhagic strokes are caused by arteriovenous malformations (AVMs), aneurysm ruptures, certain drugs, uncontrolled hypertension, hemangioblastomas, and trauma as well as by aneurysm rupture. These strokes can occur in epidural, subarachnoid, or intracerebral hemorrhage.
- Ischemic stroke can be caused by cardiovascular disease (cerebral embolism may originate in the heart) and dysrhythmia (atrial fibrillation); risk factors for coronary artery disease apply to stroke as well.
- Ischemic stroke can also be caused by vasospasm, migraines, and coagulopathies (eg, high hematocrit level).
- Excessive or prolonged fall of blood pressure may cause general cerebral ischemia.
- Drug abuse (cocaine) can cause stroke, particularly in adolescents and young adults.
- There may be a link between alcohol consumption and stroke.

Clinical Manifestations
- General signs and symptoms include numbness or weakness of face, arm, or leg; confusion or change in mental status; trouble speaking or understanding speech; visual disturbances, loss of balance, dizziness, difficulty walking, or sudden severe headache.

Motor Loss
- Hemiplegia, hemiparesis
- Flaccid paralysis and loss or decrease in the deep tendon reflexes (initial clinical feature), followed by increased muscle tone (spasticity)

Communication Loss
- Dysarthria
- Dysphasia or aphasia
- Apraxia

Perceptual Disturbances
- Visual perceptual dysfunctions (homonymous hemianopia—loss of half of the visual field)
- Disturbances in visuospatial relationships (frequently seen in patients with left hemispheric damage)
- Sensory losses: slight impairment of touch or more severe with loss of proprioception, difficulty in interrupting visual, tactile, and auditory stimuli

Impairment of Cognitive and Psychological Effects
- Frontal lobe damage: learning capacity, memory, or other higher cortical intellectual functions may be impaired. Such dysfunction may be reflected in a limited attention span, difficulties in comprehension, forgetfulness, and lack of motivation.
- Depression, other psychological problems: emotional liability, hostility, frustration, resentment, and lack of cooperation.

Bladder Dysfunction
- Transient urinary incontinence
- Persistent urinary incontinence or urinary retention (may be symptomatic of bilateral brain damage)
- Continuing bladder and bowel incontinence (may reflect extensive neurologic damage)

Diagnostic Evaluation
- Complete physical and neurologic examination
- Computed tomography (CT) or magnetic resonance imaging (MRI) scan, echocardiogram
- Carotid ultrasound
- Cerebral angiography
- Transcranial Doppler flow studies
- Electrocardiogram

Prevention
- Take steps to help patient alter predisposing risk factor for stroke

- Prepare and support patient through carotid endarterectomy
- Administer anticoagulant as ordered

Medical Management
- Recombinant tissue plasminogen activator (t-PA), unless contraindicated; monitor for bleeding
- Management of increased intracranial pressure: osmotic diuretics, maintain $PaCO_2$ at 30 to 35 mm Hg, avoid hypoxia, elevate head of bed, pulmonary toilet with supplemental oxygen, airway patency
- Maintain cardiac output 4 to 8 L/min
- Anticoagulants
- Manage complications:
  - Cerebral hypoxia: administer supplemental oxygen, maintain hemoglobin and hematocrit at acceptable levels
  - Decreased cerebral blood flow and extension of the area of injury: adequate hydration, avoid hypertension or hypotension

Nursing Management
Assessment
Maintain a neurologic flow sheet to reflect the following nursing assessment parameters:
- Change in the level of responsiveness, ability to speak, and orientation
- Presence or absence of voluntary or involuntary movements of the extremities: muscle tone, body posture, and head position
- Stiffness or flaccidity of the neck
- Eye opening, comparative size of the pupils and pupillary reactions to light, and ocular position
- Color of the face and extremities; temperature and moisture of the skin
- Quality and rates of pulse and respiration; arterial blood gases, body temperature, and arterial pressure

- Volume of fluids ingested or administered and volume of urine excreted per 24 hours
- Presence of signs of bleeding

Acute Phase
- The acute phase usually lasts 48 to 72 hours.
- Maintain the airway and adequate ventilation.
- Place patient with head of bed elevated.
- Maintain endotracheal intubation and mechanical ventilation.
- Monitor for pulmonary complications (aspiration, atelectasis, pneumonia).
- Examine heart for abnormalities in size, rhythm, and signs of congestive heart failure.

Postacute Phase
Assess the following functions:

- Mental status (memory, attention span, perception, orientation, affect, speech and language)
- Sensation and perception (usually patient has decreased awareness of pain and temperature)
- Motor control (upper and lower extremity movement); swallowing ability, nutritional and hydration status, skin integrity, activity tolerance, and bowel and bladder function
- Continue focusing nursing assessment on the impairment of function in the patient's daily activities

Major Nursing Diagnoses
- Impaired physical mobility related to hemiparesis, loss of balance and coordination, spasticity, and brain injury
- Pain related to hemiplegia and disuse
- Self-care deficits (hygiene, toileting, transfers, feeding) related to stroke sequela
- Sensory-perceptual alterations
- Impaired swallowing
- Incontinence related to flaccid bladder, detrusor instability, confusion, difficulty in communicating

- Altered thought processes related to brain damage, confusion, inability to follow instruction
- Impaired verbal communication related to brain damage, confusion, inability to follow instruction
- Risk for impaired skin integrity related to hemiparesis or hemiplegia, decreased mobility
- Sexual dysfunction
- Altered family processes related to catastrophic illness and caregiving burdens

Collaborative Problems/Potential Complications
- Decreased cerebral blood flow
- Inadequate oxygen delivery to the brain

Planning and Goals

The major goals of the patient may include improved mobility, avoidance of shoulder pain, achievement of self-care, continence, improved thought processes, achievement of a form of communication, skin integrity, restored family functioning, and absence of complications. Goals are affected by knowledge of what the patient was like before the stroke.

Nursing Interventions

MONITORING AND MANAGING
POTENTIAL COMPLICATIONS

- Assess vital signs and oxygenation status for adequate blood flow to the brain and tissues.
- Improve respiratory gas exchange with supplemental oxygen, suctioning, and chest physiotherapy.
- Maintain adequate cardiac output by medications and fluid administration.

IMPROVING MOBILITY AND
PREVENTING DEFORMITIES

- Position to prevent contractures; use measures to relieve pressure, assist in maintaining good body alignment, and prevent compressive neuropathies.

- Prevent foot drop and heel cords from shortening by using a foot board at intervals during the flaccid period.
- Apply a posterior splint at night to prevent flexion of the affected extremity.
- Prevent external rotation of hip joint with a trochanter roll.
- Prevent adduction of the affected shoulder with a pillow placed in the axilla.
- Elevate the affected arm to prevent edema and fibrosis.
- Position fingers so that they are barely flexed; place hand in slight supination. If upper extremity spasticity noted, *do not* use a hand roll.
- Use a volar resting splint to support the wrist and hand.
- Change position every 2 hours; place patient in a prone position for 15 to 30 minutes several times a day.

ESTABLISHING AN EXERCISE PROGRAM
- Provide full range of motion four or five times a day to maintain joint mobility, regain motor control, and prevent contracture development; prevent further deterioration of the neuromuscular system; enhance circulation; and prevent venous stasis. If tightness occurs in any area, perform range-of-motion exercises more frequently.
- Observe for signs of pulmonary embolus or excessive cardiac workload during exercise period (eg, shortness of breath, chest pain, cyanosis, and increasing pulse rate).
- Supervise and support patient during exercises; plan frequent short periods of exercise, not longer periods; encourage patient to exercise the unaffected side at intervals throughout the day.

PREPARING FOR AMBULATION
- Start an active rehabilitation program when consciousness returns (and all evidence of bleeding is gone, when indicated).
- Teach patient to maintain balance in a sitting position, then to balance while standing (use a tilt table if needed).

- Begin patient walking as soon as standing balance is achieved (use parallel bars and have wheelchair available in anticipation of possible dizziness).
- Keep training periods for ambulation short and frequent.

PREVENTING SHOULDER PAIN

- Never lift the patient by the flaccid shoulder or pull on the affected arm or shoulder.
- Use proper patient movement and positioning (eg, flaccid arm on a table or pillows when patient is seated, use of sling when ambulating).
- Range-of-motion exercises are beneficial, but avoid over-strenuous arm movements.
- Elevate the arm and hand to prevent dependent edema of the hand; administer analgesic agents as indicated.

ENHANCING SELF-CARE

- Encourage patient to assist in personal hygiene; select suitable self-care activities that can be carried out with one hand.
- Help to set realistic goals and add a new task daily.
- Encourage patient to carry out all self-care activities on the unaffected side as the first step.
- Make sure patient does not neglect affected side; provide assistive devices as indicated.
- Improve morale by making sure patient is fully dressed during ambulatory activities.
- Assist with dressing activities (eg, clothing fitted with Velcro closures; put garment on the affected side first); keep environment uncluttered and organized.
- Provide emotional support and encouragement to prevent overfatigue and discouragement.

MANAGING SENSORY-PERCEPTUAL DIFFICULTIES

- Approach the patient with a decreased field of vision on the side where visual perception is intact; place all visual stimuli on this side.
- Teach the patient to turn and look in the direction of the defective visual field to compensate for the loss; make eye contact with the patient, and draw attention to the affected side.

- Increase the natural or artificial lighting in the room; provide eyeglasses to improve vision.
- Remind the patient with hemianopsia of the other side of the body; place extremities so that the patient is able to see them.

MANAGING DYSPHAGIA

- Observe the patient for paroxysms of coughing, food dribbling out or pooling in one side of the mouth, food retained for long periods in the mouth, or nasal regurgitation when swallowing liquids.
- Consult with speech therapist to evaluate gag reflexes; assist in teaching alternate swallowing techniques, advise patient to take smaller boluses of food, and inform patient of foods that are easier to swallow; provide thicker liquids or puréed diet as indicated.
- Have patient sit upright, preferably in chair, when eating and drinking; advance diet as tolerated.
- Prepare for gastrointestinal feedings through a tube if indicated; elevate head of bed during feedings, check the position of the tube before feeding, administer feeding slowly, and ensure that cuff of tracheostomy tube is inflated (if applicable); monitor and report excessive residual feeding.

ATTAINING BOWEL AND BLADDER CONTROL

- Perform intermittent sterile catheterization during period of loss of sphincter control.
- Analyze voiding pattern and offer urinal or bedpan on this schedule.
- Assist the male patient to an upright posture for voiding.
- Provide high-fiber diet and adequate fluid intake (2 to 3 L/day), unless contraindicated.
- Establish a regular time (after breakfast) for toileting.

IMPROVING THOUGHT PROCESSES

- Reinforce structured training program using cognitive-perceptual retraining, visual imagery, reality orientation, and cuing procedures to compensate for losses.

- Support the patient: observe performance and progress, give positive feedback, convey an attitude of confidence and hopefulness; provide other interventions as used for improving cognitive function after a head injury.

ACHIEVING COMMUNICATION
- Reinforce the individually tailored program.
- Jointly establish goals, with the patient taking an active part.
- Make the atmosphere conducive to communication, remaining sensitive to the patient's reactions and needs and responding to them in an appropriate manner; treat the patient as an adult.
- Lend strong moral support and understanding to allay anxiety; avoid completing the patient's sentences.
- Be consistent in schedule, routines, and repetitions. A written schedule, checklists and audio tapes may help the patient's memory and concentration; a communication board may be used.
- Remember to talk to aphasic patients when providing care activities to provide social contact.
- Maintain the patient's attention when talking with the patient, speak slowly, and give one instruction at a time; allow patient time to process.

MAINTAINING SKIN INTEGRITY
- Frequently assess the skin for signs of potential breakdown, with emphasis on bony areas and dependent body parts.
- Employ pressure-relieving devices; continue regular turning and positioning (every 2 hours minimally), minimize shear and friction when positioning.
- Keep the skin clean and dry, gently massage healthy dry skin, and maintain adequate nutrition.

IMPROVING FAMILY COPING THROUGH HEALTH TEACHING
- Provide counseling and support to family.
- Ease the burden of the family in providing continuous 24-hour care with respite care or adult day care center;

encourage the caregiver to arrange for assistance, and provide information.

- Involve others in the patient's care; teach stress management techniques and maintenance of personal health for family coping.
- Give family information about the expected outcome of the stroke, and counsel them to avoid doing things for the patient that the patient can do.
- Develop attainable goals for the patient at home by involving the total health care team, patient, and family.
- Encourage everyone to approach patient with a supportive and optimistic attitude, focusing on abilities that remain; explain to the family that emotional lability usually improves with time.

REGAINING SEXUAL FUNCTION
- Encourage sexual counseling about alternative approaches to sexual expression.

Promoting Home and Community-Based Care

Teaching Patients Self-Care
- Refer to teaching checklist for topics to be covered regarding the rehabilitation process.
- Teach the patient to resume as much self-care as possible, provide assistive devices as indicated.
- Have occupational therapist make a home assessment and recommendations to help the patient become more independent.

Continuing Care
- Coordinate care provided by numerous health care professionals; help family plan aspects of care.
- Provide a speech therapist to come to the home and allow the family to be involved and to give the family practical instructions to help the patient between speech therapy sessions.

- Advise family that the patient will tire easily, will become irritable and upset by small events, and is likely to show less interest in things.
- Discuss patient's depression with the physician in relation to antidepressant therapy.
- Encourage family to support the patient and give positive reinforcement.
- Remind spouse and family members to attend to personal health problems and well-being.
- Encourage patient to attend community-based stroke clubs to give a feeling of belonging and fellowship with others.
- Encourage patient to continue with hobbies, recreational and leisure interests, and contact with friends to prevent social isolation.

Gerontologic Considerations

Do not let patient's age be a reason for failure to initiate a full rehabilitation program.

Evaluation

EXPECTED OUTCOMES
- Achieves improved mobility
- Has no complaints of pain
- Achieves self-care; turns head to see people or objects
- Demonstrates improved swallowing ability
- Achieves normal bowel and bladder elimination
- Demonstrates improved communication
- Family members demonstrate a positive attitude and coping mechanisms
- Has positive attitude regarding alternative approaches to sexual expression

---

For more information, see Chapters 10, 57, and 58 in Smeltzer and Bare: *Brunner and Suddarth's Textbook of Medical-Surgical Nursing,* 9th edition. Philadelphia: Lippincott Williams & Wilkins, 2000.

CHOLELITHIASIS (INCLUDES CHOLECYSTITIS)

Cholelithiasis (calculi or gallstones) usually form in the gallbladder from solid constituents of bile and vary greatly in size, shape, and composition. There are two major types of gallstones: pigment stones, which contain an excess of unconjugated pigments in the bile, and cholesterol stones (the most common form), which result from bile supersaturated with cholesterol due to increased synthesis of cholesterol and decreased synthesis of acids that dissolve cholesterol. Risk factors for pigment stones include cirrhosis, hemolysis, and infections of the biliary tree. These stones cannot be dissolved and must be removed surgically. Risk factors for cholesterol stones include gender (women have four times higher incidence than men); use of oral contraceptives, estrogens, and clofibrate; age (usually older than 40 years); multiparous status; and obesity. There is also an increased risk related to diabetes, gastrointestinal disease, T-tube fistula, and ileal resection or bypass.

Cholecystitis is an acute complication of cholelithiasis. Cholecystitis is an acute infection of the gallbladder. Most patients with cholecystitis have gallstones (calculous cholecystitis), in which a gallstone obstructs bile outflow and bile in the gallbladder initiates a chemical reaction, resulting in edema, compromise of the vascular supply, and gangrene. In the absence of gallstones, cholecystitis (acalculous) may occur after surgery, severe trauma, or burns, with torsion cystic duct obstruction, multiple blood transfusions, and primary bacterial infections of the gallbladder. This infection causes pain, tenderness, and rigidity of the upper right abdomen and is associated with nausea and vomiting and the usual signs of inflammation. Purulent fluid inside the gallbladder indicates an empyema of the gallbladder. See Nursing Management under Cholelithiasis for additional information.

Clinical Manifestations

- May be silent, producing no pain and only mild gastrointestinal symptoms
- May be acute or chronic with epigastric distress (fullness, abdominal distention, and vague upper right quadrant pain) after a high-fat meal
- If the cystic duct is obstructed, the gallbladder becomes distended and eventually infected; fever and palpable abdominal mass; biliary colic with excruciating upper right abdominal pain, radiating to back or right shoulder with nausea and vomiting several hours after a heavy meal; restlessness and constant or colicky pain
- Jaundice, accompanied by marked itching, with obstruction of the common bile duct, in a small percentage of patients
- Very dark urine; clay-colored stool
- Vitamin deficiencies of A, D, E, and K (fat-soluble vitamins)
- Abscess, necrosis, and perforation with peritonitis if the gallstone continues to obstruct the duct

Diagnostic Evaluation

- Abdominal radiograph, ultrasonography or cholecystography, radionuclide imaging, or cholescintigraphy
- Endoscopic retrograde cholangiopancreatography (ERCP)
- Percutaneous transhepatic cholangiography (PTC)

Medical Management

Nonsurgical Management

Major objectives of medical therapy are to reduce the incidence of acute episodes of gallbladder pain and cholecystitis by supportive and dietary management and, if possible, to remove the cause by pharmacotherapy, endoscopic procedures, or surgical intervention.

- Infusion of a solvent into the gallbladder to dissolve gallstones

- Stone removal through instrument with a basket or by ERCP endoscope
- Lithotripsy
  - Extracorporeal shock-wave lithotripsy: repeated shock waves directed at the gallstone located in the gallbladder or common bile duct to fragment the stones
  - Intracorporeal shock-wave lithotripsy: stones fragmented by ultrasound, pulsed laser, or hydraulic lithotripsy applied through an endoscope directly to the stones

Supportive and Dietary Management
- Achieve remission with rest, intravenous fluids, nasogastric suction, analgesia, and antibiotics.
- Diet immediately after an episode is usually low-fat liquids with high protein and carbohydrates followed by solid soft foods as tolerated, avoiding eggs, fatty rich foods, gas-forming vegetables, and alcohol.

Pharmacotherapy
- Analgesics, such as meperidine, may be required; avoid the use of morphine because it increases spasm of the sphincter of Oddi.
- Ursodeoxycholic acid and chenodeoxycholic acid (chenodiol, or CDCA) are effective in dissolving primarily cholesterol stones.
- Long-term follow-up and monitoring of liver enzymes are indicated.

Surgical Management
The goal of surgery is to relieve persistent symptoms, remove the cause of colic, and treat acute cholecystitis.

- Laparoscopic cholecystectomy: performed through a small incision or puncture made through the abdominal wall in the umbilicus
- Cholecystectomy: gallbladder removed after ligation of the cystic duct and artery
- Mini-cholecystectomy: gallbladder removed through a 3- to 4-cm incision

- Choledochostomy: incision into the common duct for stone removal
- Cholecystostomy (surgical or percutaneous): gallbladder is opened and the stones, bile, or purulent drainage are removed

Nursing Management: The Patient Undergoing Surgery for Gallbladder Disease

Assessment
- Assess health history: note history of smoking or prior respiratory problems.
- Assess respiratory status: note shallow respirations, persistent cough, or ineffective or adventitious breath sounds.
- Evaluate nutritional status (dietary history, general examination, and laboratory study results).

Major Nursing Diagnoses
- Pain and discomfort related to surgical incision
- Impaired gas exchange related to high abdominal surgical incision
- Impaired skin integrity related to altered biliary drainage after surgical incision
- Altered nutrition related to inadequate bile secretion
- Knowledge deficit about self-care activities related to incisional care, dietary modifications (if needed), medications, reportable signs or symptoms (fever, bleeding, vomiting)

Collaborative Problems/Potential Complications
- Bleeding
- Gastrointestinal symptoms

Planning and Goals
Goals include relief of pain, adequate ventilation, intact skin and improved biliary drainage, optimal nutritional intake, understanding of self-care routines, and absence of complications.

Nursing Interventions

POSTOPERATIVE
- Place patient in low Fowler's position.
- Provide intravenous fluids and nasogastric suction.
- Provide water and other fluids and soft diet, after bowel sounds return.

Relieving Pain
- Instruct patient to use a pillow to splint incision.
- Administer analgesics as ordered.

Improving Respiratory Status
- Remind patient to expand lungs fully to prevent atelectasis; promote early ambulation.
- Monitor elderly and obese patients most closely for respiratory problems.

Improving Nutritional Status
- Advise patient at time of discharge to maintain a nutritious diet and avoid excessive fats; fat restriction is usually lifted in 4 to 6 weeks.

Promoting Skin Care and Biliary Drainage
- Connect tubes to drainage receptacle, and secure tubing to avoid kinking (elevate above abdomen).
- Place drainage bag in patient's pocket when ambulating.
- Observe for indications of infection, leakage of bile, or obstruction of bile drainage.
- Be observant for jaundice (check the sclera).
- Note and report right upper quadrant pain, nausea, and vomiting.
- Change dressing frequently using ointment to protect the skin from irritation.
- Keep careful record of intake and output.
- Measure bile collected every 24 hours; document amount, color, and character of drainage.

Monitoring and Managing Complications
- Bleeding: assess periodically for increased tenderness and rigidity of the abdomen and report; instruct patient and family to report change in color of stools.

Monitor vital signs closely, inspect the surgical incision for bleeding.
- Gastrointestinal symptoms: assess for loss of appetite, vomiting, pain, distention of the abdomen, and temperature elevation; report promptly and instruct patient and family to report symptoms promptly; provide written reinforcement of verbal instructions.

Promoting Home and Community-Based Care

Teaching Patients Self-Care
- Instruct patient, verbally and in writing, in proper care of drainage tubes and to report to physician promptly changes in the amount or characteristics of drainage.
- Instruct about which medications are required and their actions.
- Instruct to report to the physician symptoms of jaundice, dark urine, pale-colored stools, pruritus, or signs of inflammation and infection (eg, pain or fever after laparoscopy procedure).
- Provide written and verbal instructions to patient and family about management of postoperative pain and about signs and symptoms of intraabdominal complications that should be reported. These include loss of appetite, vomiting, pain, distention of abdomen, and temperature elevation.
- Refer for home care during the first 24 to 48 hours because of drowsiness.
- Emphasize the importance of keeping follow-up appointments.

Gerontologic Considerations

- Surgical intervention for disease of the biliary tract is the most common operative procedure performed in the elderly.
- Biliary disease may be accompanied or preceded by symptoms of septic shock: oliguria, hypotension, mental changes, tachycardia, and tachypnea.

- Mortality from serious complications is high. Risk of complications and shorter hospital stays make it essential that older patients and their family members receive specific information about signs and symptoms of complications and measures to prevent them.
- Cholecystectomy is usually well tolerated and low risk if expert assessment and care are provided before, during, and after surgery.

Evaluation

EXPECTED OUTCOMES
- Reports decrease in pain
- Demonstrates appropriate respiratory function
- Exhibits normal skin integrity around biliary drainage sites
- Obtains relief of dietary intolerance
- Is free of complications

For more information, see Chapter 36 in Smeltzer and Bare: *Brunner and Suddarth's Textbook of Medical-Surgical Nursing,* 9th edition. Philadelphia: Lippincott Williams & Wilkins, 2000.

CHRONIC OBSTRUCTIVE PULMONARY DISEASE

Chronic obstructive pulmonary disease (COPD) is a disease state in which airflow is obstructed by emphysema, chronic bronchitis, or both. The airflow obstruction is usually progressive, irreversible, and associated with airway hyperreactivity. Asthma, now considered a separate disorder, overlaps with symptoms of COPD and is also discussed. Cigarette smoking, air pollution, and occupational exposure (coal, cotton, grain) are important risk factors that contribute to its development, which may occur over a 20- to 30-year span. Complications of COPD vary but include respiratory insufficiency and failure (major complications) as well as pneumonia, atelectasis, and pneumothorax.

Clinical Manifestations
- COPD is characterized by dyspnea, cough, and increased work of breathing as well as dyspnea on mild exertion, advancing to dyspnea at rest.
- Weight loss is common.
- Symptoms are specific to the disease.

See Clinical Manifestations under Asthma; Bronchiectasis; Bronchitis, Chronic; and Emphysema.

Medical Management
- Bronchodilators
- Oxygen therapy, including nighttime oxygen
- Varied treatments specific to disease

See Medical Management under Asthma; Bronchiectasis; Bronchitis, Chronic; and Emphysema.

Nursing Management

NURSING ALERT

Because hypoxemia is a stimulus for respiration in the patient with COPD, take caution to avoid depressing the respiratory drive when administering oxygen to correct hypoxemia.

Assessment
- Obtain a history about current symptoms and previous disease manifestations:
  ○ Duration of respiratory difficulty
  ○ Dyspnea, shortness of breath, wheezing, exercise tolerance, fatigue
  ○ Effect on eating and sleeping habits
- Perform a thorough physical examination to obtain baseline data:
  ○ Pulse, respiratory rate, and rhythm
  ○ Contraction of abdominal muscles during inspiration
  ○ Use of accessory muscles to breathe; prolonged expiration
  ○ Cyanosis, neck vein engorgement
  ○ Peripheral edema

○ Cough, color, amount and consistency of sputum
○ Status of patient's sensorium, increasing stupor, apprehension

Major Nursing Diagnoses

- Impaired gas exchange related to ventilation-perfusion inequality
- Ineffective airway clearance related to bronchoconstriction, increased mucus production, ineffective cough, and bronchopulmonary infection
- Ineffective breathing pattern related to shortness of breath, mucus, bronchoconstriction, and airway irritants
- Self-care deficit related to fatigue secondary to increased work of breathing and insufficient ventilation and oxygenation
- Activity intolerance due to fatigue, hypoxemia, and ineffective breathing patterns
- Ineffective individual coping related to less socialization, anxiety, depression, lower activity level, and the inability to work
- Knowledge deficit of self-care to be performed at home

Collaborative Problems/Potential Complications

- Respiratory insufficiency or failure
- Atelectasis
- Pneumonia
- Pneumothorax
- Pulmonary hypertension

Planning and Goals

The major goals of the patient include improvement of gas exchange, smoking cessation, improved breathing pattern, maximal self-management, improved activity tolerance, achievement of airway clearance, improved coping ability, improved health-related quality of life, and adherence to the therapeutic program and home care.

Nursing Interventions

IMPROVING GAS EXCHANGE
- Monitor dyspnea and hypoxia.
- Administer medications, and be alert for potential side effects.
- Assess relief of bronchospasms through patient report of experiencing less dyspnea.
- Monitor prescribed oxygen effectiveness: pulse oximetry, arterial blood gas (ABG) analysis.

ACHIEVING AIRWAY CLEARANCE
- Encourage high fluid intake to liquefy secretions.
- Instruct the patient in directed or controlled coughing.
- Provide chest physiotherapy with postural drainage and intermittent positive pressure breathing (IPPB), when ordered.
- Instruct patient in effective breathing techniques.
- Measure expiratory flow rates.

PREVENTING BRONCHOPULMONARY INFECTIONS
- Instruct patient to report signs of infection (eg, fever; change in sputum color, character, consistency, or amount), and report any worsening of symptoms.
- Instruct to avoid outdoor exposure when pollen count is high or significant air pollution because these may increase bronchospasm.
- Instruct to avoid high climate temperatures and humidity.
- Encourage immunization against *Haemophilus influenzae* and *Streptococcus pneumoniae*.

🏠 Promoting Home and Community-Based Care

- Recommend the patient adopt a lifestyle of moderate activity ideally in a climate with minimal shifts in temperature and humidity.
- Demonstrate and supervise patient and family in performing all aspects of the treatment regimen (eg, metered-dose inhaler [MDI], IPPB, chest physiotherapy,

and postural drainage) with return demonstration from patient before discharge.

- Encourage patient to avoid emotional disturbances and stressful situations.
- Recommend strategies for smoking cessation, and review progress with patient.
- Refer patient for home care.

Pulmonary Rehabilitation

- Identify potential candidates for rehabilitation, and reinforce material learned in a rehabilitation program.
- Plan individualized actions with the patient to restore the highest level of independent function and to improve the patient's quality of life; attend to both the physiologic and emotional needs of the patient; help to accept realistic short-term and long-range goals.
- Reinforce breathing exercises and retraining and exercise programs, and teach the patient methods to alleviate symptoms.
- Include information for the COPD patient, encompassing topics such as normal anatomy and physiology of the lung, pathophysiology and changes with COPD, medications and home oxygen therapy, nutrition, respiratory therapy treatments, symptom alleviation, smoking cessation, sexuality and COPD, coping with chronic disease, communicating with the health care team, and planning for the future (advance directives, living wills, informed decision making about health care alternatives).
- Instruct the patient in activity pacing (avoiding activities requiring arm lifting and movement until after the patient has been up and moving around for an hour or more).
- Participate with patient in planning self-care activities and in determining the best time for bathing and dressing.
- If prescribed, assist the patient in learning inspiratory muscle training: breathing against resistance for 10 to 15 minutes every day, and increasing the resistance gradually.

- Teach the patient to try to coordinate diaphragmatic breathing with activities such as walking, bathing, bending, or climbing stairs.
- Instruct the patient to begin gradually to bathe, dress, and take short walks, resting as needed to avoid fatigue and excessive dyspnea and to keep fluids readily available.
- If ordered, assist the patient to adhere to the oxygen prescription by explaining the proper flow rate and required number of hours for oxygen use as well as the dangers of arbitrary changes in flow rates or duration of therapy.
- Reassure the patient that oxygen is not "addictive," and explain the necessity of having regular evaluations of blood oxygenation by pulse oximetry or ABG gas analysis.
- Advise the patient that smoking with or near oxygen is extremely dangerous.
- Teach the patient coping measures (eg, remaining active up to level of symptom tolerance; how to control symptoms to increase self-esteem, sense of mastery, and well-being; and use of support groups).
- Facilitate specific services for the patient (eg, respiratory therapy education, physical therapy for exercise and breathing retraining, and occupational therapy for conservation of energy techniques during activities of daily living).
- Inform patient and family of potential resources, including the American Lung Association, American Association of Cardiovascular and Pulmonary Rehabilitation, or the American Association of Respiratory Therapy.

MONITORING AND MANAGING COMPLICATIONS
- Assess the patient for complications (respiratory insufficiency and failure, respiratory infection, and atelectasis).
- Monitor for cognitive changes, increasing dyspnea, tachypnea, and tachycardia.
- Monitor pulse oximetry values, and administer oxygen as prescribed to maintain optimal levels.

- Instruct the patient and family about signs and symptoms of infection or other complications and to report changes in physical or cognitive status.
- Emphasize that if condition worsens to the point of acute respiratory failure, intubation and mechanical ventilation will be necessary.

Gerontologic Considerations

COPD accentuates many of the physiologic changes associated with aging and is manifested in airway obstruction (in bronchitis) and excessive loss of elastic lung recoil (in emphysema). Additional changes in ventilation-perfusion ratios occur.

Evaluation

EXPECTED OUTCOMES
- Demonstrates improved gas exchange
- Achieves maximal airway clearance
- Improves breathing pattern
- Maintains maximal level of self-care and physical functioning
- Achieves activity tolerance, and exercises and performs activities with less shortness of breath
- Develops effective coping mechanisms, and participates in a pulmonary rehabilitation program
- Adheres to the therapeutic program

For more information, see Chapter 21 in Smeltzer and Bare: *Brunner and Suddarth's Textbook of Medical-Surgical Nursing,* 9th edition. Philadelphia: Lippincott Williams & Wilkins, 2000.

CIRRHOSIS, HEPATIC

Cirrhosis is a chronic disease characterized by replacement of normal liver tissue with diffuse fibrosis that disrupts the structure and function of the liver. Cirrhosis, or scarring of the liver, is divided into three types: alcoholic, most frequently due to chronic alcoholism and the most common type of cirrhosis; postnecrotic, a late result of a previous acute viral hepatitis; and biliary, a result of chronic biliary obstruction and infection (the least common type of cirrhosis).

Clinical Manifestations
- Liver enlargement early in the course (fatty liver); later in course, liver size decreases from scar tissue
- Portal obstruction and ascites: chronic dyspepsia, constipation or diarrhea, splenomegaly; spider telangiectases may be observed
- Gastrointestinal varices: distended abdominal blood vessels; varices or hemorrhoids; small hematemesis; profuse hemorrhage from the stomach; and esophageal varices in about 25% of patients
- Edema
- Vitamin deficiency (A, C, and K) and anemia
- Mental deterioration with impending hepatic encephalopathy and hepatic coma

Diagnostic Evaluation
- Liver function tests (eg, serum alkaline phosphatase, AST (SGOT), ALT (SGPT), GGT, and bilirubin), prothrombin time, ABGs, laparoscopy, in conjunction with biopsy
- Ultrasound scanning
- Computed tomography (CT) scan
- Magnetic resonance imaging (MRI)
- Radioisotopic liver scans

Medical Management

Medical management is based on presenting symptoms.

- Treatment includes antacids, vitamins, balanced diet, and nutritional supplements; potassium-sparing diuretics; avoidance of alcohol.
- Colchicine may increase the length of survival in patients with mild to moderate cirrhosis.

Nursing Management

Assessment

- Focus on diet intake, nutritional status, onset of symptoms, history of precipitating factors, including long-term alcohol abuse, exposure to toxic agents, medications.
- Assess mental status through interview and interaction with the patient; note orientation to time, place, person.
- Note relationships with family, friends, and coworkers regarding incapacitation secondary to alcohol abuse and cirrhosis.
- Note abdominal distention and bloating, gastrointestinal bleeding, bruising, and weight changes.
- Document exposure to toxic agents, such as hepatotoxic medications.

Major Nursing Diagnoses

- Activity intolerance related to fatigue, general debility, muscle wasting, and discomfort.
- Altered nutrition related to chronic gastritis, decreased gastrointestinal motility, and anorexia.
- Impaired skin integrity related to compromised immunologic status, edema, and poor nutrition.
- Risk for injury related to altered clotting mechanisms.

Collaborative Problems/Potential Complications

- Bleeding and hemorrhage
- Hepatic encephalopathy
- Fluid volume excess

C

Planning and Goals

Goals may include independence in activities, improvement of nutritional status, improvement of skin integrity, decreased potential for injury, improvement of mental status, and absence of complications.

Interventions

PROVIDING REST

- Position bed for maximal respiratory efficiency; provide oxygen if needed.
- Initiate efforts to prevent respiratory, circulatory, and vascular disturbances.
- Encourage patient to increase activity gradually and plan rest with activity and mild exercise.

IMPROVING NUTRITIONAL STATUS

- Provide a nutritious, high-protein diet supplemented by B complex vitamins and others, including A, C, and K and folic acid if there is no indication of impending coma.
- Provide small, frequent meals, consider patient preference, and encourage patient to eat; provide protein supplements, if indicated.
- Provide nutrients by feeding tube or total parenteral nutrition (TPN).
- Provide patients with fatty stools (steatorrhea) with water-soluble forms of fat-soluble vitamins A, D, and E, and give folic acid and iron to prevent anemia.
- Provide a low-protein diet temporarily if patient shows signs of impending or advancing coma; restore protein intake to normal or above when patient's condition permits.

PROVIDING SKIN CARE

- Change position frequently.
- Avoid using irritating soaps and adhesive tape.
- Provide lotion to soothe the irritated skin; take measures to prevent the patient's scratching of the skin.

REDUCING RISK OF INJURY
- Use padded side rails if patient becomes agitated or restless.
- Orient to time, place, and procedures to minimize agitation.
- Instruct patient to ask for assistance to get out of bed.
- Provide safety measures to prevent injury or cuts (electric razor, soft toothbrush).

MONITORING AND MANAGING COMPLICATIONS
Preventing bleeding due to decreased production of prothrombin and monitoring for hepatic encephalopathy are the primary concerns.

- Observe for melena, and check stools for blood.
- Take precautionary measures (eg, use padded side rails, apply pressure to injection site for long period of time, and avoid sharp objects).
- Use appropriate dietary modification and stool softeners to assist in preventing straining during defecation.
- Monitor closely for gastrointestinal bleeding.
- Keep equipment to treat hemorrhage from esophageal varices readily available: intravenous fluids, medications, Sengstaken-Blakemore tube.
- Monitor closely to identify early evidence of condition.

See Nursing Management under Hepatic Encephalopathy for additional information.

🏠 Promoting Home and Community-Based Care

Prepare for discharge by providing dietary instruction, including exclusion of alcohol.

- Refer to Alcoholics Anonymous if necessary.
- Continue sodium restriction.
- Provide necessary written instruction, teaching, support, and reinforcement to patient and family.
- Encourage rest and probably a change in lifestyle (adequate, well-balanced diet and elimination of alcohol).

- Instruct family about the symptoms of impending encephalopathy and possibility of bleeding tendencies and infection.
- Refer patient to a home care nurse to visit the patient in the home after discharge, and assist in transition from hospital to home.

Evaluation

EXPECTED OUTCOMES
- Demonstrates ability to participate in activities
- Increases nutritional intake

For more information, see Chapter 36 in Smeltzer and Bare: *Brunner and Suddarth's Textbook of Medical-Surgical Nursing,* 9th edition. Philadelphia: Lippincott Williams & Wilkins, 2000.

CONSTIPATION

Constipation refers to an abnormal infrequency or irregularity of defecation, abnormal hardening of stools that make their passage difficult and sometimes painful, decrease in stool volume, or prolonged retention of stool in the rectum. This type is referred to as colonic constipation. It can be caused by certain medications; rectal or anal disorders; obstruction; metabolic, neurologic, and neuromuscular conditions; endocrine disorders; lead poisoning, connective tissue disorders; and a variety of disease conditions. Other causative factors include weakness, immobility, debility, fatigue, and inability to increase intraabdominal pressure to facilitate the passage of stools. Constipation develops when people do not take the time to defecate or as the result of dietary habits (low consumption of fiber and inadequate fluid intake, lack of regular exercise, and a stress-filled life). Perceived constipation is a subjective problem that occurs when an individual's bowel elimination pattern is not consistent with what he or she perceives as normal. Chronic laxative use contributes to this problem, particularly in elderly people.

Clinical Manifestations

- Abdominal distention, borborygmus (intestinal rumbling), pain, and pressure
- Decreased appetite, headache, fatigue, indigestion, sensation of incomplete emptying
- Straining at stool; elimination of small-volume, hard, dry stool
- Complications, such as hypertension, hemorrhoids and fissures, fecal impaction, and megacolon

Diagnostic Evaluation

Diagnosis is based on history, physical examination, possibly a barium enema, sigmoidoscopy, stool for occult blood, anorectal manometry (pressure studies), defecography, and bowel transit studies.

Medical Management

Treatment should be aimed at the underlying cause of constipation.

- Discontinue abusive laxative use; increase fluid intake; include fiber in diet, biofeedback, and an exercise routine to strengthen abdominal muscles.
- If laxative is necessary, use bulk-forming agents, saline and osmotic agents, lubricants, stimulants, or fecal softeners.
- Specific medication therapy to increase intrinsic motor function (prokinetic agents, eg, cisapride).

Nursing Management

Assessment

Use tact and respect with patient when talking about bowel habits and obtaining health history. Note the following:

- Onset and duration of constipation, current and past elimination patterns, patient's expectation of normal bowel elimination, food and fluid intake, lifestyle, stress level, and occupation
- Current medications, history of laxative or enema use, and past medical and surgical history

- Report of presence of any of the following: rectal pressure or fullness, abdominal pain, straining at defecation, and flatulence

Major Nursing Diagnoses
- Colonic constipation or fecal impaction related to health habits or the effect of immobility on peristalsis
- Knowledge deficit about health maintenance practices to prevent constipation

Planning and Goals
The major goals of the patient may include restoration or maintenance of a regular pattern of bowel elimination, adequate intake of fluids and high-fiber foods, knowledge of methods to avoid constipation, relief of anxiety about bowel elimination patterns, and the absence of complications.

 Promoting Home and Community-Based Care

Teaching Patients Self-Care
- Teach patient to assume the normal position for defecation (semisquatting) when possible (assist patient to a bedside commode).
- Explain the physiology of defecation, and emphasize heeding the urge to defecate.
- Discuss normal variations in patterns of defecation.
- Teach how to establish a bowel routine (eg, after breakfast).
- Provide dietary information; suggest eating high-residue, high-fiber food, adding bran daily (introduce gradually), and increasing fluid intake (unless contraindicated).
- Detail the benefits of an exercise regimen, increased ambulation, and abdominal muscle toning.
- Describe abdominal toning exercises: contracting abdomen muscles four times daily and leg to chest lifts 10 to 20 times daily.
- Encourage patient confined to bed to perform range-of-motion exercises, turn frequently from side-to-side, and

lie prone (if not contraindicated) for 30 minutes every 4 hours.

For more information, see Chapter 35 in Smeltzer and Bare: *Brunner and Suddarth's Textbook of Medical-Surgical Nursing,* 9th edition. Philadelphia: Lippincott Williams & Wilkins, 2000.

CONTACT DERMATITIS

Contact dermatitis is an inflammatory reaction of the skin to physical, chemical, or biologic agents. It may be of the primary irritant type, or it may be allergic. The epidermis is damaged by repeated physical and chemical irritations. Common causes of irritant dermatitis are soaps, detergents, scouring compounds, and industrial chemicals. Predisposing factors include extremes of heat and cold, frequent use of soap and water, and a preexisting skin disease.

Clinical Manifestations
Eruptions begin when the causative agent contacts the skin.

- Itching, burning, and erythema are followed by edema, papules, vesicles, and oozing or weeping.
- In the subacute phase, the vesicular changes are less marked and alternate with crusting, drying, fissuring, and peeling.
- If repeated reactions occur or the patient continually scratches the skin, lichenification and pigmentation occur; secondary bacterial invasion may follow.

Medical Management
- Rest the involved skin, and protect it from further damage.
- Determine the distribution pattern of the reaction to differentiate between allergic type and irritant type.
- Identify and remove the offending irritant; soap is generally not used on site until healed.

- Use bland, unmedicated lotions for small patches of ery-thema; apply cool wet dressings over small areas of vesic-ular dermatitis; a corticosteroid ointment may be used.
- Medicated baths at room temperature are prescribed for larger areas of dermatitis.
- In widespread conditions, a short course of systemic steroids may be prescribed.

Promoting Home and Community-Based Care

Teaching Patients Self-Care
- Instruct the patient to adhere to the following instruc-tions for at least 4 months, until the skin appears com-pletely healed:
  ○ Think about what may have caused the problem.
  ○ Avoid contact with the irritants, or wash skin thor-oughly immediately after possible exposure to the irritants.
  ○ Avoid heat, soap, and rubbing the skin.
  ○ Avoid topical medications, lotions, or ointments, except when prescribed.
  ○ Choose bath soaps, detergents, and cosmetics that do not contain fragrance; avoid using a fabric softener dryer sheet, those added to the washer may be used.
  ○ Wear cotton-lined gloves for washing dishes, not more than 15 to 20 minutes at a time.
- Instruct the patient and family in the use of cool wet dressings to clear lesions, followed by corticosteroid ointment, as ordered.

For more information, see Chapter 52 in Smeltzer and Bare: *Brunner and Suddarth's Textbook of Medical-Surgical Nursing,* 9th edition. Philadelphia: Lippincott Williams & Wilkins, 2000.

CORONARY ATHEROSCLEROSIS AND CORONARY ARTERY DISEASE

Coronary atherosclerosis is characterized by an abnormal accumulation of lipid or fatty substances and fibrous tissue in the vessel wall. These substances create blockages or narrow the vessel in a way that reduces blood flow to the myocardium, resulting in coronary heart disease(CHD). Recent studies indicate that atherosclerosis involves repeated inflammatory response to artery wall injury and alteration in the biophysical and biochemical properties of the arterial walls. Atherosclerosis is a progressive disease. Its progress can be curtailed and in some cases reversed.

Risk Factors
Modifiable
- Cigarette smoking
- Elevated blood pressure
- High blood cholesterol (hyperlipidemia)
- Hyperglycemia (diabetes mellitus)
- Obesity
- Physical inactivity
- Use of oral contraceptives
- Behavior patterns (stress, aggressiveness, hostility)
- Geography: higher incidence in industrialized region

Nonmodifiable
- Positive family history
- Increasing age
- Gender: occurs three times more often in men than in women
- Race: higher incidence in African Americans than in Caucasians

Clinical Manifestations
Clinical features result from narrowing of the arterial lumen and obstruction of blood flow to myocardium.
- Chest pain

- Angina pectoris
- Myocardial infarction
- Electrocardiogram (ECG) changes, ventricular aneurysms
- Dysrhythmias, sudden death

Diagnostic Evaluation

Identification of risk factors for development of CHD primarily involves taking a thorough history, including family history, physical examination (note blood pressure and weight), and laboratory work (cholesterol levels, glucose).

Medical Management

See Medical Management under Angina and Myocardial Infarction for additional information.

Prevention

The major goal of medical management is prevention of CHD.

Primary prevention (taken before the development of CHD) and secondary prevention are aimed at reducing the risk factors for CHD. Four modifiable risk factors—cholesterol abnormalities, cigarette smoking, hypertension, and diabetes mellitus—have been cited as major causes of coronary artery disease (CAD) and its consequent complications.

Nursing Management

See Nursing Management under Angina and Myocardial Infarction for additional information.

Nursing Interventions

- Identify at-risk patients, and teach lifestyle modifications to prevent development of CAD.
- Teach the patient to control cholesterol levels through dietary reduction of cholesterol intake, exercise, smoking cessation, and, if needed, medications.
- Note and report findings from history, physical examination, and laboratory results that indicate hypertension

or diabetes, and teach patient to control blood pressure and blood glucose through adherence to treatment regimen.

- Encourage and help patient learn to alter behaviors and responses to stress-triggering events; teach cognitive restructuring and relaxation techniques.
- Prepare and support patient and family if patient develops CHD or complications, develops symptoms, and requires diagnostic or treatment procedures (eg, nitroglycerin, thrombolytic therapy, angiography, percutaneous transluminal coronary angioplasty [PTCA], coronary artery stent, atherectomy, transmyocardial revascularization, or coronary artery bypass).

 Gerontologic Considerations

Aging produces changes in the integrity of the lining of the walls of arteries (arteriosclerosis), impeding blood flow and tissue nutrition. These changes are often sufficient to diminish oxygenation and increase myocardial oxygen consumption (MVO_2). The result can be debilitating angina pectoris and eventually congestive heart failure.

For more information, see Chapter 25 in Smeltzer and Bare: *Brunner and Suddarth's Textbook of Medical-Surgical Nursing,* 9th edition. Philadelphia: Lippincott Williams & Wilkins, 2000.

CUSHING'S SYNDROME

Cushing's syndrome results from excessive adrenocortical activity. It may result from excessive administration of corticosteroids or adrenocorticotropic hormone (ACTH) or from hyperplasia of the adrenal cortex. It may be caused by several mechanisms, including a tumor of the pituitary gland or an ectopic malignancy that produces ACTH. Regardless of the cause, the normal feedback mechanisms that control the function of the adrenal cortex become ineffective, resulting in oversecretion of glucocorticoids, androgens, and possibly mineralocorticoid. Cushing's syndrome occurs five times more often in women ages 20 to 40 years than in men.

Clinical Manifestations
- Growth arrest, obesity, musculoskeletal changes, and glucose intolerance
- Classic features: a central-type obesity, with a fatty "buffalo hump" in the neck and supraclavicular areas, a heavy trunk, and relatively thin extremities; skin is thin, fragile, easily traumatized, with ecchymosis and striae
- Weakness and lassitude; sleep is disturbed because of altered diurnal secretion of cortisol
- Excessive protein catabolism with muscle wasting and osteoporosis; kyphosis, backache, and compression fractures of the vertebrae possible
- Retention of sodium and water, producing hypertension and congestive heart failure
- "Moon-faced" appearance, oiliness of the skin and acne
- Increased susceptibility to infection
- Hyperglycemia or overt diabetes
- Weight gain, slow healing of minor cuts and bruises
- Virilization in females (due to excess androgens) with appearance of masculine traits and recession of feminine traits (eg, excessive hair grows on face, breasts atrophy, menses cease, clitoris enlarges, and voice deepens); libido is lost in males and females
- Changes occur in mood and mental activity; psychosis may develop
- If Cushing's syndrome is the result of pituitary tumor, visual disturbances possible because of pressure on the optic chiasm

Diagnostic Evaluation
- Plasma and urinary cortisol measurements
- 24-hour urine collection for free cortisol level
- Dexamethasone suppression test (stress, obesity, depression and medications may falsely elevate results)

- Computed tomography (CT) or magnetic resonance imaging (MRI) scan or ultrasound may localize adrenal tissue and detect adrenal tumors.

Medical Management

Treatment is usually directed at the pituitary gland because most cases are due to pituitary tumors rather than tumors of the adrenal cortex.

- Surgical removal of the tumor is the primary treatment of choice (90% success rate).
- Radiation of the pituitary gland is successful but takes several months for symptom control.
- Adrenalectomy is performed in patients with primary adrenal hypertrophy.
- Postoperatively, temporary replacement therapy with hydrocortisone may be necessary until the adrenal glands begin to respond normally (may be several months).
- If bilateral adrenalectomy was performed, lifetime replacement of adrenal cortex hormones is necessary.
- Adrenal enzyme inhibitors (eg, metyrapone or mitotane) may be used with ectopic ACTH-secreting tumors that cannot be totally removed; monitor closely for inadequate adrenal function and side effects.
- If Cushing's syndrome is a result of exogenous corticosteroids, taper the drug to the minimum level or use alternate day therapy to treat the underlying disease.

Nursing Management
Assessment

Focus on the effects on the body of high concentrations of adrenal cortex hormones.

- Obtain information about the patient's level of activity and ability to carry out routine and self-care activities.
- Observe skin for trauma, infection, breakdown, bruising, and edema.
- Note changes in physical appearance and patient's responses to these changes; family is good source of

information about patient's emotional status and
changes in appearance.
- Assess patient's mental function, including mood,
response to questions, depression, and awareness of
environment.

Major Nursing Diagnoses
- Impaired skin integrity related to edema, impaired healing, and thin and fragile skin
- Risk for injury related to weakness
- Risk for infection related to altered protein metabolism
and inflammatory response
- Body image disturbance related to altered physical
appearance, impaired sexual functioning, and decrease in
activity level
- Self-care deficit related to weakness, fatigue, muscle
wasting, and altered sleep patterns
- Altered thought processes related to mood swings, irritability, and depression

Collaborative Problems/Potential Complications
- Addisonian crisis
- Adverse effects of adrenocortical activity

Planning and Goals
The major goals include decreased risk of infection, decreased risk of injury, increased ability to carry out self-care
activities, improved skin integrity, improved body image,
improved mental function, and absence of complications.

Nursing Interventions
PROMOTING FLUID AND ELECTROLYTE BALANCE
- Monitor fluid and electrolyte status.
- Weigh daily.
- Monitor and report blood glucose.

DECREASING RISK FOR INJURY
- Provide a protective environment to prevent falls, fractures, and other injuries to bones and soft tissues.

- Assist the patient who is weak in ambulating to prevent falls or colliding into furniture.
- Recommend foods high in protein, calcium, and vitamin D to minimize muscle wasting and osteoporosis; refer to dietitian for assistance.

DECREASING RISK FOR INFECTION
- Avoid unnecessary exposure to people with infections.
- Assess frequently for subtle signs of infections (corticosteroids mask signs of inflammation and infection).

PREPARING THE PATIENT FOR SURGERY
- See Preoperative Preparation under Preoperative and Postoperative Nursing Management and later in this section.
- Monitor blood glucose levels, and assess stools for blood because diabetes mellitus and peptic ulcer are common problems.

ENCOURAGING REST AND ACTIVITY
- Encourage moderate activity to prevent complications of immobility and promote increased self-esteem.
- Plan rest periods throughout the day.
- Promote a relaxing, quiet environment for rest and sleep.

PROMOTING SKIN CARE
- Use meticulous skin care to avoid traumatizing fragile skin.
- Avoid adhesive tape that can tear and irritate the skin.
- Assess skin and bony prominences frequently.
- Encourage and assist patient to change positions frequently.

IMPROVING BODY IMAGE
- Discuss the impact that changes have had on the patient's self-concept and relationships with others even though major physical changes will disappear in time if the cause of Cushing's syndrome can be treated successfully.
- Weight gain and edema may be modified by a low-carbohydrate, low-sodium diet; a high-protein intake can reduce some bothersome symptoms.

IMPROVING THOUGHT PROCESSES
- Explain to the patient and family the cause of emotional instability, and help them cope with mood swings, irritability, and depression that may occur.
- Report any psychotic behavior.
- Encourage patient and family members to verbalize feelings.

MONITORING AND MANAGING COMPLICATIONS
- Adrenal hypofunction and addisonian crisis: monitor for hypotension; rapid, weak pulse; rapid respiratory rate; pallor; and extreme weakness. Note possible trigger or factors that may have lead to crisis (eg, stress, trauma, surgery).
- Administer intravenous fluid and electrolytes and corticosteroids before, during, and after surgery or treatment as indicated.
- Monitor for circulatory collapse and shock present in addisonian crisis; treat promptly.
- Assess fluid and electrolyte status by monitoring laboratory values and daily weight.
- Monitor blood glucose, and report elevated glucose levels to physician.

🏠 Promoting Home and Community-Based Care

Teaching Patients Self-Care
- Present information about Cushing's syndrome verbally and in writing to patient and family.
- If indicated, stress to patient and family that stopping corticosteroid use abruptly and without medical supervision can result in adrenal insufficiency and reappearance of symptoms.
- Emphasize the need to keep an adequate supply of the corticosteroid to prevent running out or skipping of a dose because this could result in addisonian crisis.
- Stress the need for dietary modifications to ensure adequate calcium intake, without increasing risk for hypertension, hyperglycemia, and weight gain.

- Teach the patient and family to monitor blood pressure, blood glucose levels, and weight.
- Stress the importance of wearing a medical alert bracelet and notifying other health professionals (eg, dentist) that patient has Cushing's syndrome.

Continuing Care

- Stress the importance of follow-up care as indicated by treatment received.
- Refer for home care as indicated to ensure safe environment with minimal stress and risk for falls and other side effects.
- Emphasize the importance of regular medical follow-up, awareness of side and toxic effects of medications, and wearing the medical alert bracelet.

Evaluation

EXPECTED OUTCOMES
- Has decreased risk of injury
- Has decreased risk of infection
- Increases participation in self-care activities
- Attains or maintains skin integrity
- Achieves improved body image
- Exhibits improved mental functioning

For more information, see Chapter 38 in Smeltzer and Bare: *Brunner and Suddarth's Textbook of Medical-Surgical Nursing,* 9th edition. Philadelphia: Lippincott Williams & Wilkins, 2000.

CYSTITIS (LOWER URINARY TRACT INFECTION)

Cystitis is an inflammation of the urinary bladder. The most common route of infection is transurethral, often from fecal contamination, ureterovesical reflux, or the use of a catheter or cystoscope. Bacteria may enter the urinary tract through the blood (hematogenous spread) from a distant site of infection or through direct extension by way of a fistula from the gut. *Escherichia coli,* accounts for 80% to 90% of uncomplicated urinary tract infections (UTIs), and *Staphylococcus saprophyticus* accounts for another 10% to 15%. Cystitis occurs more often in women, particularly sexually active women. Cystitis in men is secondary to some other factor (eg, infected prostate, epididymitis, or bladder stones).

Clinical Manifestations
- Urgency, frequency, burning, and pain on urination
- Nocturia, incontinence, and back, suprapubic, or pelvic pain
- Pyuria, bacteria, and hematuria
- With complicated UTIs (eg, patients with indwelling catheters), symptoms can range from asymptomatic bacteriuria to a gram-negative sepsis with shock
- Elderly patients often lack the typical symptoms of UTI and sepsis; nonspecific symptoms, such as altered sensorium, lethargy, anorexia, new incontinence, hyperventilation, and low-grade fever may be the only clues in these patients

Diagnostic Evaluation
- Urinalysis, leukocyte esterase test, and nitrites (Griess nitrate reduction test)
- Urine culture
- Tests for sexually transmitted diseases (STDs)
- Computerized tomography (CT) scans and ultrasonography

Medical Management
- Drug therapy and patient education are the key treatment measures.
- UTIs may require 7 to 10 days of medication, or a short course (3 to 4 days) may be effective; antibiotic use in treatment of asymptomatic bacteriuria in the institutionalized elderly patient is controversial.

- Ideal treatment is an antibacterial agent that effectively eradicates bacteria from the urinary tract with minimal effects on fecal and vaginal flora.
- Medications may include sulfisoxazole (Gantrisin); co-trimoxazole (trimethoprim-sulfamethoxazole [Bactrim, Septra]), the drug of choice; or nitrofurantoin (Macrodantin).
- Occasionally, ampicillin or amoxicillin (but *E. coli* has developed resistance to these agents).

Recurrence
- About 20% of women treated for uncomplicated UTIs experience a recurrence.
- Repeated infections at close intervals suggest a cause for referral to a urologist to investigate and correct abnormalities.
- Recurrence in men is usually due to persistence of the same organism; further evaluation and treatment are indicated.
- Reinfection of women with new bacteria is more common than persistence of the initial bacteria.
- If diagnostic evaluation reveals no structural abnormalities, patient may be instructed to begin treatment on own, testing urine with a dipstick whenever symptoms occur, and to contact health care provider only with persistence of symptoms, at the occurrence of fever, or if the number of treatment episodes exceeds four in a 6-month period.
- Long-term use of antimicrobial agents decreases risk of reinfection.

Nursing Management
Assessment
- Take careful history of urinary signs and symptoms.
- Assess presence of pain, frequency, urgency, and hesitancy and changes in urine.
- Determine usual pattern of voiding to detect factors that may predispose the patient to infection.

- Assess for infrequent emptying of the bladder, association of symptoms of UTIs with sexual intercourse, contraceptive practices, and personal hygiene.
- Check urine for volume, color, concentration, cloudiness, and odor.

Major Nursing Diagnoses
- Pain related to inflammation and infection of the urethra, bladder, and other urinary tract structures
- Knowledge deficit related to factors predisposing to infection and recurrence, detection and prevention of recurrence, and pharmacologic therapy

Collaborative Problems/Potential Complications
- Renal failure due to extensive damage of kidney
- Sepsis

Planning and Goals
Major goals of the patient may include relief of pain and discomfort; increased knowledge of preventive measures and treatment modalities; and absence of complications.

Nursing Interventions
RELIEVING PAIN
- Use antispasmodic drugs to relieve bladder irritability and pain.
- Relieve pain and spasm with aspirin and heat to the perineum (hot tub baths).
- Encourage patient to drink liberal amounts of fluid (water is best); provide adequate hydration to patients at risk for dehydration (surgical patients, patients having diagnostic tests).
- Instruct patient to avoid urinary tract irritants (eg, coffee, citrus, spices, alcohol).
- Encourage frequent voiding (every 2 to 3 hours).

MONITORING AND MANAGING COMPLICATIONS
- Recognize and teach patient to recognize the signs and symptoms of UTIs early; initiate prompt treatment.

- Manage UTIs with appropriate antimicrobial therapy, liberalization of fluids, frequent voiding, and hygienic measures.
- Notify physician if fatigue, nausea, vomiting, or pruritus occurs.
- Provide for periodic monitoring of renal function.
- Avoid indwelling catheters if possible; remove at earliest opportunity.
- Provide strict aseptic technique if an indwelling catheter is necessary.
- Check vital signs and level of consciousness for impending sepsis.
- Report positive blood cultures and elevated white blood cell counts.

Promoting Home and Community-Based Care

Teaching Patients Self-Care

- Teach patient to reduce concentrations of pathogens of the vaginal opening by hygienic measures: cleanse around the perineum and urethral meatus after bowel movement with front-to-back motion.
- Advise to drink liberal amounts of fluid during the day to flush out bacteria, avoiding coffee, tea, colas, and alcohol.
- Recommend voiding every 2 to 3 hours during the day, completely emptying the bladder.
- If sexual intercourse is the initiating event for development of bacteriuria, void immediately after sexual intercourse, and take prescribed single-dose oral antimicrobial agent.
- Instruct patient to take medication after emptying bladder before going to bed to ensure adequate concentration of the drug during the night.
- Instruct patient to monitor and test urine for bacteria with dip slides (Microstix).
- Emphasize importance of seeing health care provider regularly for follow-up, recurrence of symptoms, and infection that is nonresponsive to treatment.

Evaluation

EXPECTED OUTCOMES

- Experiences relief of pain
- Understands UTIs and their treatment
- Experiences no complications

For more information, see Chapter 41 in Smeltzer and Bare: *Brunner and Suddarth's Textbook of Medical-Surgical Nursing,* 9th edition. Philadelphia: Lippincott Williams & Wilkins, 2000.

D

DIABETES INSIPIDUS

Diabetes insipidus is a disorder of the posterior lobe of the pituitary gland due to a deficiency of vasopressin, the anti-diuretic hormone (ADH). It is characterized by polydipsia and polyuria. Diabetes insipidus may be (1) secondary, related to head trauma, brain tumor, or surgical ablation or irradiation of the pituitary gland or to infections of the central nervous system or metastatic tumors (lung or breast); (2) nephrogenic (failure of the renal tubules to respond to ADH), possibly related to hypokalemia, hypercalcemia, and a variety of medications (eg, lithium, demeclocycline); (3) primary (hereditary), with symptoms possibly beginning at birth (defect in pituitary gland). The disease cannot be controlled by limiting the intake of fluids because loss of high volumes of urine continues even without fluid replacement. Attempts to restrict fluids cause the patient to experience an insatiable craving for fluid and to develop hypernatremia and severe dehydration.

Clinical Manifestations
- Polyuria: enormous daily output of very dilute urine; specific gravity 1.001 to 1.005; primary diabetes insipidus may have an abrupt onset or an insidious onset in adults.
- Polydipsia: patient experiences intense thirst, drinking 4 to 40 liters of fluid daily, with a special craving for cold water.
- Polyuria continues even without fluid replacement.

Diagnostic Evaluation
- Fluid deprivation test: fluids are withheld for 8 to 12 hours until 3% to 5% of the body weight is lost. Inability to increase specific gravity and osmolality of the urine during test is characteristic of diabetes insipidus.
- Specific gravity, serum osmolality, and serum sodium levels may be obtained.

Medical Management
The objectives of therapy are to ensure adequate fluid replacement, to replace vasopressin, and to search for and correct the underlying intracranial pathology.

Vasopressin Replacement
- Desmopressin (DDAVP), administered intranasally, two to four administrations daily to control symptoms
- Lypressin (Diapid), absorbed through nasal mucosa into blood; duration may be short for patients with severe disease
- Intramuscular administration of ADH (vasopressin tannate in oil) every 24 to 96 hours to reduce urinary volume; rotation of injection sites to prevent lipodystrophy

Fluid Conservation
- Clofibrate, a hypolipidemic agent, has an antidiuretic effect on patients who have some residual hypothalamic vasopressin.
- Chlorpropamide (Diabinese) and thiazide diuretics are used in mild forms to potentiate the action of vasopressin; may cause hypoglycemic reactions.

Nephrogenic Origin
- Thiazide diuretics, mild salt depletion, prostaglandin inhibitors (eg, ibuprofen, indomethacin), and aspirin

Nursing Management
Nursing Interventions
- Encourage and support patient while undergoing studies for possible cranial lesion.
- Instruct patient and family members about follow-up care and emergency measures.
- Advise patient to wear a medical alert bracelet and to carry medication information about this disorder at all times.
- Use caution with administration of vasopressin if coronary artery disease is present because of vasoconstriction.

For more information, see Chapter 38 in Smeltzer and Bare: *Brunner and Suddarth's Textbook of Medical-Surgical Nursing,* 9th edition. Philadelphia: Lippincott Williams & Wilkins, 2000.

DIABETES MELLITUS

Diabetes mellitus is a group of metabolic disorders characterized by elevated levels of blood glucose (hyperglycemia) resulting from defects in insulin production and secretion, decreased cellular response to insulin, or both. This leads to hyperglycemia, which may lead to acute metabolic complications, such as diabetic ketoacidosis (DKA) and hyperglycemic hyperosmolar nonketotic (HHNS) syndrome. Long-term hyperglycemia may contribute to chronic microvascular complications (kidney and eye disease) and neuropathic complications. Diabetes is also associated with an increased occurrence of macrovascular diseases, including coronary artery disease (myocardial infarction), cerebrovascular disease (stroke), and peripheral vascular disease.

Types of Diabetes
Type 1: Insulin-Dependent Diabetes Mellitus
- About 5% to 10% of diabetic patients have type 1 diabetes. Beta cells of the pancreas that normally produce insulin are destroyed by an autoimmune process.

Insulin injections are needed to control the blood glucose levels.
- Type 1 diabetes has a sudden onset, usually before the age of 30 years.

Type 2: Non–Insulin-Dependent Diabetes Mellitus
- About 90% to 95% of diabetics have type 2 diabetes. It results from a decreased sensitivity to insulin (insulin resistance) or from a decreased amount of insulin production.
- Type 2 diabetes occurs most frequently in patients older than 30 years of age and in obese patients.

Gestational Diabetes Mellitus
- Gestatational diabetes is characterized by any degree of glucose intolerance with onset during pregnancy (second or third trimester).
- It occurs in women 25 years of age or older, women younger than 25 years of age and obese, women with a family history of diabetes in first-degree relatives, or members of certain ethnic racial groups (eg, Hispanic American, native American, Asian American, African American, or Pacific Islander).

Clinical Manifestations
- Polyuria, polydipsia, and polyphagia
- Fatigue and weakness, sudden vision changes, tingling or numbness in hands or feet, dry skin, sores that heal slowly and recurrent infections. The onset of type 1 diabetes may be associated with nausea, vomiting, or stomach pains.
- Type 2 diabetes results from a slow (over years), progressive glucose intolerance and results in long-term complications if diabetes goes undetected for many years (eg, eye disease, peripheral neuropathy, peripheral vascular disease), which may have developed before the actual diagnosis is made.
- DKA causes signs and symptoms of abdominal pain, nausea, vomiting, hyperventilation, fruity odor of

breath; if untreated, altered level of consciousness, coma, and death can occur.

Diagnostic Evaluation
- Presence of abnormally high blood glucose levels: fasting plasma glucose levels equal to or above 126 mg/dL or random plasma glucose levels of more than 200 mg/dL on more than one occasion
- Glucose tolerance test: oral or intravenous

Medical Management
The main goal of treatment is to try to normalize insulin activity and blood glucose levels to reduce the development of vascular and neuropathic complications. The therapeutic goal within each type of diabetes is to achieve normal blood glucose levels (euglycemia) without hypoglycemia and without seriously disrupting the patient's usual activities. There are five components of management for diabetes: nutrition, exercise, monitoring, pharmacologic therapy, and education.
- Primary treatment of type 1 diabetes is insulin.
- Primary treatment of type 2 diabetes is weight loss.
- Exercise is important in enhancing the effectiveness of insulin.
- Use oral hypoglycemia agents if diet and exercise are not successful in controlling blood glucose levels.
- Because treatment varies throughout course because of changes in lifestyle and physical and emotional status as well as advances in therapy, continuously assess and modify treatment plan as well as daily adjustments in therapy. Also, it is essential to provide education to both patient and family.

Nutrition Management
- Provision of all the essential food constituents (eg, vitamins, minerals)
- Achievement and maintenance of ideal weight; meeting energy needs

- Prevention of wide daily fluctuations in blood glucose levels; keep as close to normal as is safe and practical
- Decrease of blood lipid levels, if elevated
- For patients who require insulin to help control blood glucose levels: maintain consistency in the number of calories and carbohydrates eaten at different mealtimes.
- For obese patients (especially type 2 diabetes): weight loss is the key to the treatment and the major preventive factor for the development of diabetes
- Consult with dietitian to plan gradual increase or addition of fiber in the meal plan (grains, vegetables)

Caloric Requirements

- Determine basic caloric requirements, taking into consideration age, gender, body weight, and height and factoring in degree of activity (Harris-Benedict formula for basal energy expenditure).
- Long-term weight reduction can be achieved (1- to 2-pound loss per week) by reducing basic caloric intake by 500 to 1000 calories from calculated basic caloric requirements.
- The American Diabetes and American Dietetic Associations recommend that for all levels of caloric intake, 50% to 60% of calories be derived from carbohydrates, 20% to 30% from fat, and the remaining 10% to 20% from protein.

Complications of Diabetes

Complications associated with both types of diabetes are classified as acute or chronic.

ACUTE

Acute complications occur from short-term imbalances in blood glucose.

- Hypoglycemia
- DKA
- HHNS syndrome

CHRONIC
- Generally occur 10 to 15 years after onset
- Macrovascular (large vessel disease): affects coronary, peripheral vascular, and cerebral vascular circulations
- Microvascular (small vessel disease): affects the eyes (retinopathy) and kidneys (neuropathy); control blood glucose levels to delay or avoid onset of both microvascular and macrovascular complications
- Neuropathic diseases: affect sensory motor and autonomic nerves and contribute to such problems as impotence and foot ulcers

Nursing Management: The Patient With Newly Diagnosed Diabetes Mellitus
Assessment
- Focus on signs and symptoms of prolonged hyperglycemia and physical, social, and emotional factors that affect ability to learn and perform diabetes self-care activities.
- Ask for a description of symptoms that preceded the diagnosis: polyuria, polydipsia, polyphagia, skin dryness, blurred vision, weight loss, vaginal itching, and nonhealing ulcers.
- Assess for signs of DKA, including ketonuria, Kussmaul respirations, orthostatic hypotension, and lethargy.
- Question regarding DKA symptoms of nausea, vomiting, and abdominal pain.
- Monitor laboratory signs for metabolic acidosis (decreased pH, decreased bicarbonate) and for signs of electrolyte imbalance.
- Assess patients with type 2 diabetes for signs of HHNS: hypotension, altered sensorium, seizures, decreased skin turgor, hyperosmolarity, and electrolyte imbalance.
- Assess physical factors that impair ability to learn or perform self-care skills: visual defects, motor coordination defects, neurologic defects.
- Evaluate patient's social situation for factors that influence diabetic treatment and education plan, such as

decreased literacy; limited financial resources or lack of health insurance; presence or absence of family support; typical daily schedule (eg, work, meals, exercise, travel plans).

- Assess emotional status through observation of general demeanor (eg, withdrawn, anxious, and body language).
- Assess coping skills by asking how the patient has dealt with difficult situations in the past.

Major Nursing Diagnoses
- Risk for fluid volume deficit related to polyuria and dehydration
- Altered nutrition related to imbalance of insulin, food, and physical activity
- Knowledge deficit about diabetes self-care skills and information
- Potential self-care deficit related to physical impairments or social factors
- Anxiety related to loss of control, fear of inability to manage diabetes, misinformation related to diabetes, and fear of diabetes complications
- Risk for complications

Collaborative Problems/Potential Complications
- Fluid overload, pulmonary edema, congestive heart failure
- Hypokalemia
- Hyperglycemia and DKA
- Hypoglycemia
- Cerebral edema

Planning and Goals
The major goals of the patient may include attainment of fluid and electrolyte balance, optimal control of blood glucose, regaining weight lost, ability to perform basic (survival) diabetes skills and self-care activities, reduction in anxiety, and absence of complications.

Nursing Interventions

MAINTAINING FLUID AND ELECTROLYTE BALANCE
- Measure intake and output.
- Administer intravenous fluids and electrolytes as ordered.
- Encourage fluid intake.
- Measure serum electrolytes (sodium, potassium), and monitor closely.
- Monitor vital signs to detect dehydration: tachycardia, orthostatic hypotension.

IMPROVING NUTRITIONAL INTAKE
- Plan the diet with glucose control as the primary goal.
- Take into consideration the patient's lifestyle, cultural background, activity level, and food preferences.
- Encourage the patient to eat full meals and snacks as per diabetic diet.
- Make arrangements for extra snacks before increased physical activity.
- Ensure that insulin orders are altered as needed for delays in eating due to diagnostic and other procedures.

REDUCING ANXIETY
- Provide emotional support; set aside time to talk with patient.
- Clear up misconceptions patient or family may have regarding diabetes.
- Assist patient and family to focus on learning self-care behaviors.
- Encourage patient to perform the skills feared most: self-injection or finger stick for glucose monitoring.
- Give positive reinforcement for self-care behaviors attempted.

MONITORING AND MANAGING
POTENTIAL COMPLICATIONS
- Fluid overload: measure vital signs and monitor central venous pressure (CVP) and total hemodynamic status at frequent intervals; assess cardiac rate and rhythm, breath

sounds, venous distention, skin turgor, and urine output; monitor intravenous fluid and other fluid intake.

D

- Hypokalemia: replace potassium cautiously, ensure that kidneys are functioning before administration; monitor cardiac rate, rhythm, electrocardiogram (ECG), and serum potassium levels.
- Hyperglycemia and DKA: monitor blood glucose levels and urine ketones; administer medications (insulin, oral hypoglycemic agents); monitor for signs and symptoms of impending hyperglycemia and DKA, administering insulin and intravenous fluids to correct.
- Hypoglycemia: treat with juice or glucose tablets; encourage patient to eat full meals or snacks as prescribed; review signs and symptoms, possible causes, and measures to prevent or treat.
- Cerebral edema: prevent by gradual reduction in the blood glucose level; monitor blood glucose level, serum electrolyte levels, urine output, mental status, and neurologic signs; minimize activities that increase intracranial pressure.

Providing Home and Community-Based Care

Teaching Patients Self-Care

- Teach patient survival skills, including simple pathophysiology, treatment modalities, recognition and prevention of acute complications, and pragmatic information (where to obtain supplies, when to call physician).
- Teach preventive behaviors for long-term diabetic complications.

Continuing Care

SPECIALIZED PATIENT EDUCATION
AND HOME HEALTH CARE

- Provide special equipment for instruction on diabetic survival skills (eg, magnifying glass for insulin preparation or injection aid device for insulin injection).
- Tailor information according to patient's ability to understand.

- Instruct family so that they may assist in diabetes management.
- Recommend follow-up education with outpatient diabetic specialist regarding optimal equipment for patients with physical impairment; recommend and arrange for home care nurse, as indicated.
- Assist in identifying community resources for education and supplies, giving consideration to financial and physical limitations.

HEALTH TEACHING ABOUT NUTRITION

- Initial education addresses the importance of consistency in eating and snacking habits, the relationship of food and insulin, and provision of individualized meal plan.
- Follow-up education focuses on more in-depth management skills, such as restaurant eating, food labeling, and adjusting meals for exercise, illness, and special occasions.
- Determine whether patient is able to learn and use the exchange system.
- Simplify information, and provide many opportunities for practice and repetition.
- Teach patients to read labels of "health" foods because they often contain sugar products (ie, honey, brown sugar, and corn syrup) and may contain saturated vegetable fats, hydrogenated vegetable fats, or animal fats that may be contraindicated with elevated blood lipids.

EXERCISE

- Exercise is extremely important because of its effects on lowering blood glucose and reducing cardiovascular risk factors.
- Exercise is useful in losing weight, easing stress, and maintaining a feeling of well-being.
- Exercise alters blood lipids, increasing levels of high-density lipoproteins (HDL) and decreasing total cholesterol and triglyceride levels.
- Teach patient with blood glucose levels of more than 250 mg/dL not to begin exercising until the urine

ketone test is negative and blood glucose levels are closer to normal. (High blood glucose levels stimulate secretion of glucagon, growth hormone, and catecholamines, resulting in release of more glucose from the liver and increase in blood glucose.)

- Teach patient to eat a 15-gram carbohydrate snack (fruit exchange) or a snack of complex carbohydrates with protein before moderate exercise to prevent hypoglycemia.
- Be aware of postexercise hypoglycemia that occurs many hours after exercise.
- Test blood glucose before, during, and after exercise and eat carbohydrate snacks as needed to maintain blood glucose; reduce dosage of insulin that peaks at the time of exercise if necessary.
- Exercise and dietary management improves glucose metabolism and enhances loss of body fat in people with type 2 diabetes.
- Exercise, coupled with weight loss, improves insulin sensitivity and may decrease need for insulin or oral agents in type 2 diabetes.
- Encourage regular daily exercise rather than sporadic exercise.
- All patients with diabetes should discuss an exercise program with their physician.

SELF-MONITORING OF BLOOD GLUCOSE

- Self-monitoring of blood glucose (SMBG) allows adjustment in the treatment regimen for optimal blood glucose and motivates patients to continue treatment.
- Provide initial training in SMBG techniques.
- Evaluate the techniques of patients "experienced" in self-monitoring.
- Discourage patient purchasing of SMBG products from stores or catalogs that do not provide direct education.
- Ensure that method used by patients is matched to their skill level, visual acuity, fine-motor coordination, cognitive ability, comfort with technology, willingness, and cost.

- Instruct patient to keep a record of blood glucose results.

GLYCOSYLATED HEMOGLOBIN

- A blood test is used that reflects average blood glucose levels over a period of about 2 to 3 months (normal values, 4% to 8%).
- Determine presence of errors in methods of SMBG if glycosylated hemoglobin is high but patient reports mostly normal results of glucose self-monitoring.

URINE TESTING FOR KETONES (ACETONE)

- Instruct patient in procedure for urine testing if patient with type 1 diabetes has glucosuria or unexplained elevated blood glucose levels (more than 250 mg/dL) and for use during illness and pregnancy.

INSULIN THERAPY

- Insulin preparations vary according to four main characteristics: time course of action, concentration, species (source), and manufacturer.
- Time course: insulins may be grouped into three categories based on onset, peak, and duration of action.
- Short-acting insulin includes regular insulin (marked "R" on the bottle), also known as crystalline zinc insulin (CZI); it is clear in appearance. Onset of regular insulin is 30 minutes to 1 hour; peak, 2 to 4 hours; duration, 6 to 8 hours.
- Intermediate-acting insulins include NPH insulin and Lente ("L") insulin and are white and milky in appearance.
- Onset of intermediate-acting insulins is 3 to 4 hours; peak, 4 to 12 hours; duration, 16 to 20 hours.
- Long-acting insulin includes Ultralente ("UL") insulin, which has a long, slow, sustained action with an onset of 6 to 8 hours; peak, 12 to 16 hours; duration, 20 to 30 hours.
- U-100 is the most common concentration of insulin in the United States (100 units of insulin per 1 cubic centimeter).

Problems With Insulin
- Local allergic reactions may occur in the form of redness, swelling, tenderness, and induration up to 1 to 2 hours after the injection is given.
- Systemic allergic reactions are rare and occasionally associated with generalized edema or anaphylaxis.
- Insulin lipodystrophy is a localized disturbance of fat metabolism, prevented by rotating injection sites and avoiding injecting insulin into the hypertrophied areas.
- Clinical insulin resistance may occur because immune antibodies develop and bind the insulin, decreasing availability for use; treat by administering a purer insulin preparation and occasionally prednisone to block the production of antibodies.
- Morning hyperglycemia may be noted. This includes the dawn phenomenon (glucose level rises after 3:00 AM), which occurs as insulin is waning, causing a progressive increase in glucose; and the Somogyi effect (nocturnal hypoglycemia followed by rebound hyperglycemia).
  - Instruct patient with insulin waning to move the evening dose of NPH insulin to bedtime (from before dinner).
  - Instruct patient and family to test blood glucose levels at bedtime, at 3:00 AM, and on awakening.

ORAL HYPOGLYCEMIC AGENTS
- Oral hypoglycemic agents may be effective for type 2 diabetic patients who cannot be treated by diet and exercise. A functioning pancreas is necessary for these agents to be effective, and they cannot be used in the treatment of type 1 diabetes, in patients prone to DKA, or during pregnancy.
- Hypoglycemia may occur when an excessive dose of an oral hypoglycemic is used, meals are omitted, or food intake is decreased.
- Avoid ingestion of alcohol because a disulfiram (Antabuse) type of reaction may occur.
- Oral hypoglycemic drugs may be discontinued temporarily when insulin is needed if the patient

develops hyperglycemia due to infection, trauma, or surgery.

PROMOTING COMPLIANCE

- Avoid the use of "scare" tactics (blindness or amputation) if patient does not comply with the treatment plan.
- Do not judge the patient; it only promotes feelings of guilt and low self-esteem.
- Distinguish among problems of compliance, knowledge deficit, and self-care deficit, and do not assume that problems with diabetes are related to nonadherence.
- Recognize that physical (eg, visual acuity) and emotional factors may impair the patient's ability to perform self-care skills.
- Assess for signs of infection or emotional stress that lead to elevated glucose levels despite adherence to treatment regimen.

❧ Gerontologic Considerations

- Elevation of blood glucose increases in frequency with advancing age.
- Physical activity that is consistent and realistic is beneficial to the elderly with diabetes.
- Advantages of exercise include a decrease in hyperglycemia, general sense of well-being, use of ingested calories, and weight reduction. Consider physical impairment from other chronic diseases when planning an exercise regimen.

For more information, see Chapter 37 in Smeltzer and Bare: *Brunner and Suddarth's Textbook of Medical-Surgical Nursing,* 9th edition. Philadelphia: Lippincott Williams & Wilkins, 2000.

DIABETIC KETOACIDOSIS

Diabetic ketoacidosis (DKA) is caused by an absence or inadequate amount of insulin. This results in disorders in the metabolism of carbohydrates, protein, and fat. The three main clinical features of DKA are (1) hyperglycemia, due to decreased use of glucose by the cells and increased production of glucose by the liver; (2) dehydration and electrolyte loss, resulting from polyuria, with a loss of up to 6.5 liters of water and up to 400 to 500 mEq each of sodium, potassium, and chloride over 24 hours; and (3) acidosis, due to an excess breakdown of fat to fatty acids and production of ketone bodies, which are also acids. Three main causes of DKA are (1) decreased or missed dose of insulin, (2) illness or infection, and (3) initial manifestation of undiagnosed or untreated diabetes.

Clinical Manifestations
- Polyuria and polydipsia (increased thirst)
- Blurred vision, weakness, and headache
- Orthostatic hypotension in patients with volume depletion
- Weak, rapid pulse
- Gastrointestinal symptoms, such as anorexia, nausea, and abdominal pain (may be severe)
- Acetone breath (fruity odor)
- Kussmaul respirations: hyperventilation with very deep, but not labored, respirations
- Mental status changes, which vary widely from patient to patient (alert to lethargic or comatose)

Laboratory Values
- Blood glucose: 300 to 800 mg/dL (may be lower or higher)
- Low serum bicarbonate: 0 to 15 mEq/L
- Low pH: 6.8 to 7.3; low pCO_2: 10 to 30 mm Hg
- Sodium and potassium levels may be low, normal, or high depending on amount of water loss (dehydration)

- Elevated creatinine, blood urea nitrogen (BUN), hemoglobin, and hematocrit may be seen with dehydration

Medical Management
Treatment of DKA is aimed at correcting hyperglycemia, dehydration, electrolyte loss, and acidosis.

Dehydration
- Patients may need up to 6 to 10 liters of intravenous fluid (0.9% normal saline is administered at a high rate of 0.5 to 1 L/h for 2 to 3 hours) to replace fluid loss caused by polyuria, hyperventilation, diarrhea, and vomiting.
- Hypotonic normal saline of 0.45% may be used for hypertension or hypernatremia or congestive heart failure.
- 0.45% normal saline (200 to 500 mL/h for several additional hours) is fluid of choice after the first few hours provided blood pressure is stable and sodium level is not low.
- Use plasma expanders for correction of severe hypotension that does not respond to intravenous fluid treatment.

Electrolyte Loss
- Potassium is the main electrolyte of concern in treating DKA.
- Cautious replacement of potassium is vital for avoidance of severe cardiac dysrhythmias that occur with hypokalemia.

Acidosis
- Acidosis of DKA is reversed with insulin, which inhibits the fat breakdown.
- Infuse insulin (regular insulin only) at a slow, continuous rate (eg, 5 units per hour).
- Add dextrose to intravenous fluids (D5W) when blood glucose reaches 300 mg/dL or less to avoid too rapid a drop in blood glucose.

- Intravenous insulin must be infused continuously until subcutaneous administration of insulin is resumed.
- Intravenous insulin must be continued until the serum bicarbonate improves and patient can eat; normalized blood glucose levels are not an indication that acidosis has resolved.

Nursing Management
Nursing Interventions
PROMOTING FLUID BALANCE
- Administer fluids as ordered, and monitor infusion carefully.
- Monitor fluid volume status (including checking for orthostatic changes of blood pressure and heart rate), lung assessment, and intake and output (initial urine output will lag behind intravenous fluid intake until dehydration is corrected).
- Monitor for signs of fluid overload in elderly patients and those at risk for congestive heart failure.

PROMOTING ELECTROLYTE AND
ACID–BASE BALANCE
- Observe frequently for signs of hyperkalemia (ie, tall, peaked T waves on the electrocardiogram [ECG]) and obtain frequent (every 2 to 4 hours) potassium values during first 8 hours of treatment.
- Withhold potassium only if hyperkalemia is present and patient is not urinating; notify physician.
- Administer continuous insulin drip as ordered, and monitor blood glucose values hourly.

Promoting Home and Community-Based Care

Teaching Patients Self-Care
- Teach prevention: sick-day rules.
  - Teach patient not to eliminate insulin doses when sick and nausea and vomiting occur.

- ○ Teach patient to take usual insulin dose or previously prescribed sick-day doses, and attempt to consume frequent small portions of carbohydrates.
- ○ Teach patient to drink fluid every hour including broth for avoidance of dehydration.
- ○ Check blood glucose level every 3 to 4 hours.
- ○ Notify physician if unable to take fluids without vomiting or if elevated glucose level persists.
- ○ Teach patients how to contact their physician 24 hours a day.
- Teach self-management skills.
  - ○ Insulin administration
  - ○ Blood glucose and urine ketone testing
- Assess skills to ensure that accidental error in insulin administration or blood glucose testing did not occur.
- Recommend psychological counseling for patient and family if intentional alteration in insulin dosing was the cause of DKA.

For more information, see Chapter 37 in Smeltzer and Bare: *Brunner and Suddarth's Textbook of Medical-Surgical Nursing,* 9th edition. Philadelphia: Lippincott Williams & Wilkins, 2000.

DIARRHEA

Diarrhea is a condition defined by an increased frequency of bowel movements (more than three per day), increased amount of stool (more than 200 per day), and altered consistency (liquid stool). It is usually associated with urgency, perianal discomfort, incontinence, or a combination of these factors. Diarrhea can result from any condition that causes increased intestinal secretions, decreased mucosal absorption, or altered (increased) motility. It can be acute (self-limiting and often associated with infection) or chronic (persists for a long period and may return sporadically). It is classified as secretory (high volume), osmotic (nonabsorbed particles), or mixed (includes inflammatory bowel disease). It can be caused by certain medications, tube feedings, metabolic and endocrine disorders, and viral and bacterial infections. Other causes are nutritional and malabsorptive disorders, anal sphincter deficit, Zollinger-Ellison syndrome, paralytic ileus, acquired immunodeficiency syndrome (AIDS), and intestinal obstruction.

Clinical Manifestations
- Increased frequency and fluid content of the stool
- Abdominal cramps, distention, intestinal rumbling (borborygmus), anorexia, and thirst
- Painful spasmodic contractions of the anus and ineffectual straining (tenesmus) with each defecation
- Other symptoms, depending on the cause and severity and related to dehydration and fluid and electrolyte imbalances
- Watery stools, which may indicate small bowel disease
- Loose, semisolid stools, which are associated with disorders of the colon
- Voluminous greasy stools, which suggest intestinal malabsorption
- Mucus and pus in the stools, which denote inflammatory enteritis or colitis
- Oil droplets on the toilet water, which are diagnostic of pancreatic insufficiency
- Nocturnal diarrhea, which may be a manifestation of diabetic neuropathy
- Complications: cardiac dysrhythmias due to fluid and electrolyte (potassium) imbalance, urinary output less than 30 mL/h, muscle weakness, paresthesia, hypotension, anorexia, drowsiness (report if potassium level is less than 3 mEq/L), and death if imbalances become severe

Diagnostic Evaluation
When cause is unknown: stool examination for infectious or parasitic organisms, complete blood count, chemical profile, endoscopy, or barium enema.

Medical Management

- Primary medical management is directed at controlling symptoms, preventing complications, and eliminating or treating the underlying disease.
- Certain medications (eg, antibiotics, antiinflammatory agents) may reduce the severity of diarrhea and the disease.
- Increase oral fluids; oral glucose and electrolyte solution may be prescribed.
- Antidiarrheals, such as diphenoxylate (Lomotil) and loperamide (Imodium), may be prescribed to decrease motility from a noninfectious source.
- Antimicrobials are prescribed when the infectious agent has been identified or diarrhea is severe.
- Intravenous therapy is used for rapid hydration in very young or elderly patients.

Nursing Management

Assessment

- Elicit a complete health history to identify character and pattern of diarrhea, and the presence of the following: any related signs and symptoms; current medication therapy; daily dietary patterns and intake; past related medical and surgical history; and recent exposure to an acute illness or travel to another geographic area.
- Perform a complete physical assessment, paying special attention to auscultation (characteristic bowel sounds), palpation for abdominal tenderness, inspection of stool (obtain a sample for testing).
- Inspect mucous membranes and skin to determine hydration status, and assess blood pressure (postural hypotension).
- Inspect perianal skin for irritation; note intake and output and weight.

Major Nursing Diagnoses

- Diarrhea related to infection, ingestion of irritating foods, or disorder of the bowel.

D

- Risk for fluid volume deficit related to frequent passage of stools and insufficient fluid intake.
- Anxiety related to frequent, uncontrolled elimination.
- Risk for impaired skin integrity related to frequent, loose stools.

Collaborative Problems/Potential Complications
- Dehydration
- Fluid and electrolyte imbalance
- Cardiac dysrhythmias

Planning and Goals
The major goals may include regaining normal bowel patterns, avoidance of fluid and electrolyte deficit, reduction of anxiety, maintenance of perianal skin integrity, and absence of potential complications.

Nursing Interventions
CONTROLLING DIARRHEA
- Encourage bed rest, liquids, and foods low in bulk until acute period subsides.
- Recommend bland diet (semisolids to solids) when food intake is tolerated.
- Limit caffeine and carbonated beverage, and avoid very hot and cold foods because these increase intestinal motility.
- Restrict milk products, fat, whole grain products, fresh fruits, and vegetables for several days.
- Administer antidiarrheal drugs as prescribed.

MAINTAINING FLUID AND ELECTROLYTE BALANCE
- Assess for dehydration (decreased skin turgor, tachycardia, decreased pulse volume, decreased serum sodium, thirst).
- Administer intravenous fluids if ordered for rapid rehydration (in elderly patients or those with preexisting gastrointestinal disturbance).

- Encourage oral fluid replacement in the form of water, juices, bouillon, and commercial preparations, such as Gatorade; give parenteral fluids as ordered.
- Monitor serum electrolyte levels closely.
- Report evidence of dysrhythmias or change in level of consciousness immediately.

NURSING ALERT

Older people can quickly become dehydrated and suffer from low potassium levels (hypokalemia) as a result of diarrhea. Teach the older patient taking digitalis about how quickly dehydration and hypokalemia can occur with diarrhea. Instruct the patient to recognize the signs of hypokalemia (which intensifies the action of digitalis, leading to digitalis toxicity).

REDUCING ANXIETY

- Provide opportunity for patient to express fears or worry about being embarrassed by lack of control over bowel elimination.
- Assist to identify any factors that precipitate diarrhea. Teach patient to be sensitive to body clues, use absorbent underwear, and take prescribed antianxiety medications.

PROVIDING SKIN CARE

- Instruct patient to follow a perianal care routine, such as wiping or patting the area dry after defecation, cleansing with mild soap and warm water, and patting dry.
- Apply lotion or ointment as a skin barrier; a skin sealant may be used.
- Treat all patients with diarrhea as potentially infectious; use gloves and standard precautions, as with all patients.

🍁 Gerontologic Considerations

Skin in elderly people is sensitive to rapid perianal excoriation because of decreased turgor and reduced subcutaneous fat layers.

For more information, see Chapter 35 in Smeltzer and Bare: *Brunner and Suddarth's Textbook of Medical-Surgical Nursing,* 9th edition. Philadelphia: Lippincott Williams & Wilkins, 2000.

D

DISSEMINATED INTRAVASCULAR COAGULOPATHY (DIC)

Disseminated intravascular coagulopathy (DIC) is a potentially life-threatening sign (not a disease itself) of a serious underlying disease mechanism. The normal hemostatic mechanisms are altered, so that tiny clots form within the microcirculation of the body. These clots consume platelets and clotting factors, eventually causing coagulation to fail and bleeding to result. This bleeding disorder is characterized by low fibrinogen levels; prolonged prothrombin time (PT), partial thromboplastin time (PTT), and thrombin time; low platelet counts (thrombocytopenia); and elevated fibrin split products. Many serious illnesses may predispose a patient to DIC, including septicemia, premature separation of the placenta in pregnancy, metastatic malignancies, hemolytic transfusion reactions, massive tissue trauma, and shock.

Clinical Manifestations

The clinical manifestations of DIC are reflected in the organs affected either by excessive clot formation (with resultant ischemia to that organ or part of organ) or bleeding.

- Patients with DIC may bleed from mucous membranes, venipuncture sites, and the gastrointestinal and urinary tracts.
- The bleeding can range from minimal occult internal bleeding to profuse hemorrhage from all orifices.
- Patients may also develop organ dysfunction, such as renal failure and pulmonary and multifocal central nervous system infarctions due to microthrombosis, macrothrombosis, or hemorrhage.

- Initially, the only manifestation is a progressive decrease in the platelet count, then progressively, the patient exhibits signs and symptoms of thrombosis in the organs involved. Eventually bleeding occurs (at first subtle, advancing to frank hemorrhage). Signs depend on the organs involved.

Medical Management

- The most important management issue is treating the underlying cause of DIC.
- A second goal is to correct the secondary effects of tissue ischemia by improving oxygenation, replacing fluids, and administering vasopressor medications.
- If serious hemorrhage occurs, the depleted coagulation factors and platelets may be replaced (cryoprecipitate to replace fibrinogen and factors V and VII; fresh-frozen plasma to replace other coagulation factors).
- A controversial method may be used to interrupt the thrombosis process by the use of heparin infusion.
- An even more controversial management method involves administering fibrinolytic inhibitors, such as aminocaproic acid, which reduces the fibrin degradation products by decreasing the lysis of microthrombi.

Nursing Management

Assessment

- Be aware of those patients at risk for DIC (sepsis and acute promyelocytic leukemia are the most common causes).
- Assess patients thoroughly and frequently for signs and symptoms of thrombi or bleeding, and monitor for any progression of these signs.

Major Nursing Diagnoses

- Potential for fluid volume deficit related to bleeding
- Potential for impaired skin integrity related to ischemia or bleeding
- Potential for fluid volume excess

- Potential for diminished tissue perfusion related to microthrombi
- Fear of the unknown and possible death

Collaborative Problems/Potential Complications
- Renal failure
- Gangrene
- Pulmonary embolism or hemorrhage
- Altered level of consciousness, stroke
- Acute respiratory distress syndrome

Planning and Goals
The major goals of the patient include maintenance of hemodynamic status, intact skin and oral mucosa, maintenance of fluid balance, maintenance of tissue perfusion, enhanced coping, and prevention of complications.

Nursing Interventions
MAINTAINING FLUID VOLUME
- Avoid procedures and activities that can increase intracranial pressure, such as coughing and straining.
- Closely monitor vital signs, including neurologic checks, and for amount of external bleeding.
- Avoid medications that interfere with platelet function, if possible (eg, beta-lactam antibiotics, acetylsalicylic acid, nonsteroidal antiinflammatory drugs).
- Avoid rectal probes and rectal or intramuscular injection medications.
- Use low pressure with any suctioning.
- Administer oral hygiene carefully: use sponge-tipped swabs, salt or soda mouth rinses; avoid lemon-glycerine swabs, hydrogen peroxide, commercial mouthwashes.
- Avoid dislodging any clots, including those around intravenous sites, injection sites, and so forth.

MAINTAINING SKIN INTEGRITY
- Assess skin, with particular attention to bony prominences and skin folds.

- Reposition carefully; use pressure-reducing mattress and lamb's wool between digits and around ears and soft absorbent material in skin folds, as needed.
- Perform skin care every 2 hours; administer oral hygiene carefully (see earlier).
- Use prolonged pressure (5 minutes minimum) after essential injection procedures.

MONITORING FOR FLUID VOLUME EXCESS
- Auscultate breath sounds every 2 to 4 hours.
- Monitor extent of edema.
- Monitor volume of intravenous medications and blood products; decrease volume of intravenous medications if possible.
- Administer diuretics as prescribed.

ASSESSING FOR DIMINISHED TISSUE PERFUSION RELATED TO MICROTHROMBI
- Assess neurologic, pulmonary, and skin systems.
- Monitor response to heparin therapy; monitor fibrinogen levels.
- Assess extent of bleeding.
- Stop epsilon-aminocaproic acid if symptoms of thrombosis occur.

REDUCING ANXIETY
- Identify previous coping mechanisms, if possible; encourage patient to use them as appropriate.
- Explain all procedures and rationale in terms that the patient and family can understand.
- Assist family in supporting patient.
- Use services from behavioral medicine and clergy, if desired.

MONITORING AND MANAGING POTENTIAL COMPLICATIONS
- If dialysis is required, place dialysis catheter with extreme caution, and prepare for transfusion of adequate platelets and plasma.

- Monitor for and implement measures to address potential complications as indicated (see specific condition).

For more information, see Chapter 30 in Smeltzer and Bare: *Brunner and Suddarth's Textbook of Medical-Surgical Nursing,* 9th edition. Philadelphia: Lippincott Williams & Wilkins, 2000.

D

DIVERTICULAR DISORDERS

A diverticulum is a saclike out-pouching or herniation of the mucosa and submucosa that protrudes through a weak portion of the muscle layer. Diverticula may occur anywhere along the gastrointestinal tract. Diverticulosis exists when multiple diverticula are present without inflammation or symptoms. *Diverticulitis* results when food and bacteria retained in the diverticulum produce infection and inflammation that can impede draining and lead to perforation or abscess. It may occur in acute attacks or persist as a long-continued, smoldering infection. Diverticulitis is more common in the sigmoid colon. A congenital predisposition is likely when the disorder is present in those younger than 40 years of age. Diverticulosis is more common in people older than 60 years of age. A low intake of dietary fiber is considered a major predisposing factor. Complications of diverticulitis include peritonitis, abscess formation, and bleeding.

Clinical Manifestations
Diverticulosis
- Frequently, no problematic symptoms noted; constipation from spastic colon syndrome often precedes development
- Bowel irregularity and diarrhea
- Crampy pain in the left lower quadrant
- Low-grade fever
- Nausea and anorexia and some bloating or abdominal distention

Diverticulitis
- Narrowing of the large bowel with fibrotic stricture
- Cramps, narrow stools, and increased constipation
- Occult bleeding
- Weakness, fatigue, and anorexia
- Tenderness, a palpable mass, fever, and leukocytes, which may indicate abscess development
- Abdominal pain, a rigid boardlike abdomen, loss of bowel sounds, and signs and symptoms of shock, which may indicate peritonitis
- Septicemia if condition remains untreated

Diagnostic Evaluation
- Computed tomography (CT) scan (procedure of choice)
- Radiographic studies (barium enema, unless peritoneal irritation)
- Colonoscopy
- Complete blood count (white blood cell count and sedimentation rate elevated)

Medical Management
- Diverticulosis: a high-fiber diet is prescribed to prevent constipation.
- Diverticulitis: can treat at home with clear liquid until inflammation subsides, then high-fiber, low fat diet is recommended.
- Antibiotics are prescribed for 7 to 10 days.
- A bulk-forming laxative is also prescribed.
- Patient with significant symptoms and often those who are elderly, immunocompromised, or on steroids are hospitalized.
- The bowel is rested by withholding oral intake; administer intravenous fluids, institute nasogastric suctioning; broad-spectrum antibiotics and analgesics are prescribed.
- Oral intake is increased as symptoms subside. A low-fiber diet may be necessary until signs of infection decrease.

- For spastic pain, antispasmodics are taken before meals and at bedtime; sedatives and tranquilizers and bowel antimicrobials may be required.
- Normal stools can be achieved by bulk preparations (Metamucil), stool softeners, warm oil enemas, and evacuant suppositories.
- Surgery (resection) is usually necessary only if perforation, peritonitis, abscess formation, hemorrhage, or obstruction occur; recurrence of diverticula is common. Type of surgery performed varies according to the extent of complications found during surgery.

Nursing Management
Assessment
- Assess health history, including onset and duration of pain, dietary habits (fiber intake), and past and present elimination patterns (straining at stool, constipation with diarrhea, tenesmus [spasm of the anal sphincter with pain and persistent urge to defecate]).
- Auscultate for the presence and character of bowel sounds; palpate for tenderness, pain, or firm mass over left lower quadrant; inspect stool for pus, mucus, or blood. Monitor blood pressure, temperature, and pulse for abnormal variations.

Major Nursing Diagnoses
- Constipation related to narrowing of the colon secondary to thickened muscular segments and strictures.
- Pain related to inflammation and infection.

Collaborative Problems/Potential Complications
- Peritonitis
- Abscess formation
- Bleeding

Planning and Implementation
The major goals of the patient may include attainment and maintenance of normal elimination, reduction in pain,

improvement in gastrointestinal tissue perfusion, and absence of potential complications.

Nursing Interventions

MAINTAINING NORMAL ELIMINATION PATTERNS
- Increase fluid intake to 2 L/day within limits of patient's cardiac and renal reserve.
- Promote foods that are soft but have increased fiber diet.
- Encourage individualized exercise program to improve abdominal muscle tone.
- Review patient's routine to establish a set time for meals and defecation.
- Increase daily intake of bulk laxatives (eg, Metamucil, stool softeners, or oil-retention enemas).

RELIEVING PAIN
- Administer analgesics for pain and antispasmodics.
- Record and monitor intensity, duration, and location of pain.

MONITORING AND MANAGING
POTENTIAL COMPLICATIONS
- Identify patients at risk.
- Assess for indicators of perforations: tender, rigid abdomen; elevated white blood cell count; elevated sedimentation rate; increased temperature; tachycardia and hypotension.
- Perforation constitutes a surgical emergency: monitor vital signs and urine output, and administer intravenous fluids as ordered.

🍁 Gerontologic Considerations

The incidence of diverticular disease increases with age because of degeneration and structural changes in the circular muscle layers of the colon and cellular hypertrophy. Symptoms are less pronounced among elderly patients, who may not experience abdominal pain until infection occurs. They delay reporting symptoms because they fear surgery or cancer. Blood in stool may frequently be over-looked because of failure to examine the stool or inability to see changes because of diminished vision.

D

Evaluation

EXPECTED OUTCOMES
• Attains a normal pattern of elimination
• Experiences no pain or discomfort

For more information, see Chapter 35 in Smeltzer and Bare: *Brunner and Suddarth's Textbook of Medical-Surgical Nursing,* 9th edition. Philadelphia: Lippincott Williams & Wilkins, 2000.

E

EMPHYSEMA, PULMONARY

Pulmonary emphysema is defined as a nonuniform pattern of abnormal, permanent distention of the air spaces with destruction of the alveolar walls and eventually a reduced pulmonary capillary bed. It appears to be the end stage of a process that has progressed slowly for many years. Smoking is the major cause. In a small percentage of patients, there is a familial predisposition associated with a plasma protein abnormality (deficiency of alpha-1-antitrypsin), making a person sensitive to environmental factors (air pollution, infectious agents, allergens). It manifests commonly in the fifth decade of life and is classified as follows:

Panlobular (panacinar): characterized by destruction of the respiratory bronchiole, alveolar duct, and alveoli; air spaces within the lobule are enlarged, with little inflammatory disease

Centrilobular (centriacinar): causes pathologic changes in the center of the secondary lobule, producing chronic hypoxemia, hypercapnia, polycythemia, and episodes of right-sided heart failure.

Both types of emphysema can occur together.

Clinical Manifestations
Dyspnea With Insidious Onset
- History of cigarette smoking, chronic cough, wheezing, dyspnea, fatigue, and tachypnea
- Insidious dyspnea progressing to occurrence with slight exertion (major symptom)
- On inspection, "barrel chest" due to air trapping, muscle wasting, and pursed-lip breathing

- On auscultation, diminished breath sounds with crackles, wheezes, rhonchi, and prolonged expiration
- Hyperresonance with percussion and a decrease in fremitus
- Anorexia, weight loss, weakness, and inactivity
- Hypoxemia and hypercapnia, morning headaches in advanced stages
- Inflammatory reactions and infections from pooled secretions

Diagnostic Evaluation

Evaluation entails primarily chest radiographs, chest computed tomography (CT) scans, pulmonary function tests, pulse oximetry, blood gases, and complete blood count.

Medical Management

The major goals of medical management are to improve quality of life, slow progression of the disease, and treat obstructed airways to relieve hypoxia.

- Treatment to improve ventilation and decrease work of breathing.
- Prevention and prompt treatment of infection
- Physical therapy to conserve and increase pulmonary ventilation
- Maintenance of proper environmental conditions to facilitate breathing
- Supportive and psychological support
- Ongoing program of patient education and rehabilitation
- Bronchodilators and metered dose inhalers (aerosol therapy, dispensing particles in fine mist)
- Treatment of infection (antimicrobial therapy at the first sign of respiratory infection)
- Benefits of corticosteroid use unclear
- Oxygenation in low concentrations for severe hypoxemia

See Nursing Management under Chronic Obstructive Pulmonary Disease for additional information.

For more information, see Chapter 21 in Smeltzer and Bare: *Brunner and Suddarth's Textbook of Medical-Surgical Nursing,* 9th edition. Philadelphia: Lippincott Williams & Wilkins, 2000.

EMPYEMA

Empyema is a collection of purulent (infected) liquid or pus in the pleural cavity. At first, pleural fluid is thin, but it progresses to a fibropurulent stage then to a stage at which it encloses the lung with a thick exudative membrane.

Clinical Manifestations
- Fever, night sweats, pleural pain, cough, dyspnea, anorexia, and weight loss
- Absence of breath sounds; flatness on chest percussion; decreased fremitus

Diagnostic Evaluation
- Chest auscultation, which demonstrates decreased or absent breath sounds over the affected area; flatness on chest percussion; decreased fremitus
- Chest radiographs and thoracentesis
- Symptoms vague (immunocompromised patient) or less obvious if patient has received antimicrobial therapy

Medical Management
The objectives of management are to drain the pleural cavity and to achieve full expansion of the lung; accomplished by adequate drainage, antibiotics (large doses), streptokinase, or a combination of these. Drainage of the pleural fluid depends on the stage of the disease and is accomplished as follows:

- Needle aspiration (thoracentesis) if fluid is not too thick
- Tube thoracostomy water-seal chest drainage, with fibrinolytic agents instilled through chest tube when indicated

- Open chest drainage to remove thickened pleura, pus, and debris and to remove the underlying diseased pulmonary tissue
- Decortication, surgical removal, if inflammation has been long-standing

Nursing Management
See Preoperative and Postoperative Nursing Management for additional information.

Nursing Interventions
- Provide care specific to method of drainage of pleural fluid.
- Help patient cope with condition; instruct in lung expansion breathing exercises (pursed lip and diaphragmatic breathing).

Promoting Home and Community-Based Care

Teaching Patients Self-Care
- Instruct patient and family about care of the drainage system and drain site and measurement and observation of drainage.
- Teach patient and family the signs and symptoms of infection and how and when to contact the health care provider.

For more information, see Chapter 21 in Smeltzer and Bare: *Brunner and Suddarth's Textbook of Medical-Surgical Nursing,* 9th edition. Philadelphia: Lippincott Williams & Wilkins, 2000.

ENDOCARDITIS, INFECTIVE

Infective endocarditis (bacterial endocarditis) is an infection of the valves and the endothelial surface of the heart. It is caused by direct invasion of bacteria or other organisms leading to deformity of the valve leaflets. Causative organisms include many bacteria (eg, streptococci, pneumococci, staphylococci) and fungi. Risk factors include valvular heart disease, rheumatic heart disease, mitral valve prolapse, and prosthetic valve surgery. It is more common in older people because of their decreased immunologic response, the metabolic changes of aging, and increased invasive diagnostic procedures. There is a high incidence of staphylococcal endocarditis among intravenous drug users. Hospital-acquired endocarditis occurs most often in patients with debilitating disease or indwelling catheters and in those receiving prolonged intravenous or antibiotic therapy. Patients taking immunosuppressive medications or steroids may develop fungal endocarditis.

Clinical Manifestations

- Insidious onset; signs and symptoms develop from toxicity of infection, destruction of heart valves, and embolization of fragments of vegetative growths on the heart.
- General manifestations include vague complaints of malaise, anorexia, weight loss, and back and joint pain.
- Fever is intermittent; may be absent in patients who are receiving antibiotics or corticosteroids, elderly patients, and patients with congestive heart failure or renal failure.
- Splinter hemorrhages under the fingernails and toenails and petechiae in the conjunctiva and mucous membranes are seen.
- Hemorrhages with pale centers (Roth's spots) in the fundi of the eyes can occur.
- Cardiac manifestations include heart enlargement, congestive heart failure, and heart murmurs (may be absent initially); progressively changing murmurs indicate valvular damage.
- Central nervous system manifestations include headache, transient cerebral ischemia, focal neurologic lesions, and stroke.
- Emboli involving other organ systems manifest in the lung (recurrent pneumonia, pulmonary abscesses), kidney (hematuria, renal failure), spleen (left upper quad-

rant pain), heart (myocardial infarction), brain (stroke), and peripheral vessels.

Medical Management

The objectives of treatment are to eradicate the invading organism through adequate doses of an appropriate antimicrobial agent (continuous intravenous infusion for 4 to 6 weeks at home).

- Isolate causative organism through serial blood cultures. Blood cultures are taken to monitor the course of therapy.
- After recovery from the infectious process, seriously damaged valves may require replacement.
- Patient's temperature is monitored for treatment effectiveness.
- Treat complications: congestive heart failure, cerebral vascular complications, valve stenosis or regurgitation, myocardial damage, and mycotic aneurysms.
- Surgical valve replacement is required for development of congestive heart failure; more than one serious systemic embolic episode; and uncontrolled infection, recurrent infection, or fungal endocarditis.

Nursing Management

Additional nursing may involve postsurgical care. See Preoperative and Postoperative Patient Nursing Management .

🏠 Promoting Home and Community-Based Care

- Reinforce that antibiotic prophylaxis is recommended for people at risk undergoing invasive procedures.
- Refer to home care nurse to supervise and monitor intravenous antibiotic therapy in the home.

For more information, see Chapter 26 in Smeltzer and Bare: *Brunner and Suddarth's Textbook of Medical-Surgical Nursing,* 9th edition. Philadelphia: Lippincott Williams & Wilkins, 2000.

ENDOCARDITIS, RHEUMATIC

Rheumatic endocarditis is directly attributed to rheumatic fever caused by group A streptococcal infection. Rheumatic fever affects all bony joints, producing a polyarthritis. The most serious damage occurs in the heart. Rheumatic endocarditis manifests as tiny, translucent vegetations that resemble beads about the size of a pinhead, arranged in a row along the free margins of the valve flaps. The flaps gradually become shorter and thicker than normal, which prevents them from closing the valve orifice completely. The result is valvular regurgitation (leakage); most common is mitral regurgitation. Valvular stenosis may also occur. A small percentage of patients become critically ill with intractable heart failure, serious dysrhythmias, and rheumatic pneumonia. The myocardium can compensate for these valvular defects very well for a time. Sooner or later, however, decompensation occurs and is manifested by congestive heart failure.

Clinical Manifestations
- Eventually, the heart murmurs characteristic of valvular stenosis, regurgitation, or both become audible on auscultation; "thrills" may be detectable on palpation.
- Cardiac symptoms depend on which side of the heart is involved. Severity of symptoms depends on size and location of the lesion.
- The mitral valve is most often affected, producing symptoms of left-sided heart failure: shortness of breath, crackles, and wheezes.

Medical Management
- The objectives of medical management are aggressive eradication of the causative organism and prevention of additional complications, such as a thromboembolic event.
- Long-term antibiotic therapy is the treatment of choice. Parenteral penicillin remains the medication of choice.

- If valve function is faulty and the disease is quiet, no therapy is required so long as the heart pumps effectively.
- Prevention is achieved through early and adequate treatment of streptococcal infection in all patients.
- A throat culture is the only method by which accuracy of diagnosis can be determined.

E

Nursing Management

 Promoting Home and Community-Based Care

- Educate patient and community regarding recognition of streptococcal infections and the need to treat them adequately and to control community epidemics.
- Teach susceptible patients that they may require long-term oral antibiotic therapy and may be required to take prophylactic antibiotics before procedures, such as dental checkups or cystoscopy.
- Emphasize that less common diagnostic procedures, such as cystoscopy, also require prophylactic antibiotic therapy.

For more information, see Chapter 26 in Smeltzer and Bare: *Brunner and Suddarth's Textbook of Medical-Surgical Nursing,* 9th edition. Philadelphia: Lippincott Williams & Wilkins, 2000.

ENDOMETRIOSIS

Endometriosis is a benign lesion with cells similar to those lining the uterus, growing aberrantly in the pelvic cavity outside the uterus. During menstruation, the lesion bleeds (pseudocyst), mostly in areas without outlet, resulting in adhesions, cysts, scar tissue, pain, and infertility. There is a high incidence among patients who bear children later and have fewer children. It is usually found in young, nulliparous woman aged 25 to 35 years. There appears to be a familial predisposition to endometriosis. It is a major cause of infertility.

Clinical Manifestations
- Symptoms vary with the location of endometrial tissue.
- The chief symptom is a type of dysmenorrhea: deep-seated aching in the lower abdomen, vagina, posterior pelvis, and back, occurring 1 or 2 days before the menstrual cycle and lasting 2 or 3 days.
- Some patients have no pain.
- Abnormal uterine bleeding and dyspareunia (painful intercourse) can occur.
- Nausea and diarrhea can occur.

Diagnostic Evaluation
Laparoscopy confirms the diagnosis and helps to stage the disease.

Medical Management
Treatment depends on patient's symptoms, desire for pregnancy, and extent of the disease. In asymptomatic cases, routine examination may be all that is required. Other therapies include palliative measures (eg, analgesics, hormone administration, prostaglandin inhibitors, and surgery). Pregnancy alleviates symptoms because no ovulation or menstruation occurs.

Pharmacologic Therapy
- Oral contraceptives are used to suppress menstruation and relieve menstrual pain.
- Synthetic androgen, danazol (Danocrine), causes atrophy of the endometrium and subsequent amenorrhea. (Danazol is expensive and may cause troublesome side effects, such as fatigue, depression, weight gain, oily skin, decreased breast size, mild acne, hot flashes, and atrophy of the vagina.)
- Gonadotropin-releasing hormone (GnRH) agonist or GnRH blocker (nafarelin acetate [Synarel]) results in decreased estrogen production and subsequent amenor-

rhea. This agent is administered by nasal spray twice a day for 6 months. Side effects related to low estrogen levels.

Surgical Management

- Laparoscopy to fulgurate endometrial implants and to lyse (release) adhesions
- Laser surgery to vaporize endometrial implants or to coagulate the implant and destroy the endometriosis
- Other surgical procedures may include laparotomy, uterine suspension, abdominal hysterectomy, bilateral salpingo-oophorectomy, and appendectomy

Nursing Management

Nursing Interventions

- Obtain health history and physical examination, concentrating on identifying when and how long specific symptoms have been bothersome and on defining woman's reproductive desires.
- Assess for pain, and evaluate techniques and prescribed medications that provide relief.
- Explain various diagnostic procedures to alleviate anxiety.
- Provide emotional support to the woman and her partner who wish to have children.
- Respect and address psychosocial impact of realization that pregnancy is not easily possible.
- Discuss alternatives, such as in vitro fertilization (IVF) or adoption, and offer referrals.
- Encourage patient to seek care of dysmenorrhea or abnormal bleeding patterns.
- Direct patient to the Endometriosis Association for more information and support.

For more information, see Chapter 43 in Smeltzer and Bare: *Brunner and Suddarth's Textbook of Medical-Surgical Nursing,* 9th edition. Philadelphia: Lippincott Williams & Wilkins, 2000.

EPIDIDYMITIS

Epididymitis is an infection of the epididymis that usually results from an infected prostate or urinary tract. It may also develop as a complication of gonorrhea. In men younger than 35 years of age, the major cause is *Chlamydia trachomatis* infection.

Clinical Manifestations
- Unilateral pain and soreness in the inguinal canal along the course of the vas deferens
- Pain and swelling in the scrotum and groin
- Extremely painful and swollen epididymis; temperature elevated
- Pyuria and bacteriuria with resulting chills and fever

Medical Management
- If seen within first 24 hours after onset of pain, spermatic cord may be infiltrated with a local anesthetic agent for relief.
- If chlamydial in origin, patient and patient's sexual partners must be treated with antibiotics.
- Observe for abscess formation.
- If no improvement within 2 weeks, underlying testicular tumor should be considered.
- Epididymectomy (excision of the epididymis from the testes) is done for recurrent, incapacitating episodes or chronic, painful conditions.

Nursing Management
Nursing Interventions
- Place patient on bed rest with scrotum elevated with a scrotal bridge or folded towel to prevent traction on spermatic cord and improve venous drainage and relieve pain.
- Give antimicrobials as prescribed.

- Provide intermittent cold compresses to scrotum to help ease pain; later, local heat or sitz baths may hasten resolution of inflammatory process.
- Give analgesics as prescribed for pain relief.

🏠 Promoting Home and Community-Based Care

Teaching Patients Self-Care
- Instruct patient to avoid straining, lifting, and sexual excitement until the infection is under control.
- Instruct to continue with analgesics and antibiotics as prescribed and to use ice packs as necessary for discomfort.
- Explain that it may take 4 weeks or longer for the epididymis to return to normal.

For more information, see Chapter 45 in Smeltzer and Bare: *Brunner and Suddarth's Textbook of Medical-Surgical Nursing*, 9th edition. Philadelphia: Lippincott Williams & Wilkins, 2000.

EPILEPSIES

The epilepsies are a symptom complex of several disorders of brain function characterized by recurring seizures. There may be associated loss of consciousness, excess movement, or loss of muscle tone or movement and disturbances of behavior, mood, sensation, and perception. The basic problem is an electrical disturbance (dysrhythmia) in the nerve cells in one section of the brain, causing them to emit abnormal, recurring, uncontrolled electrical discharges. The characteristic epileptic seizure is a manifestation of this excessive neuronal discharge. In most cases, the cause is unknown (idiopathic). There is evidence that susceptibility to some types may be inherited. Epilepsies often follow many medical disorders, traumas, and drug or alcohol intoxication. They are also associated with brain tumors, abscesses, and congenital malformations. Epilepsy begins before 20 years of age in more than 75% of patients. Epilepsy is not synonymous with mental retardation or illness; it is not associated with intellectual level.

Clinical Manifestations

Seizures range from simple staring episodes to prolonged convulsive movements with loss of consciousness. Seizures are classified as partial, generalized, and unclassified according to the area of brain involved. *Aura,* a premonitory or warning sensation, occurs before seizure (eg, seeing a flashing light, hearing a sound).

Simple Partial Seizures

Only a finger or hand may shake; the mouth may jerk uncontrollably; the patient may talk unintelligibly, may be dizzy, or may experience unusual or unpleasant sights, sounds, odors, or taste—all without loss of consciousness.

Complex Partial Seizures

The patient remains motionless or moves automatically but inappropriately for time and place; may experience excessive emotions of fear, anger, elation, or irritability; does not remember episode when it is over.

Generalized Seizures (Grand Mal Seizures)

Grand mal seizures involve both hemispheres of the brain. There is intense rigidity of the entire body, followed by jerky alternations of muscle relaxation and contraction (generalized tonic-clonic contraction).

- Simultaneous contractions of diaphragm and chest muscles produce characteristic epileptic cry.
- Tongue is chewed; patient is incontinent of urine and stool.
- Convulsive movements last 1 or 2 minutes.
- The patient then relaxes and lies in deep coma, breathing noisily.

Postictal State

After the seizure, the patient is often confused and hard to arouse and may sleep for hours. Many complain of headache or sore muscles.

Diagnostic Evaluation

- A developmental history and physical and neurologic examinations are done to determine the type, frequency, and severity of seizures; biochemical, hematologic, and serologic studies are included.
- Computed tomography (CT) imaging is performed to detect lesions, focal abnormalities, cerebral vascular abnormalities, and cerebral degenerative changes.
- Electroencephalograms (EEG) aid in classifying the type of seizure.

Medical Management

The management of epilepsy and status epilepticus is planned according to immediate and long-range needs and is tailored to meet the individual patient because some cases arise from brain damage and others are due to altered brain chemistry.

The goals of treatment are to stop the seizures as quickly as possible, to ensure adequate cerebral oxygenation, and to maintain the patient in a seizure-free state.

- Establish an airway and adequate oxygenation (intubate if necessary); establish an intravenous line for medications and blood work.
- Give intravenous diazepam, lorazepam, or fosphenytoin slowly in an attempt to halt the seizures.
- Give other anticonvulsant medications (phenytoin, phenobarbital) as prescribed after the diazepam to maintain a seizure-free state.
- Monitor vital signs and neurologic signs continuously.
- Monitor EEG to determine the nature of epileptogenic activity.
- Use general anesthesia with a short-acting barbiturate, if initial treatment is unsuccessful.

- Measure serum concentration of the anticonvulsant medication the patient was taking.
- Patient may die from cardiac involvement or respiratory depression.
- Assess potential for postictal cerebral swelling.

Pharmacologic Management

Medication therapy is used to achieve seizure control.

- The usual treatment is single-drug therapy.
- Major anticonvulsant medications include carbamazepine, primidone, phenytoin, phenobarbital, ethosuximide, and valproate.
- Perform periodic physical examinations and laboratory tests for patients receiving medications known to have toxic hematopoietic, genitourinary, or hepatic effects.

Surgical Management

- Surgery is indicated when epilepsy results from intracranial tumors, abscess, cysts, or vascular anomalies.
- Surgical removal of the epileptogenic focus is done for seizures that originate in a well-circumcised area of the brain that can be excised without producing significant neurologic defects.

Nursing Management

Assessment

- Obtain a complete seizure history; ask about factors or events that may precipitate the seizures; document alcohol intake.
- Assess effects of epilepsy on lifestyle.
- Observe and assess neurologic condition during and after a seizure.

Major Nursing Diagnoses

- Fear related to the ever-present possibility of having seizures
- Ineffective coping related to stresses imposed by epilepsy
- Knowledge deficit about epilepsy and its control

Collaborative Problems/Potential Complications
• Status epilepticus

Planning and Goals
The major goals of the patient may include control of seizures, achievement of a satisfactory psychosocial adjustment, acquisition of knowledge, understanding of the condition, and absence of complications.

Nursing Interventions
• Provide ongoing assessment and monitoring of respiratory and cardiac function.
• Monitor the seizure type and general condition of the patient.
• Turn patient to side-lying position to assist in draining pharyngeal secretions.
• Have suction equipment available for risk of aspiration.
• Monitor intravenous line closely for dislodgment during seizures.
• Protect patient from injury during seizures with padded side rails, and keep under constant observation.
• Do not restrain patient's movements during seizure activity.

CONTROLLING SEIZURES
• Reduce fear that a seizure may occur unexpectedly by patient's compliance to prescribed treatment.
• Emphasize that the prescribed antiepileptic medication must be taken on a continuing basis and is not habit forming.
• Prevent or control gingival hyperplasia with thorough oral hygiene, regular dental care, and gum massage for patients taking phenytoin (Dilantin).
• Assess lifestyle and environment to determine factors that precipitate seizures, such as emotional disturbances, new environmental stressors, onset of menstruation in female patients, or fever.
• Encourage patient to follow a regular and moderate routine in lifestyle, diet (avoiding excessive stimulants), exercise, and rest (regular sleep patterns).

- Avoid photic stimulation (eg, bright flickering lights, television viewing); dark glasses or covering one eye may help.
- Provide classes in stress management; avoid stimuli that precipitate seizures.

IMPROVING COPING MECHANISMS
- Understand that epilepsy imposes feelings of fear, alienation, depression, and uncertainty.
- Provide counseling to the patient and family to understand the condition and limitations imposed.
- Provide social and recreational opportunities.
- Instruct patient to avoid over-the-counter medications unless approved by the patient's physician.
- Provide comprehensive mental health services to patients who exhibit symptoms of schizophrenia or impulsive or irritable behavior.

MONITORING AND MANAGING POTENTIAL
COMPLICATIONS (STATUS EPILEPTICUS)
Status epilepticus (acute prolonged seizure activity) is a series of generalized seizures that occur without full recovery of consciousness between attacks.
- Continuous clinical or electrical seizures lasting at least 30 minutes, even without impairment of consciousness
- Considered a major medical emergency
- Repeated episodes of cerebral anoxia and swelling, which may lead to irreversible and fatal brain damage
- Common factors that precipitate status epilepticus include withdrawal of antiepileptic medication, fever, and intercurrent infection

🏠 Promoting Home and Community-Based Care

Teaching Patients Self-Care
- Instruct patient and family about medication side effects and toxicity.
- Provide specific guidelines to assess and report signs and symptoms of overdose.

- Instruct patient to notify physician if unable to take medications due to illness.
- Teach patient to keep a "drug and seizure chart," noting when medications are taken and any seizure activity.
- Instruct patient to take showers rather than tub baths to avoid drowning and never to swim alone.
- Educate patient to exercise in moderation in a temperature-controlled environment to avoid excessive heat.
- Mental outlook: modify the attitudes of the patient and family toward the disease itself; provide factual information concerning epilepsy.
- Instruct patient to carry an emergency medical identification card or wear an identification bracelet.
- Genetic counseling: advise patient to seek preconception and genetic counseling if desired (inherited transmission of epilepsy has not been proved).

Continuing Care

- Financial considerations: the Epilepsy Foundation of America offers a mail-order program for medications at minimum cost and access to life insurance as well as information on vocational rehabilitation and coping with epilepsy.
- Vocational rehabilitation: the State Vocational Rehabilitation Agency, Epilepsy Foundation of America, and federal and state agencies may be of assistance.

Evaluation

EXPECTED OUTCOMES
- Maintains control of seizures
- Exhibits psychosocial adjustments
- Gains knowledge and understanding of epilepsy
- Is free of seizures and complications of status epilepticus

---

For more information, see Chapter 59 in Smeltzer and Bare: *Brunner and Suddarth's Textbook of Medical-Surgical Nursing,* 9th edition. Philadelphia: Lippincott Williams & Wilkins, 2000.

EPISTAXIS (NOSEBLEED)

Epistaxis is a hemorrhage from the nose caused by the rupture of tiny, distended vessels in the mucous membrane. The anterior septum is the most common site. Causes include trauma, infection, drugs, cardiovascular diseases, blood dyscrasias, nasal tumors, low humidity, foreign body, and a deviated nasal septum. Vigorous nose blowing and nose picking are additional causes.

Medical Management
- A nasal speculum or headlight is used to determine site.
- Apply direct pressure.
- Sit patient upright with the head tilted forward to prevent swallowing and aspiration of blood.
- Compress the soft outer portion of the nose against the midline septum for 5 or 10 minutes continuously.
- Anterior nosebleeds are cauterization by chemical agents (eg, silver nitrate and Gelfoam) or electrocautery; topical vasoconstrictors (eg, adrenaline [1:1000], cocaine [0.5%], phenylephrine).
- For posterior nosebleeds, drug-moistened cotton pledgets are inserted into the nostril to reduce blood flow; suction is used to remove excess blood and clots from the field of inspection.
- Nose is packed with petrolatum-impregnated gauze when origin of bleed cannot be identified. Keep packing in place for 48 hours or up to 5 or 6 days if necessary to control bleeding.
- Antibiotics may be given.

Nursing Management

🏠 Promoting Home and Community-Based Care
- Monitor vital signs and assist in control of bleeding.
- Provide tissues and an emesis basin for expectoration of blood.

E

- Reassure patient that bleeding can be controlled.
- Maintain a calm, efficient manner.

Teaching Patients Self-Care
- Review ways to prevent epistaxis, including avoiding forceful nose blowing, straining, high altitudes, and nasal trauma (including nose picking).
- Provide adequate humidification to prevent drying of nasal passages.
- Instruct patient how to apply direct pressure to nose with thumb and index finger for 15 minutes if nosebleed recurs.
- Instruct patient to seek medical attention if recurrent bleeding cannot be stopped.

For more information, see Chapter 20 in Smeltzer and Bare: *Brunner and Suddarth's Textbook of Medical-Surgical Nursing,* 9th edition. Philadelphia: Lippincott Williams & Wilkins, 2000.

ESOPHAGEAL VARICES, BLEEDING

Bleeding or hemorrhage from esophageal varices is one of the major causes of death in patients with cirrhosis. Esophageal varices are dilated tortuous veins usually found in the submucosa of the lower esophagus; they may develop higher in the esophagus or extend into the stomach. The condition nearly always is caused by portal hypertension. Risk factors for hemorrhage include muscular strain from heavy lifting; straining at stool, sneezing, coughing, or vomiting; esophagitis or irritation of vessels; and salicylates or any drug that erodes the esophageal mucosa.

Clinical Manifestations
- Hematemesis and melena occur, mainly in those who have abused alcohol.
- Dilated veins usually cause no symptoms unless portal pressure increases and mucosa becomes thin (then massive hemorrhage takes place).

Diagnostic Evaluation
- Endoscopy, barium swallow, ultrasound, computed tomography (CT) scan, and angiography.
- Neurologic and portal hypertension assessment.
- Liver function tests.

Medical Management
The goals of management are aggressive medical care and expert nursing care.
- Evaluate extent of bleeding, and monitor vital signs continuously when hematemesis and melena are present.
- Note signs of potential hypovolemia.
- Monitor blood volume with central venous pressure or arterial catheter.
- Give oxygen to prevent hypoxia and to maintain adequate blood oxygenation.
- Provide intravenous fluids and volume expanders to restore fluid volume and replace electrolytes.
- Assess for need of blood transfusion.
- Monitor intake and output.

Nonsurgical Management
Nonsurgical treatment is preferable because of high mortality of emergency surgery for control of bleeding of esophageal varices and because of poor physical condition of the patient with severe liver dysfunction.
- Pharmacologic therapy: vasopressin (Pitressin), propranolol (Inderal), somatostatin
- Balloon tamponade, saline lavage, endoscopic sclerotherapy
- Transjugular intrahepatic portosystemic shunting (TIPS)
- Esophageal banding therapy, variceal band ligation

Surgical Management
- Surgical bypass procedures (eg, portacaval shunts, splenorenal shunt, mesocaval shunt)
- Devascularization and transection

Nursing Management

NURSING ALERT

Postoperative care is similar to that for any abdominal surgery, but the risk for complications (hypovolemic or hemorrhagic shock, hepatic encephalopathy, electrolyte imbalance, metabolic and respiratory alkalosis, alcohol withdrawal syndrome, and seizures) is high. In addition, bleeding may recur as new collateral vessels develop.

Nursing Interventions

- Monitor the patient's physical condition, and evaluate emotional responses and cognitive status.
- Monitor and record vital signs, and assess the patient's nutritional status.
- Perform a neurologic assessment, monitoring for signs of hepatic encephalopathy (findings may range from drowsiness to encephalopathy and coma).
- Treat bleeding by complete rest of the esophagus; initiate total parenteral nutrition (TPN) as ordered.
- Assist patient to avoid straining and vomiting. Maintain gastric suction to keep the stomach as empty as possible.
- Provide frequent oral hygiene and moist sponges to the lips, to relieve the patient's thirst.
- Closely monitor the patient's blood pressure.
- Provide vitamin K therapy and multiple blood transfusions as ordered for blood loss.
- Provide a quiet environment and calm reassurance to help to relieve the patient's anxiety and reduce agitation.
- Provide support and pertinent explanations regarding medical and nursing interventions.
- Monitor the patient closely to detect and manage complications.
- Provide support before and during examination by endoscopy to relieve stress.
  - Monitor carefully to detect early signs of cardiac dysrhythmias, perforation, and hemorrhage.

- ○ Do not give fluids after the examination until the gag reflex returns.
- ○ Use lozenges and gargles to relieve throat discomfort.
- ○ No oral intake is permitted if patient is actively bleeding.
- Provide support and explanations regarding care and procedures.
- Give postoperative care similar to that for any thoracic or abdominal operation (see Preoperative and Postoperative Nursing Management for additional information).
- Assess closely for complications, including hypovolemic or hemorrhagic shock, hepatic encephalopathy, electrolyte imbalance, metabolic and respiratory alkalosis, alcohol withdrawal syndrome, and seizures.
- Monitor closely to prevent accidental removal or displacement of tube, subsequent airway obstruction, and aspiration related to balloon tamponade.
  - ○ Explain procedure to patient briefly to obtain cooperation with insertion and maintenance of esophageal-tamponade tube.
  - ○ Provide frequent oral hygiene.
  - ○ Ensure patency of nasogastric tube to prevent aspiration. Observe gastric aspirate for blood and cessation of bleeding.
- Observe for aspiration, perforation of esophagus, and recurrence of bleeding related to endoscopic sclerotherapy or variceal binding.

🍁 Gerontologic Considerations

Bleeding esophageal varices can quickly lead to hemorrhagic shock and should be considered an emergency.

For more information, see Chapter 36 in Smeltzer and Bare: *Brunner and Suddarth's Textbook of Medical-Surgical Nursing,* 9th edition. Philadelphia: Lippincott Williams & Wilkins, 2000.

EXFOLIATIVE DERMATITIS

Exfoliative dermatitis is a serious condition characterized by a progressive inflammation in which erythema and scaling occur in a more or less generalized distribution. This condition starts acutely as either a patchy or a generalized erythematous eruption. Exfoliative dermatitis has a variety of causes. It is considered to be a secondary or reactive process to an underlying skin or systemic disease. It may appear as a part of the lymphoma group of diseases and may precede the appearance of lymphoma. Preexisting skin disorders implicated as a cause include psoriasis, atopic dermatitis, and contact dermatitis. It also appears as a severe medication reaction, including penicillin and phenylbutazone reactions. The cause is unknown in about 25% of cases.

Clinical Manifestations

- Chills, fever, prostration, occasional gastrointestinal symptoms, severe toxicity, and an itchy scaling of the skin
- Profound loss of stratum corneum (outermost layer of the skin), capillary leakage, hypoproteinemia, negative nitrogen balance
- Widespread dilation of cutaneous vessels, resulting in large amounts of body heat loss
- Skin color changes from pink to dark red; after a week, exfoliation (scaling) begins in the form of thin flakes that leave the underlying skin smooth and red, with new scales forming as the older ones come off
- Possible hair loss
- Relapse common
- Systemic effects: high-output congestive heart failure, intestinal disturbances, gynecomastia (breast enlargement), hyperuricemia, and temperature disturbances

Medical Management

Goals of management are to maintain fluid and electrolyte balance and to prevent infection. Treatment is individualized and supportive and is started as soon as condition is diagnosed.

- Hospitalize patients and place on bed rest.
- Discontinue all medications that may be implicated.
- Maintain a comfortable room temperature because of patient's abnormal thermoregulatory control.
- Maintain fluid and electrolyte balance because of considerable water and protein loss from the skin surface.
- Give plasma expanders as indicated.

Nursing Management
Nursing Interventions

NURSING ALERT

Observe for signs and symptoms of high-output congestive heart failure due to hyperemia and increased blood flow.

- Carry out continual nursing assessment to detect infection.
- Administer prescribed antibiotics on the basis of culture and sensitivity.
- Assess for hypothermia because of increased skin blood flow coupled with increased heat and water loss through the skin.
- Use topical therapy to give symptomatic relief.
- Use soothing baths, compresses, and lubrication with emollients to treat extensive dermatitis.
- Give prescribed oral or parenteral steroids when disease is not controlled by more conservative therapy.
- Advise patient to avoid all irritants, particularly medications.

For more information, see Chapter 52 in Smeltzer and Bare: *Brunner and Suddarth's Textbook of Medical-Surgical Nursing,* 9th edition. Philadelphia: Lippincott Williams & Wilkins, 2000.

F

FRACTURES

A fracture is a break in the continuity of bone and is defined according to type and extent. Fractures occur when the bone is subjected to stress greater than it can absorb. Fractures can be caused by a direct blow, crushing force, sudden twisting motion, or even extreme muscle contraction. When the bone is broken, adjacent structures are also affected, resulting in soft tissue edema, hemorrhage into the muscles and joints, joint dislocations, ruptured tendons, severed nerves, and damaged blood vessels. Body organs may be injured by the force that caused the fracture or by the fracture fragments.

Types of Fractures
- *Complete fracture*: a break across the entire cross-section of the bone, which is frequently displaced
- *Incomplete fracture*, also called *greenstick fracture:* break occurs through only part of the cross-section of the bone
- *Comminuted fractures*: a break with several bone fragments
- *Closed fracture*, or *simple fracture*: does not produce a break in the skin
- *Open fracture*, or *compound or complex fracture:* a break in which the skin or mucous membrane wound extends to the fractured bone. Open fractures are classified as follows:
  - *Grade I:* a clean wound less than 1 cm long
  - *Grade II:* a larger wound without extensive soft tissue damage

○ *Grade III:* wound is highly contaminated, has extensive soft tissue damage (most severe type).

Fractures may also be described according to anatomic placement of fragments, particularly if they are displaced or nondisplaced.

Early complications of fracture include shock, fat embolism, compartment syndrome, thromboembolism (pulmonary embolism), disseminated intravascular coagulopathy (DIC), and infection. Delayed complications include delayed union and nonunion, avascular necrosis of bone, reaction to external-fixation devices, reflex sympathetic dystrophy, and heterotrophic ossification.

Clinical Manifestations
Not all of the clinical manifestations are present in every fracture.

- The patient experiences muscle spasm and continuous pain that increases in severity until bone fragments are immobilized.
- Loss of function, deformity, and shortening of the extremity may be noted.
- Crepitus, local swelling, and discoloration may also be seen.
- If fat embolism syndrome occurs, with blockage of the small blood vessels that supply the brain, lungs, kidneys, and other organs (sudden onset, usually occurring within 24 to 72 hours, but may occur up to a week after injury), the following may be noted: hypoxia, tachypnea, tachycardia, and pyrexia, mental status changes varying from mild agitation and confusion to delirium and coma, dyspnea, crackles, wheezes, precordial chest pain, cough, large amounts of thick white sputum, hypoxia and blood gas values with PO_2 below 60 mm Hg, with an early respiratory alkalosis and later respiratory acidosis. The chest radiograph exhibits a typical "snowstorm" infiltrate. Eventually, acute pulmonary

edema, adult respiratory distress syndrome (ARDS), and heart failure develop.

- With systemic embolization, the patient appears pale. Petechiae are noted in the buccal membranes and conjunctival sacs, on the hard palate, on the fundus of the eye, and over the chest and anterior axillary folds. Fever, with a temperature above 39.4°C (103°F), develops. Free fat may be found in the urine when emboli reach the kidneys. Kidney failure may develop.

- Compartment syndrome (develops when tissue perfusion in the muscles is less than that required for tissue viability) may reveal a patient complaint of deep, throbbing, unrelenting pain, which is not controlled by opioids (can be due to a tight cast or constrictive dressing or an increase in muscle compartment contents because of edema or hemorrhage). Cyanotic (blue-tinged) nail beds, pale or dusky and cold fingers or toes, and nail bed capillary refill time are prolonged (greater than 3 seconds); pulse may be diminished (Doppler) or absent; motor weakness, paralysis, and paresthesia may occur.

- Manifestations of DIC include ecchymoses, unexpected bleeding after surgery, and bleeding from the mucous membranes, venipuncture sites, and gastrointestinal and urinary tracts.

- Symptoms of infection may include tenderness, pain, redness, swelling, local warmth, elevated temperature, and purulent drainage.

- Manifestation of other complications may be noted (deep vein thrombosis [DVT], thromboembolism, and pulmonary embolus). See specific disorders for additional information.

NURSING ALERT

Subtle personality changes, restlessness, irritability, or confusion in a patient who has sustained a fracture are indications for immediate blood gas studies.

Diagnostic Evaluation

- The diagnosis of a fracture depends on the patient's symptoms, the physical signs, and radiographic examination.
- Usually, the patient reports having sustained an injury to the area.

Medical Management

Emergency Management of Fractures

- Immediately after injury, immobilize the body part before the patient is moved, or if an injured patient must be moved before splints can be applied, support the extremity above and below the fracture site to prevent rotation or angular motion.
- Splint the fracture, including joints adjacent to the fracture, to prevent damage to the soft tissue.
- Apply temporary, well-padded splints, firmly bandaged over clothing, to immobilize the fracture.
- Assess vascular status distal to the injury to determine adequacy of peripheral tissue perfusion and nerve function.
- Cover the wound of an *open fracture* with a clean (sterile) dressing to prevent contamination of deeper tissues.

Medical Management of Fractures

The principles of fracture treatment include reduction, immobilization, and regaining of normal function and strength through rehabilitation.

- Reduction of a fracture ("setting" the bone) through closed method (manipulation and manual traction, eg, splint or cast); or open method (surgical placement of internal-fixation devices, eg, pins, wires, screws, plates, nails) to restore the fracture fragments into anatomic alignment and rotation; specific method depends on nature of the fracture.
- Immobilization, after the fracture has been reduced, holds the bone in correct position and alignment until union occurs, (accomplished by external or internal fixation).

• Maintaining and restoring function by controlling swelling by elevating the injured extremity and applying ice as prescribed; controlling restlessness, anxiety, and discomfort with a variety of approaches (eg, reassurance; position changes; pain relief strategies, including analgesics). Isometric and muscle setting exercises are done to minimize disuse atrophy and to promote circulation. With internal fixation, the surgeon determines the amount of movement and weight-bearing stress the extremity can withstand and prescribes the level of activity.

Management of Complications

• Treatment of shock consists of restoring blood volume and circulation, relieving the patient's pain, providing adequate splinting, and protecting the patient from further injury and other complications. See Nursing Management under Hypovolemic Shock for additional information.
• Prevention and management of fat embolism includes immediate immobilization of fractures and adequate support for fractured bones during turning and positioning. Prompt initiation of respiratory support is essential. Corticosteroids may be given as well as vasoactive medications, fluid replacement therapy, and morphine for pain and anxiety.
• Compartment syndrome is managed by controlling swelling by elevation of the extremity to the heart level or by releasing restrictive devices (dressings or cast). A *fasciotomy* (surgical decompression with excision of the fibrous membrane covering and separating muscles) may be needed to relieve the constrictive muscle fascia.
• Other complications are treated as indicated (see specific disorders).

Nursing Management
Nursing Interventions
PROMOTING FRACTURE HEALING
• Provide pharmacologic and nonpharmacologic measures for pain management.

- Monitor the client for signs of infection (if grafts were done, monitor the donor and recipient sites).
- Provide patient education, and reinforce information concerning the objectives of the bone graft, immobilization, avoidance of weight bearing, wound care, signs of infection, and follow-up care with the orthopedic surgeon.
- For the patient with electrical stimulation for nonunion (prolonged therapy), provide emotional support and encouragement to the patient, and encourage compliance with the treatment regimen. Include patient education regarding daily use of the stimulator as prescribed and need for follow-up evaluation by the orthopedist, who evaluates the progression of bone healing with periodic radiographic studies.

Closed Fractures

- Encourage patients with closed (simple) fractures to return to their usual activities as rapidly as possible, within the limits of the fracture immobilization.
- Teach patients how to control swelling and pain associated with the fracture and soft tissue trauma.
- Teach exercises to maintain the health of unaffected muscles and to increase strength of muscles needed for transferring and for using assistive devices (eg, crutches, walker).
- Teach patients how to use assistive devices safely.
- Arrange to help patients modify their home environment as needed and to secure personal assistance if necessary.
- Provide patient teaching, including self-care, medication information, monitoring for potential complications, and the need for continuing health care supervision.

Open Fractures

- The objectives of management are to prevent infection of the wound, soft tissue, and bone and to promote healing of soft tissue and bone. In an open fracture, there is risk of osteomyelitis, tetanus, and gas gangrene.
- Administer tetanus prophylaxis.

- Perform serial irrigation and débridement to remove anaerobic organisms.
- Administer intravenous antibiotics to prevent or treat infection.
- Perform aseptic dressing changes with sterile gauze to permit swelling and wound drainage, with wound irrigation and débridement as ordered.
- Provide, or teach patient and family to perform, wound care to flap or skin graft after the wound is closed in 5 to 7 days.
- Elevate and teach patient and family to elevate the extremity to minimize edema.
- Assess neurovascular status frequently.
- Measure the patient's temperature at regular intervals, and monitor for signs of infection.
- Promote intake of adequate nutrition to promote wound healing.

Fractures of Specific Sites
- Maximum functional recovery is the goal of management.
- With a *clavicle fracture*, head or cervical spine injuries may be seen. Caution the patient not to elevate the arm above shoulder level until the ends of the bone have united (about 6 weeks). Encourage the patient to exercise the elbow, wrist, and fingers as soon as possible and, when prescribed, to perform shoulder exercises. Tell the patient that vigorous activity is limited for 3 months.
- With *humeral neck* fractures (seen most frequently in older women after a fall on an outstretched arm), perform neurovascular assessment of the involved extremity to evaluate the extent of injury and possible involvement of the neurovascular bundle (nerves and blood vessels) of the arm. Provide and teach the patient to support the arm and immobilize it by a sling and swathe that secure the supported arm to the trunk. Place a soft pad in the axilla to absorb moisture and avoid skin breakdown. Begin pendulum exercises as soon as tolerated by the

patient. Instruct the patient to avoid vigorous activity, such as tennis, for an additional 10 to 14 weeks. Inform the patient that residual stiffness, aching, and some limitation of range of motion may persist for 6 or more months. When a humeral neck fracture is displaced with required fixation, exercises are started only after a prescribed period of immobilization.

- With *humeral shaft* fractures, the nerves and brachial blood vessels may be injured. Monitor for wrist drop, which is indicative of radial nerve injury. With an oblique, spiral, or displaced fracture that has resulted in shortening of the humeral shaft, instruct patient in care of a hanging cast, if used. Emphasize that a hanging cast must be dependent (hang free without support) because the weight of the cast provides the continuous traction to the arm. Advise the patient to sleep in an upright position so that traction from the weight of the cast is maintained. Teach patient to perform finger exercises as soon as the cast is applied, pendulum-shoulder exercises as prescribed, and isometric exercises. Instruct patient to use a sling after the cast is removed and to begin exercises to the shoulder, elbow, and wrist. For elderly patients who do not tolerate a cast, provide a sling and swathe for comfort and immobilization. If ordered, provide and teach patient about functional bracing. Instruct patient regarding a shoulder spica cast if used for early treatment of unstable humerus fracture or skeletal traction (eg, over-the-face traction, balanced side-arm traction).

- *Elbow* fractures (distal humerus) may result in injury to the median, radial, or ulnar nerves. Evaluate the patient for paresthesia and signs of compromised circulation in the forearm and hand. Monitor closely for Volkmann's ischemic contracture (a compartment syndrome) as well as for hemarthrosis (blood in the joint). Reinforce information regarding reduction and fixation of the fracture and planned active motion when swelling has subsided and healing has begun. Explain care if the arm is immobilized in a cast or posterior splint with a sling. Encour-

age active finger exercises. Teach and encourage patient
to do gentle range-of-motion exercise of the injured
joint about 1 week after internal fixation and after 2
weeks with closed reduction.

- *Radial head* fractures are usually produced by a fall on
  the outstretched hand with the elbow extended. Instruct
  patient in use of a splint for immobilization. If the fracture is displaced, reinforce the need for postoperative
  immobilization of the arm in a posterior plaster splint
  and sling. Encourage the patient to carry out a program
  of active motion of the elbow and forearm when
  prescribed.
- *Wrist* fractures (distal radius—Colles' fracture) are frequently seen in elderly women with osteoporotic bones
  and weak soft tissues that do not dissipate the energy of
  a fall. Reinforce care of the cast, or with more severe
  fractures with wire insertion, teach incision care.
  Instruct patient to keep the wrist and forearm elevated
  for 48 hours after reduction. Begin active motion of the
  fingers and shoulder promptly by teaching the patient to
  do the following exercises to reduce swelling and prevent
  stiffness:
  ○ Hold the hand at the level of the heart.
  ○ Move the fingers from full extension to flexion. Hold
    and release. (Repeat at least 10 times every hour when
    awake.)
  ○ Use the hand in functional activities.
  ○ Actively exercise the shoulder and elbow, including
    complete range-of-motion exercises of both joints.
    Assess the sensory function of the median nerve by
    pricking the distal aspect of the index finger, and assess
    the motor function by testing the patient's ability to
    touch the thumb to the little finger. If diminished cir-
    culation and nerve function is noted, prepare to treat
    with prompt release of constricting bandages.
- *Hand* trauma often requires extensive reconstructive surgery. The objective of treatment is always to regain maximum function of the hand. With a nondisplaced fracture, the finger is splinted for 3 to 4 weeks to relieve

pain and protect the fingertip from further trauma, but displaced fractures and open fractures may require open reduction with internal fixation, using wires or pins. Evaluate the neurovascular status of the injured hand. Teach the patient to control swelling by elevating the hand. Encourage functional use of the uninvolved portions of the hand.

- *Rib* fracture (uncomplicated fractures of the ribs) occur frequently in adults and usually result in no impairment of function but produce painful respirations. Assist the patient to cough and take deep breaths by splinting the chest with hands or pillow during cough. Reassure the patient that pain associated with rib fracture diminishes significantly in 3 or 4 days, and the fracture heals within 6 weeks. Monitor for complications, which may include a *flail chest*, *pneumothorax*, and *hemothorax.* (See specific disorders for nursing management).

- *Pelvic* fractures may be caused by falls, motor vehicle crashes, or crush injuries and are serious because at least two thirds of these patients have significant and multiple injuries. Monitor for symptoms, including ecchymosis; tenderness over the symphysis pubis, anterior iliac spines, iliac crest, sacrum, or coccyx; local swelling; numbness or tingling of pubis, genitals, and proximal thighs; and inability to bear weight without discomfort. Complete a neurovascular assessment of the lower extremities to detect injury to pelvic blood vessels and nerves. Monitor for hemorrhage and shock, two of the most serious consequences that may occur. Palpate the peripheral pulses of both lower extremities for absence of pulses, which may indicate a torn iliac artery or one of its branches. Assess for injuries to the bladder, rectum, intestines, other abdominal organs, and pelvic vessels and nerves; examine urine for blood to assess for urinary tract injury. In male patients, do not insert a catheter until the status of the urethra is known. Monitor for abdominal pain and signs of peritonitis as well as signs of a paralytic ileus. If patient has a stable pelvic fracture, maintain the patient on bed rest for a few days, and provide symptom management until the pain and discomfort are controlled. Provide fluids, dietary fiber, ankle and leg exercises, log rolling, coughing and deep breathing, and skin care to reduce the risk for complications and to increase the patient's comfort. Monitor bowel sounds. If the patient has a fracture of the coccyx and experiences pain on sitting and with defecation, assist with sitz baths as prescribed to relieve pain, and administer stool softeners to prevent the need to strain on defecation. As pain resolves, instruct patient to resume activity gradually, using ambulatory aids for protected weight bearing. Patients with unstable pelvic fractures may be treated with external fixation or open reduction and internal fixation (ORIF). Promotes hemodynamic stability and comfort, and encourage early mobilization. Teach and encourage patient to perform exercises (leg, respiratory, range-of-motion, and strengthening). Apply and encourage use of elastic pressure stockings and elevation of the foot of the bed (without the bed gatched at the knee) to aid venous return and to help diminish the effects of bed rest. When prescribed, assist the patient in mobility with progressive weight bearing, usually with crutches.

- *Femoral shaft* fractures are most often seen in young men involved in a motor vehicle crash or falls from a high place. Frequently, these patients have associated multiple trauma and develop shock from a loss of 2 to 3 units of blood. Assess neurovascular status of the extremity, especially circulatory perfusion of the foot (popliteal, posterior tibial, and pedal pulses and toe capillary refill as well as Doppler ultrasound monitoring). Note signs of dislocation of the hip and knee, and knee effusion, which may suggest ligament damage and possible instability of the knee joint. Apply and maintain skin traction for comfort and immobilization of the fracture or skeletal traction to achieve muscle relaxation and alignment of the fracture fragments before ORIF procedures, and later a cast brace. Assist patient in minimal partial weight bearing when indicated and progress to full weight bearing as tolerated. Reinforce that the cast brace is worn for 12 to 14 weeks. Instruct in and encourage patient to exercise the lower leg, foot, and toes on a regular basis. Assist the patient in performing active and passive knee exercises as soon as possible, depending on the management approach and the stability of the fracture and knee ligaments.

- *Tibia* and *fibula* fractures (most common fractures below the knee) result from a direct blow, falls with the foot in a flexed position, or a violent twisting motion. Provide instruction on care of the long leg-walking or patellar-tendon-bearing cast. Monitor for an anterior compartment syndrome (pain unrelieved by medications and increasing with plantar flexion, tense and tender muscle lateral to tibial crest, and paresthesia). Instruct patient and assist with partial weight bearing, usually in 7 to 10 days. Instruct patient on care of a short leg cast or brace (in 3 to 4 weeks), which allows for knee motion. Instruct patient in care of skeletal traction, if applicable. Encourage patient to perform foot and knee exercises within the limits of the immobilizing device. Instruct patient to begin weight bearing when prescribed (usually in about 4 to 6 weeks). Instruct patient to elevate extremity to control edema. Perform continuous neurovascular evaluation.

Nursing Management: The Elderly Patient With a Hip Fracture

Hip fractures occur with high incidence among elderly people, who have brittle bones from osteoporosis (particularly women) and who tend to fall frequently. The patient who has sustained a hip fracture frequently has a comorbid disease (ie, cardiovascular, pulmonary, renal, endocrine). Fractures of the neck of the femur may destroy blood vessels, disrupting blood supply to the head and the neck of the femur and resulting in bone death and commonly nonunion or aseptic necrosis.

Gerontologic Considerations

Hip fractures are a frequent contributor to death after the age of 75 years. Stress and immobility related to the trauma predispose the older adult to pneumonia, sepsis, and reduced ability to cope with other health problems.

F

Many elderly people hospitalized with hip fracture are confused as a result of the stress of the trauma, unfamiliar surroundings, sleep deprivation, medications, and systemic illness. Preoperative predictors of postoperative delirium include age over 70 years, alcohol abuse, poor cognitive or functional status, and marked electrolyte imbalance.

Assess the elderly patient for chronic conditions that require close monitoring. Examine the legs for edema due to congestive heart failure, and assess for peripheral pulselessness from arteriosclerotic vascular disease.

Treatment includes ORIF of fracture with temporary skin traction, or Buck's extension, to reduce muscle spasm, to immobilize the extremity, and to relieve pain and apply and maintain sandbags or a trochanter roll.

Major Nursing Diagnoses
- Pain related to fracture, soft tissue damage, muscle spasm, and surgery
- Impaired physical mobility related to fractured hip
- Actual impairment of skin integrity related to surgical incision
- Potential alteration in patterns of urinary elimination related to immobility
- Potential alteration in thought process related to age, stress of trauma, unfamiliar surroundings, and drug therapy
- Risk for ineffective individual coping related to injury, anticipated surgery, and dependence
- Risk for impaired home maintenance related to fractured hip and impaired mobility

Collaborative Problems/Potential Complications
- Hemorrhage
- Pulmonary complications

- Neurovascular compromise
- Deep vein thrombosis
- Pressure ulcers

Planning and Goals

Major goals may include relief of pain, achievement of a functional stable hip, wound healing, maintenance of normal urinary elimination patterns, use of effective coping mechanisms to modify stress, oriented and participatory in decision making, ability to care for self at home, and absence of complications.

Nursing Interventions

Postoperatively, after ORIF or replacement of the femoral head with a prosthesis (hemiarthroplasty), provide routine postoperative monitoring and interventions. (See Postoperative Nursing Management for additional information).

RELIEVING PAIN

- Assess type, degree (pain scale), and location of patient's pain
- Inform patient of available analgesics.
- Handle extremity gently, supporting it with hands or pillow.
- Use pain-modifying strategies (eg, modify environment, administer analgesics, evaluate response to medications).
- Position for comfort and function, and assist with frequent changes in position.

PROMOTING HIP FUNCTION AND STABILITY

- Maintain neutral positioning of hip.
- Maintain temporary skin traction, or Buck's extension, to reduce muscle spasm, to immobilize the extremity, and to relieve pain; apply and maintain sandbags or a trochanter roll to control the external rotation.
- Place a pillow between the legs to maintain abduction and alignment and to provide needed support when turning.
- Turn the patient on the affected or unaffected extremity as prescribed by the physician.

- Encourage the patient to exercise as much as possible by means of the over-bed trapeze.
- Arrange for physical therapists to work with the patient on transfers, ambulation, and the safe use of walker and crutches.
- Instruct in and supervise safe use of ambulatory aids.

PROMOTING WOUND HEALING
- Monitor vital signs.
- Use aseptic dressing changes.
- Assess wound appearance and character of drainage.
- Assess complaint of pain.
- Administer prescribed intravenous prophylactic antibiotics.
- Suspect infection if the patient complains of moderate hip discomfort and has mildly elevated sedimentation rate.

PROMOTING NORMAL URINARY ELIMINATION PATTERNS
- Monitor intake and output.
- Avoid or minimize use of indwelling catheter.
- Monitor clients for loss of bladder control (incontinence) or urinary retention.
- Assess the patient's voiding patterns.
- Encourage liberal fluid intake within the cardiovascular tolerance of the patient.

PROMOTING SKIN INTEGRITY
- Apply elastic tape in a vertical fashion to reduce the incidence of tape blisters.
- Provide proper skin care, especially to the heels, back, sacrum, and shoulders.
- Obtain and apply a high-density foam, static air, or other special mattress to provide protection and distribute pressure more evenly.

PROMOTING EFFECTIVE COPING MECHANISMS
- Encourage patient to express concerns and to discuss the possible impact of fractured hip.

- Support use of coping mechanisms. Involve significant others and support services as needed.
- Contact social services, if needed.
- Encourage patient to participate in planning.
- Explain anticipated treatment regimen and routines to facilitate positive attitude in relation to rehabilitation.

PROMOTING PATIENT ORIENTATION AND PATIENT
PARTICIPATION IN DECISION MAKING
- Assess orientation status.
- Interview family regarding patient's orientation and cognitive abilities before injury.
- Assess patient for auditory and visual deficits.
- Orient to and stabilize environment.
- Encourage participation in hygiene and nutritional activities.
- Provide for safety (eg, keep side rails up when patient is in bed, keep light on at night, have call bell available).
- Assess mental responses to medications, especially sedatives and analgesics.

MONITORING AND PREVENTING
POTENTIAL COMPLICATIONS
- Pulmonary complications: monitor chronic respiratory problems, if present, and encourage coughing and deep-breathing exercises. Monitor elderly patients who are taking cardiac, antihypertensive, or respiratory medications for their response to these medications. Assess breath sounds at least every 4 to 8 hours to detect adventitious or diminished sounds.
- Pressure ulcers and deep vein thrombosis: monitor and promote treatment of dehydration and poor nutrition by encouraging patient to consume adequate fluids and a balanced diet; monitor urine output. Encourage the patient to move all joints except the involved hip and knee and to use arms and the overhead trapeze for repositioning and to strengthen the arms and shoulders to facilitate walking with assistive devices; promote early mobilization. Encourage foot flexion exercises every 1 to 2 hours. Apply thigh-high elastic compression stockings

and pneumatic compression devices to prevent venous stasis. On the first postoperative day, transfer the patient to a chair with assistance and begin assisted ambulation. Assess the patient's legs at least every 4 hours for signs of DVT.

🏠 Promoting Home and Community-Based Care

Teaching Patients Self-Care

- Arrange for a home environment assessment, and refer patient for home care as needed.
- Assist patient as needed to make modifications in the home to permit safe use of walkers and crutches and for the patient's continuing care.
- Teach patient to monitor for neurovascular complications by monitoring the neurovascular status of the affected leg.
- Instruct patient in measures to prevent DVT; encourage fluids and ankle and foot exercises. Encourage use of elastic stockings, sequential compression devices, and prophylactic anticoagulant therapy as prescribed.
- Instruct patient to perform deep-breathing exercises, to change position at least every 2 hours, and to use of an incentive spirometer help to prevent respiratory complications.
- Teach patient and family to monitor or prevent delayed complications of hip fractures, including infection, nonunion, avascular necrosis of the femoral head (particularly with femoral neck fractures), and fixation device problems (eg, protrusion of the fixation device through the acetabulum; loosening of hardware).

Evaluation

EXPECTED OUTCOMES
- Reports pain relief
- Engages in therapeutic positioning
- Maintains normal urinary elimination pattern
- Exhibits normal wound healing
- Demonstrates use of effective coping mechanisms

- Remains oriented and participates in decision making
- Establishes effective communication
- Experiences no complications

For more information, see Chapter 63 in Smeltzer and Bare: *Brunner and Suddarth's Textbook of Medical-Surgical Nursing,* 9th edition. Philadelphia: Lippincott Williams & Wilkins, 2000.

G

GASTRITIS

Acute gastritis is inflammation of the stomach mucosa lasting several hours to a few days. It is most often due to dietary indiscretion, that is, eating irritating food that is too highly seasoned or food that is infected. Other causes include excessive alcohol, aspirin, or other nonsteroidal antiinflammatory drug (NSAID) use; bile reflux; or radiation therapy. A more severe form of acute gastritis is caused by strong acids or alkalies, which may cause the mucosa to become gangrenous or to perforate. Gastritis may also be the first sign of acute systemic infection.

Chronic gastritis is a prolonged inflammation of the stomach that may be caused by either benign or malignant ulcers of the stomach or by the bacteria, such as *Helicobacter pylori*. Chronic gastritis may be associated with autoimmune diseases, such as pernicious anemia and with dietary factors, such as hot drinks, spices, drug use (eg, NSAIDs), alcohol, smoking, or reflux of intestinal contents into the stomach. It occurs in the fundus or body of the stomach.

Clinical Manifestations
Acute Gastritis
- Abdominal discomfort with headache, lassitude, nausea, anorexia, vomiting, and hiccuping
- Can be asymptomatic
- Superficial ulceration, which can lead to hemorrhage
- Colic and diarrhea resulting from irritating food that is not vomited but reaches the bowel

- Recovery in about 1 day, although appetite may be diminished for 2 to 3 days

Chronic Gastritis
- May be asymptomatic except for symptoms of vitamin B_{12} deficiency, when present
- Anorexia, heartburn after eating, belching, sour taste in mouth, or nausea and vomiting

Diagnostic Evaluation
- Gastritis is associated with absence or low levels of hydrochloric acid or with high acid levels.
- Gastroscopy, upper gastrointestinal radiographic series, and biopsy with histologic examination are performed.
- Serologic testing for antibodies to the *H. pylori* antigen and a breath test may be performed.

Medical Management
Acute Gastritis
- The patient should refrain from alcohol and eating until symptoms subside; progress to nonirritating diet.
- If symptoms persist, intravenous fluids may be necessary.
- If bleeding is present, management is similar to that of upper gastrointestinal tract hemorrhage.
- If gastritis is due to ingestion of strong acids or alkalies, dilute and neutralize the acid with common antacids (eg, aluminum hydroxide); neutralize alkali with diluted lemon juice or diluted vinegar.
- If corrosion is extensive or severe, avoid emetics and lavage because of danger of perforation.
- Supportive therapy may include nasogastric intubation, analgesics, and sedatives.
- Emergency surgery may be required to remove gangrenous or perforated tissue; gastric resection (gastrojejunostomy) may be necessary to treat pyloric obstruction.

Chronic Gastritis
- Diet modification, rest, stress reduction, and pharmacotherapy are key treatment measures.

- *H. pylori* may be treated with antibiotics (ie, tetracycline or amoxicillin) and bismuth salts (Pepto-Bismol).

Nursing Management
Assessment
- Ask about presenting signs and symptoms: heartburn, indigestion, nausea, vomiting. When do symptoms occur? Are symptoms related to anxiety, stress, allergies, eating or drinking too much or too quickly?
- How are symptoms relieved?
- Inquire about whether others in the patient's environment have similar symptoms and whether blood has been vomited or any caustic element has been swallowed.
- Perform complete physical assessment. Note abdominal tenderness, dehydration, and evidence of systemic disorder that may be responsible for symptoms.

Major Nursing Diagnoses
- Anxiety related to treatment
- Altered nutrition: less than body requirements related to inadequate intake of nutrients.
- Risk for fluid volume deficit related to insufficient fluid intake and excessive fluid loss subsequent to vomiting.
- Pain related to irritated stomach mucosa.
- Knowledge deficit about dietary management and disease process.

Collaborative Problems/Potential Complications
- Perforation
- Hemorrhage
- Pyloric obstruction

Planning and Goals
The major goals of the patient may include reduced anxiety, adequate nutritional intake, maintenance of fluid balance, increase awareness of dietary management, and absence or minimal pain experience.

Nursing Interventions

REDUCING ANXIETY

- Carry out emergency measures for ingestion of acids or alkalies.
- Offer support therapy to patient and family during treatment and after the ingested acid or alkali has been neutralized or diluted.
- Prepare patient for additional diagnostic studies (endoscopy) or surgery.
- Use a calm approach and answer questions as completely as possible; explain all procedures and treatments.

PROMOTING OPTIMAL NUTRITION

- Provide physical and emotional support for patients with acute gastritis.
- Avoid foods and fluids by mouth for hours or days until acute symptoms subside.
- Provide intravenous therapy as necessary and monitor serum electrolyte values daily.
- Offer ice chips and clear liquids when symptoms subside.
- Encourage patient to report any symptoms suggesting a repeat episode of gastritis as food is introduced.
- Discourage caffeinated beverages (caffeine increases gastric activity and pepsin secretion).
- Discourage alcohol and cigarette smoking (nicotine inhibits neutralization of gastric acid in the duodenum). Instruct patient that nicotine increases muscular activity in the bowel, leading to nausea and vomiting (parasympathetic stimulation).
- Refer patient for alcohol counseling and smoking cessation when appropriate.

PROVIDING ADEQUATE FLUID INTAKE

- Monitor daily intake and output for dehydration (minimal intake of 1.5 L/day and urine output of 30 mL/h). Infuse intravenous fluids if prescribed.
- Assess electrolyte values every 24 hours for fluid imbalance.

- Be alert for indicators of hemorrhagic gastritis (hematemesis, tachycardia, hypotension), and notify physician.

RELIEVING PAIN
- Instruct patient to avoid foods and beverages that may be irritating to the gastric mucosa.
- Instruct patient in the use of medications to relieve chronic gastritis.
- Assess level of pain and attainment of comfort through use of medications and avoidance of irritating substances.

Promoting Home and Community-Based Care

Teaching Patients Self-Care
- Assess knowledge about gastritis and develop an individualized teaching plan that incorporates the patient's pattern of eating, daily caloric needs, and food preferences.
- Provide a list of substances to avoid (caffeine, nicotine, spicy foods, irritating or highly seasoned foods, alcohol); plan consult with nutritionist if indicated.
- Educate about antibiotics, antacids, bismuth salts, sedatives, or anticholinergics that may be prescribed.
- Give patients with pernicious anemia instructions regarding need for long-term vitamin B_{12} injections (teach self-administration or arrange for patient to receive injections from health care provider).

For more information, see Chapter 34 in Smeltzer and Bare: *Brunner and Suddarth's Textbook of Medical-Surgical Nursing,* 9th edition. Philadelphia: Lippincott Williams & Wilkins, 2000.

GLAUCOMA

Glaucoma refers to a group of ocular conditions character-ized by visual field loss caused by damage to the optic nerve. Damage is related to the level of intraocular pressure (IOP), which is too high for proper functioning of the optic nerve. Glaucoma is one of the leading causes of blindness among adults in the United States. When it is diagnosed early and managed properly, blindness is almost always preventable. Most cases are asymptomatic until extensive and irreversible damage has occurred. Glaucoma affects people of all ages but is more prevalent with increasing age. Others at risk are patients with diabetes, African Americans, those with a family history of glaucoma, and people with previous eye trauma or surgery or those who have had long-term steroid treatment.

Classification

There are two major categories of glaucoma: open angle and angle closure. The categories are further divided into the following:

- *Primary glaucomas*: cause unknown; usually bilateral and thought to have a hereditary component
- *Secondary glaucomas*: cause known; often unilateral

Causes of Secondary Open-Angle Glaucoma

- Long-term corticosteroid use
- Intraocular tumors
- Uveitis from diseases such as herpes simplex and herpes zoster
- Trabecular meshwork blockage by lens material, vis-coelastic substance (used in cataract surgery), blood, or pigment

Clinical Manifestations

- Glaucoma is often asymptomatic until late in its course; it is insidious in onset, slowly progressive, and small areas of peripheral vision loss may go unnoticed

- One eye frequently is involved earlier and more severely than the other.
- Symptoms include pain (aching or discomfort around eyes and headache), halo vision, blurred vision, difficulty seeing in low light, redness, and change in the eye's appearance (pallor and cupping of the optic nerve disc).
- Ocular pain caused by rapid rise in IOP by inflammation or medication-induced side effects.
- Severe ocular pain accompanied by nausea, vomiting, sweating, or bradycardia.

Diagnostic Evaluation
- Routine eye examinations and screening clinics are vital to detection.
- Ocular and medical histories (exposes predisposing factors) and tonometry, ophthalmoscopy, gonioscopy, and perimetry are major diagnostic tests.

Medical Management
- The objective of treatment is to lower the IOP and maintain it at a level consistent with retaining vision.
- Treatment varies depending on classification of the disease and response to therapy.
- Medication therapy, laser surgery, and conventional surgery may be used to control progressive damage; first one eye is treated, then the second eye.
- Lifelong medication therapy is almost always necessary.

Pharmacotherapy
- Pharmacotherapy is the initial and principal treatment for glaucoma.
- Acute angle-closure glaucoma is treated with medication (including miotics) to reduce IOP before laser or incisional iridectomy.
- Commonly used agents include the following:
  ○ Beta-adrenergic antagonists, most widely used hypotensive agents, effective in many types of glaucoma
  ○ Cholinergic agents (topical), used in short-term management of glaucoma with pupillary block

○ Alpha-2-adrenergic agonists (topical), which reduce IOP by increasing aqueous humor outflow
○ Carbonic anhydrase inhibitor (systemically), which lowers IOP by reducing aqueous humor formation
○ Osmotic diuretics, which reduce IOP by increasing the osmolality of the plasma to draw water from the eye into the vascular circulation

Surgical Management

• Ophthalmic laser surgery is indicated as the primary treatment for glaucoma or is required when medication therapy is poorly tolerated or ineffective in lowering IOP.
• Conventional surgery procedures are performed when laser techniques are unsuccessful or when the patient is not a good candidate for laser surgery (eg, a patient who is unable to sit still or follow instructions).
• Filtering procedures: an opening or a fistula in the trabecular meshwork (trabeculectomy) is made to allow drainage, or drainage implant surgery may be performed.

🏠 Promoting Home and Community-Based Care

Teaching Patients Self-Care

• Teach that optimum reduction of IOP and control of glaucoma damage depend on adherence to medication regimen and attendance at follow-up examinations.
• Give written instructions that identify name of medications, description of containers, frequency and times of administration. Check for understanding of the expected action and possible side effects. Verify accuracy of eye-drop instillation, even with "experienced" patients with glaucoma.
• Suggest that patient review all medications with ophthalmologist and mention side effects at each visit.
• Stress importance of making medication administration a part of daily routine so that doses are not missed.

Stress that medication is to be continued even when IOP is under control. Patient may ask if generic form of medication is available for cost savings.

- Make patient aware that glaucoma medications may cause focus problems, and advise them to be cautious.
- Teach patient to note how the eyes look and feel and report unusual changes to the physician: excessive irritation, watering, blurring, cloudy vision, discharge, rainbows around lights at night, flashes of light, and floating objects in the field of vision.
- Inform patient of possible drug interactions with glaucoma medications and other medications.

G

Continuing Care

- Refer patients with severe impairment to assistive services.
- When patients meet the criteria for legal blindness, refer to agencies that assist in obtaining benefits from federally assisted programs.
- Encourage maintaining good health and limiting stress: proper nutrition, salt restriction, avoiding excessive fluid intake, maintaining appropriate weight level, exercising, and taking time for fun and relaxation.
- Encourage sharing feelings and concerns with family and friends or talking with other patients with glaucoma; support family caregivers.

🍁 Gerontologic Considerations

Most patients with glaucoma are in the older age group. Often, dimming vision is accepted as part of aging, and medical assistance is not sought. For people older than 35 years of age, tonometry is recommended, with periodic checking of eye pressure thereafter.

Help the elderly patient to understand that eyedrops must be continued to keep glaucoma from worsening. Discontinuation of the medication allows glaucoma to continue insidiously until blindness occurs.

Recognize when caring for the elderly patient with glaucoma that other problems must be considered, such as arthritis, depression, potential for falling, and accidents.

For more information, see Chapter 54 in Smeltzer and Bare: *Brunner and Suddarth's Textbook of Medical-Surgical Nursing,* 9th edition. Philadelphia: Lippincott Williams & Wilkins, 2000.

GLOMERULONEPHRITIS, ACUTE

Acute glomerulonephritis is a disease of the kidney in which there is an inflammation of the glomerular capillaries. In most cases, the stimulus of the reaction is group A streptococcal infection, which ordinarily precedes the onset of glomerulonephritis by an interval of 2 to 3 weeks. Antigen—antibody complexes in the blood are trapped in the glomeruli, stimulating inflammation and producing injury to the kidney. Glomerulonephritis may also follow scarlet fever, impetigo, and acute viral infections, including upper respiratory infections, mumps, varicella zoster virus infection, Epstein-Barr virus infection, hepatitis B, and human immunodeficiency virus (HIV) infection. It is predominantly a disease of youth.

Clinical Manifestations
- Urine is cola colored as a result of hematuria and proteinuria.
- In the more severe form of the disease, headache, malaise, facial edema, flank pain, and renal failure with oliguria occur.
- Mild to severe hypertension, some degree of edema (circulatory overload possible in elderly patients), and tenderness of the costovertebral angle are common.

Diagnostic Evaluation
- Primary presenting feature is microscopic or gross (macroscopic) hematuria.

- Proteinuria, increased antistreptolysin-O titer, elevated blood urea nitrogen (BUN) and serum creatinine levels, and anemia are found.
- Kidney biopsy is performed for definitive diagnosis.

Medical Management

The goals of management are to preserve kidney function and to treat complications promptly.

G

- Penicillin for residual streptococcal infection
- Diuretics and antihypertensive agents
- Plasma exchange (plasmapheresis) and treatment with steroids and cytotoxic drugs to reduce inflammatory response, in rapid progressive disease
- Dialysis occasionally necessary
- Bed rest, during the acute phase until the urine clears and BUN and creatinine levels and blood pressure return to normal

Nutritional Management

- Dietary protein restricted with elevated BUN level
- Sodium restricted with hypertension, edema, and congestive heart failure
- Carbohydrates for energy and to reduce protein catabolism
- Fluids according to fluid losses and daily body weight; intake and output

🏠 Promoting Home and Community-Based Care

- Instruct patient to schedule follow-up evaluations of blood pressure, urinalysis for protein, and BUN and creatinine studies to determine if disease has exacerbated.
- Instruct patient to notify the physician if infection is noted or symptoms of renal failure occur: fatigue, nausea, vomiting, diminishing urinary output.
- Review fluid and diet restrictions.
- Refer to home care nurse as indicated for patient assessment and detection of early symptoms.

For more information, see Chapter 41 in Smeltzer and Bare: *Brunner and Suddarth's Textbook of Medical-Surgical Nursing,* 9th edition. Philadelphia: Lippincott Williams & Wilkins, 2000.

GLOMERULONEPHRITIS, CHRONIC

Chronic glomerulonephritis may have its onset as acute glomerulonephritis or some other type of antigen–antibody reaction that is overlooked. After repeated occurrences of these reactions, the kidneys are reduced to as little as one fifth of their normal size and consist largely of fibrous tissue. As chronic glomerulonephritis progresses, the signs and symptoms of renal insufficiency and chronic renal failure occur. The result is severe glomerular damage that results in end-stage renal disease (ESRD).

Clinical Manifestations

Symptoms are variable. Some patients with severe disease have no symptoms for many years.

- First indications may be sudden, severe nosebleed, stroke, or convulsions.
- Many patients merely notice that their feet are slightly swollen at night.
- Other symptoms include loss of weight and strength, increasing irritability, and nocturia.
- Headaches, dizziness, and digestive disturbances are common.

Signs and Symptoms of Renal Insufficiency and Chronic Renal Failure

- Patient appears poorly nourished with a yellow-gray pigmentation of the skin and periorbital and peripheral edema.
- Blood pressure is normal or severely elevated.
- Retinal findings include hemorrhage, exudate, narrowed tortuous arterioles, and papilledema.

- Pale mucous membranes are seen.
- Neck veins may be distended from fluid overload.
- Cardiomegaly, gallop rhythm, and other signs of congestive heart failure may be present.
- Crackles are heard in lungs.
- Peripheral neuropathy with diminished deep tendon reflexes may be present.
- Neurosensory changes occur late in the illness, resulting in confusion and limited attention span.
- Late findings include pericarditis with pericardial friction rub and pulsus paradoxus.

Diagnostic Evaluation
Laboratory Abnormalities
- Urinalysis reveals fixed specific gravity of 1.010, variable proteinuria, and urinary casts.
- Blood studies related to renal failure progression show hyperkalemia, metabolic acidosis, anemia, hypoalbuminemia, decreased serum calcium and increased serum phosphorus, and hypermagnesemia.
- Chest films may show cardiac enlargement and pulmonary edema.
- Electrocardiogram may be normal or may reflect left ventricular hypertrophy.

Medical Management
The treatment of ambulatory patients is guided by symptoms.

- If hypertension is present, the blood pressure is lowered with sodium and water restriction.
- Proteins of high biologic value are provided to support good nutritional status.
- Urinary tract infections are treated promptly.
- If severe edema develops, patient is placed on bed rest with head of bed elevated to promote comfort and diuresis.
- Patient's weight is monitored daily.
- Diuretics are administered to reduce fluid overload.

- Sodium and fluid intake are adjusted according to the ability of the patient's kidneys to excrete water and sodium.
- Dialysis is considered early in the course of disease to keep the patient in optimal physical condition, prevent fluid and electrolyte imbalances, and minimize the risk of complications of renal failure.

Nursing Management
Nursing Interventions
- Observe for signs of deterioration of renal function; report changes in fluid and electrolyte status and in cardiac and neurologic status.
- Give emotional support throughout the course of the disease and treatment by providing opportunity for patient and family to verbalize concerns and have questions answered and options discussed.

🏠 Promoting Home and Community-Based Care

- Educate the patient and family about prescribed treatment plan and the risk of noncompliance. Instructions include explanations and scheduling for follow-up evaluations of blood pressure, urinalysis for protein and casts, blood for BUN, and creatinine. Instruct in recommended diet and fluid modifications, and provide medication teaching.
- Refer to community health or home care nurse for careful assessment of patient progress and continued education about problems to report to health care provider.
- Give patient and family assistance and support regarding dialysis and long-term implications.

For more information, see Chapter 41st in Smeltzer and Bare: *Brunner and Suddarth's Textbook of Medical-Surgical Nursing,* 9th edition. Philadelphia: Lippincott Williams & Wilkins, 2000.

GOUT

Gout is a heterogeneous group of conditions related to a genetic defect of purine metabolism and resulting hyperuricemia. There is either an oversecretion of uric acid or a renal defect resulting in decreased excretion of uric acid or a combination of both. Primary hyperuricemia may be due to severe dieting or starvation, excessive intake of foods high in purines (shellfish, organ meats), or heredity. In secondary hyperuricemia, the gout is a minor clinical feature secondary to any of a number of genetic or acquired processes, including conditions with an increase in cell turnover (leukemias, some anemias) and an increase in cell breakdown.

Clinical Manifestations

Four stages of gout can be identified: asymptomatic hyperuricemia, acute gouty arthritis, intercritical gout, and chronic tophaceous gout.

Manifestations of Acute Gouty Arthritis

- Acute arthritis of gout is the most common early sign.
- The metatarsophalangeal (MTP) joint of the big toe is the most commonly affected; the tarsal area, ankle, or knee may also be targeted.
- The acute attack may be triggered by trauma, alcohol ingestion, dieting, medication, surgical stress, or illness.
- Abrupt onset occurs at night, causing severe pain, redness, swelling, and warmth over the affected joint.
- Early attacks tend to subside spontaneously over 3 to 10 days without treatment.
- The next attack may not come for months or years; in time, attacks tend to occur more frequently, involve more joints, and last longer.

Hyperuricemia

- Fewer than one in five hyperuricemic people develop clinically apparent urate crystal deposits.

- Subsequent development of gout is directly related to duration and magnitude of hyperuricemia.

Tophi
- Tophi, a chalky deposit of sodium urate, are noted an average of 10 years after the onset of gout.
- Tophi are generally associated with frequent and severe inflammatory episodes.
- Higher serum concentrations of uric acid are associated with tophus formation.
- Tophi occur in the synovium, olecranon bursa, subchondral bone, infrapatellar and Achilles' tendons, subcutaneous tissue, and overlying joints.
- Tophi have also been found in aortic walls, heart valves, nasal and ear cartilage, eyelids, cornea, and sclerae.
- Joint enlargement may cause loss of motion.

Increased Risk for Urolithiasis
- Incidence of renal stones is two times higher in patients with secondary gout than in those with primary gout.
- Stone formation is related to increased serum uric acid, acidity of urine, and urinary concentration.

Medical Management
- Hyperuricemia, tophi, joint destruction, and renal problems are treated after the acute inflammatory process has subsided.
- Uricosuric agents, such as probenecid, correct hyperuricemia and dissolve deposited urate.
- Colchicine (oral or parenteral) or a nonsteroidal anti-inflammatory drug (NSAID), such as indomethacin, is used to relieve acute attacks.
- Allopurinol is effective, but it is limited because of the risk of toxicity.
- Aspiration and intraarticular corticosteroids are used to treat large-joint acute attacks.

Nursing Management

See Nursing Management under Arthritis for additional information.

- Review medications with patient and family members.
- Stress the importance of continuing medications to maintain effectiveness.

For more information, see Chapter 50 in Smeltzer and Bare: *Brunner and Suddarth's Textbook of Medical-Surgical Nursing,* 9th edition. Philadelphia: Lippincott Williams & Wilkins, 2000.

G

GUILLAIN-BARRÉ SYNDROME (POLYRADICULONEURITIS)

Guillain-Barré is a clinical syndrome of unknown cause involving the peripheral, spinal, and cranial nerves. In most patients, the syndrome is preceded by an infection (respiratory or gastrointestinal) 1 to 4 weeks before the onset of neurologic deficits. In some instances, it has occurred after vaccination or surgery. It may be due to a primary viral infection, immune reaction, some other process, or a combination of processes. One hypothesis is that a viral infection induces an autoimmune reaction that attacks the myelin of the peripheral nerves.

Clinical Manifestations

- Initial neurologic symptoms are paresthesia (tingling and numbness) and muscle weakness of the legs, which may progress to upper extremities, trunk, and facial muscles. Muscle weakness may be followed quickly by complete paralysis.
- Cranial nerves are frequently affected, leading to paralysis of the ocular, facial, and oropharyngeal muscles, causing difficulty in talking, chewing, and swallowing.

- Autonomic dysfunction frequently occurs in the form of overreactivity or underreactivity of the sympathetic or parasympathetic nervous system. It is manifested by disturbances of heart rate and rhythm, blood pressure changes, and a variety of other vasomotor disturbances.
- There may be severe, persistent pain in the back and calves.
- Frequently, there is loss of position sense and diminished or absent tendon reflexes.
- Sensory changes are manifested by paresthesias.
- Most patients make a full recovery after several months to a year; about 10% have residual disability.

Diagnostic Evaluation
- Clinical presentation, history of recent viral infection, and results of laboratory and diagnostic studies provide key information for diagnosis.
- Spinal fluid shows an increased protein concentration with normal cell count.
- Electrophysiologic testing shows marked slowing of nerve conduction velocity.

Medical Management
- The syndrome is considered a medical emergency and the patient is managed in an intensive care unit.
- Respiratory problems require mechanical ventilation.
- Plasmapheresis (plasma exchange) may be used in the severely affected patient to limit deterioration and demyelinization.
- Continuous electrocardiogram (ECG) monitoring: observe and treat cardiac dysrhythmias. Atropine may be administered to avoid episodes of bradycardia during endotracheal suctioning and physical therapy.

Nursing Management
Assessment
- Assess for acute respiratory failure, a life-threatening problem.

• Assess for complications, including ECG monitoring for cardiac dysrhythmias, deep vein thrombosis (DVT), and pulmonary embolism.

Major Nursing Diagnoses
• Ineffective breathing pattern and gas exchange related to rapidly progressive weakness and impending respiratory failure
• Impaired physical mobility related to paralysis
• Altered nutrition: less than body requirements related to inability to swallow, which is secondary to cranial nerve dysfunction
• Impaired verbal communication related to cranial nerve dysfunction
• Fear related to loss of control and paralysis

Collaborative Problems/Potential Complications
• Respiratory failure
• Autonomic dysfunction

Planning and Goals
The major goals of the patient may include improved respiratory function, increased mobility, improved nutritional status, effective communication, decreased fear and anxiety, and absence of complications.

Nursing Interventions
MAINTAINING RESPIRATORY FUNCTION
• Assess carefully for difficulty in coughing and swallowing, which may cause aspiration of saliva and precipitate acute respiratory failure.
• Provide chest physical therapy, and elevate head of bed to facilitate respirations and promote effective coughing.
• Suction to maintain a clear airway.

MONITORING FOR RESPIRATORY FAILURE
• Assess for difficulty in coughing and swallowing or decreasing vital capacity, indicating deterioration of respiratory function.

- Watch for breathlessness while talking, shallow and irregular breathing, increasing pulse rate, use of accessory muscles while breathing, and change in respiratory pattern.

PREVENTING COMPLICATIONS FROM IMMOBILITY

- Monitor for and institute preventive measures related to urinary retention, transient hypertension, orthostatic hypotension, or other threats to the immobilized or paralyzed patient.
- Provide passive range-of-motion exercises at least twice daily; support the paralyzed extremities in functional positions.
- Collaborate with physical therapist to prevent contracture deformities.
- Ensure adequate hydration and administer prescribed anticoagulant regimen to prevent DVT and pulmonary embolism; assist with physical therapy; and use antiembolism stockings.
- Place padding over elbows and head of the fibula to prevent compression neuropathies of the ulnar and peroneal nerves.
- Use principles of nursing management of the unconscious patient.
- Use tilt table to help assume upright posture when recovery begins to prevent orthostatic hypotension.

PROVIDING ADEQUATE NUTRITION

- Provide adequate nutrition to prevent muscle wasting.
- Provide intravenous feedings as prescribed, and monitor bowel sounds.
- Provide nasogastric tube feedings if patient is unable to swallow.
- Resume oral feeding when patient can swallow normally.

IMPROVING COMMUNICATION

- Establish communication through lip reading, use of picture cards, and a system of blinking eyes to indicate yes or no if patient is on ventilator or otherwise unable to speak; obtain referral for speech therapy as indicated.

- Provide diversional therapy, such as television, tapes, and visits, to alleviate some of the frustrations that are encountered.

RELIEVING FEAR AND ANXIETY
- Involve family and friends with selected patient care activities and diversion to reduce sense of isolation.
- Provide patient with information about condition, emphasizing a positive appraisal of coping resources.
- Encourage relaxation exercises and distraction techniques, giving positive feedback.
- Create a positive attitude and atmosphere.
- Give expert nursing care, explanations, and reassurance to help patient gain control over situation.

Promoting Home and Community-Based Care

Teaching Patients Self-Care
- Teach patient and family about the disorder and its generally favorable prognosis.
- During the acute phase, instruct patient and family about strategies they can implement to minimize the effects of immobility and other complications.
- Explain the care of the patient and the roles of the patient and family in the rehabilitation process.
- Use an interdisciplinary effort for family or caregiver education.

Continuing Care
- Provide care in a comprehensive inpatient program, an outpatient program, if patient able to travel by car, or encourage a home program of physical and occupational therapy.
- Support patient and family through long recovery phase, and promote involvement for return of former abilities.

- Inform patient and caregivers of the Guillain-Barré support group.

Evaluation

EXPECTED OUTCOMES
- Maintains effective respirations and airway clearance
- Shows increasing mobility
- Demonstrates ability to swallow
- Demonstrates recovery of speech
- Shows lessening fear and anxiety
- Is free of complications

For more information, see Chapters 22 and 59 in Smeltzer and Bare: *Brunner and Suddarth's Textbook of Medical-Surgical Nursing,* 9th edition. Philadelphia: Lippincott Williams & Wilkins, 2000.

H

HEAD INJURY

Injuries to the head involve trauma to the scalp, skull, and brain. Head injuries are among the most common and serious sources of neurologic impairment and have reached epidemic proportions as a result of motor vehicle crashes. Other causes include falls, assaults, and sports injuries. A major risk to the patient who experiences a head injury is damage to the brain from bleeding or swelling that causes increased intracranial pressure (ICP). Two thirds of people with head injury are younger than 30 years of age, with a 3:1 male-to-female incidence ratio. The second highest incidence of head injury occurs in the elderly population.

SCALP AND SKULL INJURIES
- Scalp trauma may result in an abrasion (brush wound), contusion, laceration, or hematoma. The scalp bleeds profusely when injured. Scalp wounds are a portal entry for intracranial infections.
- Fracture of the skull is a break in the continuity of the skull caused by trauma. Fractures may occur with or without damage to the brain. They are classified as linear, comminuted, depressed, or basilar and may be open (dura is torn) or closed (dura is not torn).

Clinical Manifestations
Symptoms, other than local, depend on amount and distribution of brain injury.

- Persistent, localized pain usually suggests fracture.

- Fractures of the cranial vault produce swelling in that region.
- Fractures of the base of the skull frequently produce hemorrhage from the nose, pharynx, or ears, and blood may appear under the conjunctiva.
- Ecchymosis may be seen over the mastoid (Battle's sign).
- Drainage of cerebral spinal fluid (CSF) from the ears and the nose suggests basal skull fracture.
- Drainage of CSF may cause serious infection (eg, meningitis) through a tear in the dura mater.
- Bloody spinal fluid suggests brain laceration or contusion.
- Brain injury may have various signs, including altered level of consciousness, pupillary abnormalities, altered or absent gag reflex or corneal reflex, neurologic deficits, change in vital signs (eg, respiration pattern, hypertension, bradycardia), hyperthermia or hypothermia, and sensory, vision, or hearing impairment.
- Signs of a postconcussion syndrome may include headache, dizziness, anxiety, irritability, and lethargy.
- In acute or subacute subdural hematoma, changes in level of consciousness, pupillary signs, hemiparesis, coma, hypertension, bradycardia, and slowing respiratory rate are signs of expanding mass.
- Chronic subdural hematoma may result in severe headache, alternating focal neurologic signs, personality changes, mental deterioration, and focal seizures.

Diagnostic Evaluation
- Physical examination and evaluation of neurologic status
- Radiographic studies: computed tomography (CT), magnetic resonance imaging (MRI)
- Cerebral angiography, spinal tap

Medical Management
- Nondepressed skull fractures generally do not require surgical treatment but require close observation of the patient.

- Depressed skull fractures may be managed conservatively; contaminated or deforming fractures require surgery.

BRAIN INJURY
CONCUSSION

A cerebral concussion after head injury is a temporary loss of neurologic function with no apparent structural damage. Concussion generally involves a period of unconsciousness lasting from a few seconds to a few minutes. Jarring of the brain may be so slight as to cause only dizziness and spots before the eyes, or severe enough to cause complete loss of consciousness. If the frontal lobe is affected, the patient may exhibit bizarre irrational behavior. If the temporal lobe is affected, patient may exhibit temporary amnesia or disorientation.

Nursing Management
- Give information, explanations, and encouragement to reduce postconcussion syndrome.
- Instruct family to look for the following signs and notify physician or clinic: difficulty in awakening, difficulty in speaking, confusion, severe headache, vomiting, or weakness of one side of the body.
- Advise patient to resume normal activities slowly.

CONTUSION

A cerebral contusion is a more severe cerebral injury. The brain is bruised, with possible surface hemorrhage. The patient is unconscious, may exhibit symptoms of shock (eg, cool, pale skin, subnormal blood pressure and temperature), and may be incontinent of bowel or bladder. The patient may be aroused with effort but soon slips back into unconsciousness. In general, patients with widespread injury who have abnormal motor function, abnormal eye movements, and elevated ICP have a poor outcome (brain damage, disability, or death). Conversely, these patients may recover consciousness completely, may pass into a stage of cerebral irritability (ie, easily disturbed by any form of stimulation, such as noise and light), and may become hyperactive. Recovery is often delayed, and residual headache and vertigo are common; impaired mentality or seizures may occur.

INTRACRANIAL HEMORRHAGE

Hematomas that develop within the cranial vault are the most serious results of brain injury. A hematoma may be epidural, subdural, or intracerebral, depending on location. Its main effects are frequently delayed until the hematoma is large enough to cause distortion and herniation of the brain and increased ICP.

EPIDURAL HEMATOMA (EXTRADURAL HEMATOMA OR HEMORRHAGE)

Blood collects in the epidural space between the skull and dura mater. Symptoms are caused by the expanding hematoma: usually, a momentary loss of consciousness at time of injury, followed by an interval of apparent recovery. Sudden signs of compression may appear, including deterioration of consciousness and signs of focal neurologic deficits (dilation and fixation of a pupil or paralysis of an extremity); patient deteriorates rapidly.

Medical Management
Extreme Emergency
• Marked neurologic deficit or respiratory arrest may occur within minutes. Burr holes are made to remove the clots, and the bleeding point is controlled (craniotomy; drain insertion).

SUBDURAL HEMATOMA

Blood collects between the dura and the underlying brain and is more frequently venous in origin. The most common cause is trauma, but it may also be associated with various bleeding tendencies and rupture of an aneurysm. Subdural hematoma may be acute (major head injury), subacute (sequelae of less severe contusions), or chronic (minor head injuries in the elderly may be cause; signs and symptoms fluctuate and may be mistaken for neurosis, psychosis, or stroke).

INTRACEREBRAL HEMORRHAGE OR HEMATOMA

Bleeding occurs into the substance of the brain. Hematoma is commonly seen when forces are exerted to the head over a small area (missile injuries or bullet wounds; stab injury). It may also result from systemic hypertension causing degeneration and rupture of a vessel. Its onset may be insidious with neurologic deficits followed by headache.

Medical Management

- Management involves supportive care, control of ICP, maintenance of fluid and electrolyte balance, administration of antihypertensive medications, or craniotomy.
- Increased ICP is managed by adequate oxygenation, mannitol administration, ventilatory support, hyperventilation, elevation of the head of bed, maintenance of fluid and electrolyte balance, nutritional support, pain and anxiety management, or neurosurgery.

See Medical Management and Nursing Management under Increased Intracranial Pressure for additional information.

Nursing Management for the Patient With a Head Injury

Assessment

Obtain health history, including time of injury, cause of injury, direction and force of the blow; loss of consciousness, and condition following injury. Detailed neurologic and system assessments provide baseline data. The Glasgow Coma Scale serves as an excellent guide for assessing levels of consciousness based on the three criteria of (1) eye opening, (2) verbal responses, and (3) motor responses to a verbal command or painful stimuli. The Rancho Los Amigos Level of Cognitive Function is another useful evaluation scale.

MONITORING VITAL SIGNS

- Monitor at frequent intervals to assess intracranial status.
- Assess for increasing ICP, including slowing of pulse, increasing systolic pressure, and widening of pulse pressure. As brain compression increases, vital signs are reversed, pulse and respirations become rapid, and blood pressure may decrease.
- Monitor for rapid rise in body temperature; keep temperature below 38°C (100.4°F) to avoid increased metabolic demands on the brain.
- Tachycardia and hypotension may indicate bleeding elsewhere in the body.

ASSESSING MOTOR FUNCTION

- Observe spontaneous movements; ask patient to raise and lower extremities; compare strength of hand grasp at periodic intervals.
- Note presence or absence of spontaneous movement of each extremity.
- Assess responses to painful stimuli in absence of spontaneous movement; abnormal response carries a poorer prognosis.
- Determine patient's ability to speak; note quality of speech.

EVALUATING EYE SIGNS

- Evaluate spontaneous eye opening.
- Evaluate size of pupils and reaction to light (unilaterally dilated and poorly responding pupils may indicate developing hematoma). If both pupils are fixed and dilated, it usually indicates overwhelming injury and poor prognosis.

MONITOR FOR COMPLICATIONS (CEREBRAL EDEMA AND HERNIATION)

- Deterioration in condition may be due to expanding intracranial hematoma, progressive brain edema, and herniation of the brain.
- Peak swelling occurs about 72 hours after injury, with resulting elevation of ICP.

MONITORING FOR OTHER COMPLICATIONS
- Assess for complications, including systemic infections or neurosurgical infections: wound infection, osteomyelitis, or meningitis.
- After injury, some patients develop focal nerve palsies, such as anosmia (lack of sense of smell) or eye movement abnormalities and focal neurologic defects, such as aphasia, memory defects, and posttraumatic seizures or epilepsy.
- Patients may be left with organic psychosocial deficits and may lack insight into their emotional responses.

H

Major Nursing Diagnoses
- Ineffective airway clearance and ventilation related to hypoxia
- Fluid volume deficit related to disturbances of consciousness and hormonal dysfunction
- Altered nutrition: less than body requirements related to metabolic changes, fluid restrictions, and inadequate intake
- Risk for injury (self-directed and directed to others) related to disorientation, restlessness, and brain damage
- Risk for altered body temperature: increased related to damage to temperature regulating mechanism
- Potential for impaired skin integrity related to bed rest, hemiparesis, hemiplegia, and immobility
- Altered thought processes (deficits in intellectual function, communication, memory, information processing) related to results of brain injury
- Potential for sleep pattern disturbance related to head injury and frequent neurologic checks
- Potential for ineffective family coping related to unresponsiveness of patient, unpredictability of outcome, prolonged recovery period, and patient's residual physical and emotional deficit
- Knowledge deficit about rehabilitation process

See Nursing Management under the Unconscious Patient and Increased Intracranial Pressure for additional information.

Collaborative Problems
- Cerebral edema and herniation
- Decreased cerebral perfusion
- Impaired oxygenation and ventilation
- Impaired fluid, electrolyte, and nutritional balance

Planning and Goals
Goals may include maintenance of a patent airway, adequate cerebral perfusion pressure, fluid and electrolyte balance, and adequate nutritional status; prevention of injury; maintenance of skin integrity; improvement of cognitive function; effective family coping; increased knowledge about rehabilitation process; and absence of complications.

Nursing Interventions

MAINTAINING THE AIRWAY
- Position the unconscious patient to facilitate drainage of secretions; elevate head of bed 30 degrees to decrease intracranial venous pressure.
- Establish effective suctioning procedures.
- Guard against aspiration and respiratory insufficiency.
- Monitor arterial blood gases to assess adequacy of ventilation.
- Monitor the patient on mechanical ventilation.

MAINTAINING FLUID AND ELECTROLYTE BALANCE
This is particularly important in patients receiving osmotic diuretics, those with inappropriate antidiuretic hormone secretion, and those with posttraumatic diabetes insipidus.

- Monitor serum electrolytes, blood glucose values, and intake and output; test urine regularly for acetone.
- Record daily weights.

PROVIDING ADEQUATE NUTRITION
- Start nasogastric feedings as soon as condition has stabilized unless there is discharge of CSF from the nose; oral feeding tubes may be used.
- Give small, frequent feedings to lessen the possibility of vomiting and diarrhea (continuous-drip infusion or

controlling pump to regulate the feeding); elevate head of bed, and check residual feeding before feedings.

PREVENTING INJURY
- Observe for restlessness that may be due to hypoxia, fever, pain, or a full bladder.
- Know that restlessness may also be a sign that the unconscious patient is regaining consciousness.
- Protect from self-injury (padded side rails, hands wrapped in mitts).
- Avoid restraints when possible because straining can increase ICP.
- Avoid narcotics for restlessness because the medications depress respiration, constrict pupils, and alter level of consciousness.
- Keep environmental stimuli to a minimum.
- Provide adequate lighting to prevent visual hallucinations.
- Do not disrupt sleep–wake cycles.
- Use an external sheath catheter for incontinence because an indwelling catheter may produce infection.

MAINTAINING SKIN INTEGRITY
- Assess all body surfaces, and document skin integrity every 8 hours.
- Turn and reposition patient every 2 to 4 hours.
- Provide skin care every 4 hours; use skin lubricant to prevent irritation due to rubbing against the sheet.
- Assist patient to get out of bed three times a day (when appropriate).

IMPROVING COGNITIVE FUNCTIONING
- Redevelop the patient's ability to devise new problem-solving strategies through cognitive rehabilitation over time; use a multidisciplinary approach.
- Be aware that there are fluctuations in the orientation and memory and that these patients are easily distracted.
- Do not push to a level greater than patient's impaired cortical functioning allows because fatigue, headache, and stress (headache, dizziness) may occur.

H

PREVENTING SLEEP PATTERN DISTURBANCE
- Group nursing activities so that the patient is disturbed less frequently.
- Decrease environmental noise, and dim room lights.
- Provide strategies (eg, back rubs) to increase patient comfort.

SUPPORTING FAMILY COPING
- Provide family members with accurate and honest information.
- Encourage family to continue to set well-defined, mutual, short-term goals.
- Encourage family counseling to deal with feeling of loss and helplessness, and provide guidance in the management of inappropriate behaviors.
- Refer family to support groups that provide a forum for networking, sharing problems, and gaining assistance in maintaining realistic expectations and hope.

MONITORING AND MANAGING
POTENTIAL COMPLICATIONS
- Monitor for a patent airway, altered breathing pattern, and occurrence of hypoxemia and pneumonia. Assist with intubation and mechanical ventilation.
- Provide enteral feedings, intravenous fluids, or insulin as prescribed.
- Initiate total parenteral nutrition as ordered if patient is unable to eat.
- Monitor for systemic or neurosurgical infection and heterotropic ossification.
- Take measures to control ICP: elevate head of bed 30 degrees, maintain head and neck in alignment (no twisting), prevent Valsalva maneuver, use medications to decrease ICP, maintain normal body temperature, hyperventilate on mechanical ventilation, maintain fluid restriction, avoid noxious stimuli (suctioning), administer sedation to reduce metabolic demands.

Promoting Home and Community-Based Care

Teaching Patients Self-Care

- Reinforce information given to the family about the patient's condition and prognosis early in the course of head injury.
- As patient's status changes over time, focus teaching on interpretation and explanation of changes in the patient's responses.
- Instruct the patient and family about limitations that can be expected and complications that may occur if patient is to be discharged.
- Identify and teach the complications that merit contacting the neurosurgeon.
- Teach about self-care management strategies, if patient's status indicates.
- Instruct about side effects of medications and importance of taking them as prescribed.

Continuing Care

- Encourage to continue rehabilitation program after discharge. Improvement may take up to 3 or more years after discharge, during which time the family and their coping skills need frequent assessment.
- Inform patient and family that posttraumatic seizures occur frequently and that anticonvulsants may be prescribed for 1 to 2 years after injury.
- Encourage to return to normal activities gradually.
- Continue support and teaching for patient and family with frequent assessment of coping abilities during long-term rehabilitation.

Evaluation

EXPECTED OUTCOMES

- Attains or maintains effective airway clearance, ventilation, and brain oxygenation

- Achieves normal blood gas values and has normal breath sounds
- Attains adequate nutritional status
- Avoids injury
- Has no fever
- Demonstrates intact skin integrity
- Shows improvement in cognitive function and improved memory
- Demonstrates normal sleep–wake cycle
- Family members demonstrate adaptive coping mechanisms
- Patient and family members participate in rehabilitation process as indicated
- Demonstrates absence of complications

For more information, see Chapter 58 in Smeltzer and Bare: *Brunner and Suddarth's Textbook of Medical-Surgical Nursing,* 9th edition. Philadelphia: Lippincott Williams & Wilkins, 2000.

HEADACHE

Headache (cephalgia) is one of the most common of all human physical complaints. Headache is actually a symptom rather than a disease entity and may indicate organic disease (neurologic), a stress response, vasodilation (migraine), skeletal muscle tension (tension headache), or a combination of these factors. Headaches are classified as *primary headaches*, which include the following:

- Migraine (with and without aura)
- Tension-type headache
- Cluster headache and paroxysmal hemicrania
- Headaches are also classified as *secondary headaches*, such as the following:
- Miscellaneous headaches associated with structural lesion
- Headache associated with head trauma

- Headache associated with vascular disorders (eg, subarachnoid hemorrhage)
- Headache associated with nonvascular intracranial disorders (eg, brain tumor)
- Headache associated with use of chemical substances or their withdrawal
- Headache associated with noncephalic infection
- Headache associated with metabolic disorder (eg, hypoglycemia)
- Headache or facial pain associated with disorder of the head, neck, or their structures (eg, acute glaucoma)
- Cranial neuralgias (persistent pain of cranial nerve origin)

MIGRAINE HEADACHE

This symptom complex is characterized by periodic and recurrent attacks of severe headache. The cause of migraine has not been clearly demonstrated, but it is primarily a vascular disturbance that occurs more commonly in women and has strong familial tendencies. Onset typically occurs in puberty, with highest incidence between 20 and 35 years of age.

Clinical Manifestations

Headache often begins in early morning (headache on awakening). The classic migraine attack can be divided into four phases: the prodrome, the aura, the headache, and the recovery phases.

Prodrome Phase

- This phase is present in 60% of patients with migraine headache.
- Symptoms may occur consistently hours to 2 days before onset of migraine.
- Depression, irritability, feeling cold, food cravings, anorexia, change in activity level, increased urination, diarrhea, or constipation may be noted with each migraine.

Aura Phase

- This phase occurs in about 20% of patients and lasts for up to 30 minutes.
- Focal neurologic symptoms, predominantly visual disturbances (light flashes) occur and may be hemianoptic (occurring in half of the visual field).
- Numbness and tingling of the face or hands, mild confusion, slight weakness of an extremity, and drowsiness and dizziness may be present.

Headache Phase

- This phase, occurring in 60% of patients, involves unilateral, throbbing headache that intensifies over several hours.
- The pain is severe and incapacitating, often associated with photophobia, nausea, and vomiting.
- Its duration varies from about 4 to 72 hours.

Recovery Phase (Termination and Postdrome)

- The pain gradually subsides.
- There is a period of muscle contraction in the neck and scalp with associated muscle ache and point (localized) tenderness, exhaustion, and mood changes.
- Any physical exertion exacerbates the headache pain.
- Patients may sleep for extended periods.

Diagnostic Evaluation

- Physical assessment of the head and neck
- Neurologic examination
- Detailed health and headache assessment and history
- Cerebral angiography, CT, or MRI if abnormalities on neurologic examination
- Electromyography (EMG) and laboratory tests (complete blood count, electrolytes, glucose), creatinine, erythrocyte sedimentation rate, and thyroid panel

Medical Management

Therapy is divided into abortive (symptomatic) and preventive approaches.

- Abortive approach is used for frequent attacks and is aimed at relieving or limiting a headache at onset or while in progress.
- Preventive approach is used for those who have frequent attacks at regular or predictable intervals and may have medical conditions that preclude abortive therapies.

Management of Acute Attack

Treatment varies greatly; close monitoring is indicated.

- Ergotamine preparations may be effective if taken early. Cafergot is a combination of ergotamine and caffeine. Dihydroergotamine (DHE) is highly effective in attacks lasting more than 72 hours (contraindicated in patients with coronary or peripheral vascular disease).
- The patient should lie quietly in a darkened room with head slightly elevated.
- Drinking black coffee may be helpful.
- Sumatriptan (Imitrex) is used for acute migraine and cluster headaches; Cafergot is used to relieve moderate to severe migraines.
- Symptomatic therapy includes analgesics, sedatives, antianxiety agents, and antiemetics.

Prevention

PHARMACOLOGIC THERAPY
- Daily use of medications at 3- to 6-month intervals with gradual tapering
- Beta-blockers, such as propranolol (Inderal), most widely used
- Antidepressants, barbiturates, tranquilizers (use cautiously and on short-term basis)
- Calcium antagonists used frequently (require several weeks until effective); methysergide (Sansert) or anticonvulsants (divalproex sodium [Dapakote]) may be used; lidocaine nose drops effective in treating cluster headaches and migraine

Nursing Management

Assessment

- Obtain a detailed history and physical assessment; data obtained for the health history should reflect the patient's own words. Include medications, toxic substance exposure, stress, insomnia, and family history.
- Focus health history on assessment of the headache (location, quality, frequency, precipitating factors, time, associated symptoms).

Major Nursing Diagnosis

- Pain related to vascular changes

Planning and Goals

The goals include treating the acute event of the headache and preventing recurrent episodes.

Nursing Interventions

RELIEVING PAIN

- Attempt to abort headache early.
- Provide comfort measures (eg, a quiet, dark environment); elevate the head of the bed 30 degrees.
- Provide symptomatic treatment, such as antiemetics, as indicated.

🏠 Promoting Home and Community-Based Care

Teaching Patients Self-Care

- Teach that migraine headaches are likely to occur when a person is ill, overtired, or feeling stressed.
- Instruct about the importance of proper diet, adequate rest, and coping strategies.
- Help patient identify circumstances that precipitate headache, and assist in development of alternate means of coping.
- Help patients develop insight into their feelings, behaviors, and conflicts to make necessary lifestyle modifications.

- Suggest regular periods of exercise and relaxation and avoidance of offending factors.
- Avoid long intervals between meals.
- Advise patient to awaken at the same time each day; disruption of normal sleeping pattern provokes a migraine in many patients.

Continuing Care

The National Headache Foundation provides a list of clinics in the United States and the names of physicians who are members of the American Association for the Study of Headaches.

Evaluation

EXPECTED OUTCOMES
- Demonstrates relief of pain
- Verbalizes techniques to prevent or minimize headache

CLUSTER HEADACHE

Cluster headaches are another severe form of vascular headache seen most frequently in men between 20 and 40 years of age. The attacks come in clusters of one to eight daily, with excruciating pain localized in the eye and orbit and radiating to the facial and temporal regions. The pain is accompanied by watering of the eye and nasal congestion lasting from 15 minutes to 3 hours and may have a crescendo–decrescendo pattern, penetrating and steady. The headaches may be precipitated by alcohol, nitrites, vasodilators, and histamines.

CRANIAL ARTERITIS

Inflammation of the cranial arteries is characterized by a severe headache localized in the region of the temporal artery. The inflammation may be generalized or focal. This is a cause of headache in the older population, particularly those older than 70 years of age. Clinical manifestations include inflammation (eg, heat, redness, swelling, and tenderness or pain over the involved artery). A tender, swollen, or nodular temporal artery may be visible. Visual problems are caused by ischemia of the involved structures. The headache is treated with corticosteroid drugs *(do not stop abruptly)* and analgesic agents.

TENSION HEADACHE (MUSCLE CONTRACTION HEADACHE)

Emotional or physical stress may cause contraction of the muscles in the neck and scalp, resulting in tension headache. This is characterized by a steady, constant feeling of pressure that usually begins in the forehead, the temple, or the back of the neck. Tension headaches tend to be more chronic than severe and are probably the most common type of headache. Relief may be obtained by local heat, massage, analgesics, antidepressants, and muscle relaxants. Reassure the patient that the headache does not indicate a brain tumor, and teach stress reduction techniques (biofeedback, exercise, medication).

For more information, see Chapter 59 in Smeltzer and Bare: *Brunner and Suddarth's Textbook of Medical-Surgical Nursing,* 9th edition. Philadelphia: Lippincott Williams & Wilkins, 2000.

HEMOPHILIA

Hemophilia is a relatively rare disease. There are two hereditary bleeding disorders that are clinically indistinguishable but can be separated by laboratory tests: hemophilia A and hemophilia B. Hemophilia A is due to a deficiency of factor VIII clotting activity. Hemophilia B stems from a deficiency of factor IX. Factor VIII deficiency is about three times more common. Both types are inherited as X-linked traits. All ethnic groups are affected. Almost all affected people are male; their mothers and some sisters are carriers but do not have symptoms. The disease is usually recognized in early childhood, usually in toddlers. Mild hemophilia may not be diagnosed until the onset of trauma or surgery.

Clinical Manifestations

The frequency and severity of bleeding depend on the degree of factor deficiency and intensity of trauma.

- Hemorrhage occurs into various body parts (large, spreading bruises and bleeding into muscles, joints, and soft tissues) after even minimal trauma.
- Pain in joints may occur before swelling and limitation of motion are apparent; pain occurs most often in knees, elbows, ankles, shoulders, wrists, and hips.
- Chronic pain or ankylosis (fixation) of the joint may occur with recurrent hemorrhage; many patients are crippled by joint damage before adulthood.
- Spontaneous hematuria and gastrointestinal bleeding can occur. Hematomas within the muscle can cause peripheral nerve compression with decreased sensation, weakness, and atrophy of the area.
- Some patients have a milder deficiency and bleed only after dental extractions or surgery; such hemorrhages can prove fatal if the cause is not recognized quickly. The most dangerous hemorrhage is within the head.

Diagnostic Evaluation

Laboratory tests include clotting factors and complete blood count.

Medical Management

- Factor VIII and IX concentrates are given when active bleeding occurs or as a prophylactic measure before dental extractions, lumbar puncture, or surgery.
- Aminocaproic acid (Amicar) may slow the dissolution of blood clots; DDAVP (desmopressin) induces transient increase in factor VIII.
- Avoid aspirin or intramuscular injections.
- Encourage good dental hygiene as a preventive measure.
- Use splints or other orthopedic devices in patients who have suffered joint or muscle hemorrhage.

Nursing Management

Assessment
- Assess for evidence of internal bleeding, muscle hematomas, and hemorrhage into joint spaces.
- Monitor vital signs and hemodynamic pressure readings for hypovolemia.
- Assess all joints for swelling, mobility limitation, and pain. Perform range-of-motion exercises slowly, with care to avoid more damage.
- Assess surgical sites frequently and carefully for bleeding.
- Question how patient and family are coping with the condition and any limitations imposed on lifestyle and daily activities.

Major Nursing Diagnoses
- Pain related to joint hemorrhage and subsequent ankylosis
- Altered health maintenance related to ongoing need for preventive health practices and coping with chronic illness
- Ineffective coping related to the chronicity of the condition and its effect on lifestyle

Collaborative Problems/Potential Complications
- Bleeding

Planning and Goals
The major goals of the patient may include relief or minimization of pain, compliance with measures to prevent bleeding, coping with chronicity and altered lifestyle, and absence of complications.

Nursing Interventions
RELIEVING OR MINIMIZING PAIN
- Give analgesics to alleviate pain.
- Encourage patient to move slowly and prevent stress on involved joints.

- Encourage warm baths to promote relaxation, improved mobility, and lessened pain.
- Avoid heat during bleeding episodes because it potentiates further bleeding.
- Use splints, canes, or crutches to shift body weight off painful joints.

MONITORING AND MANAGING COMPLICATIONS

- Assess frequently for signs and symptoms of hypoxia to vital organs: restlessness, anxiety, confusion, pallor, cool and clammy skin, chest pain, and decreased urinary output.
- Assess for hypotension and tachycardia as a result of volume depletion.
- Monitor hemodynamic parameters; perform blood studies.
- Observe for bleeding from the skin, mucous membranes, and wounds and for internal bleeding.
- Apply cold compresses to bleeding sites when indicated.
- Administer parenteral medications with small-gauge needles to decrease trauma and bleeding.
- Administer blood, blood components, and medications as prescribed.
- Use safety precautions to prevent patient injury.

Promoting Home and Community-Based Care

Preventive Bleeding Measures

- Inform patient and family of risk of bleeding and necessary safety precautions.
- Teach families how to administer the concentrate at home at the first sign of bleeding.
- Encourage patient and family to alter the home environment to prevent physical trauma.
- Encourage electric razor for shaving and soft toothbrush for oral hygiene.
- Teach patient to avoid forceful nose blowing, coughing, and straining at stool; use stool softener as necessary.

- Teach patient to avoid aspirin and aspirin-containing drugs.
- Encourage noncontact sports such as swimming, hiking, and golf, and discourage engagement in contact sports.
- Encourage regular checkups and laboratory studies.

Coping With Chronicity and Altered Lifestyle

- Assist in coping with the condition because it is chronic and places restrictions on lifestyle. It is an inherited disorder that can be passed to future generations.
- Encourage patient to be self-sufficient and to maintain independence.
- Encourage working through feelings about condition to accept more responsibility for maintaining optimal health.
- In cases in which patient has the human immunodeficiency virus (HIV), support patient's and family's efforts to deal with anger. (The percentage of patients with hemophilia who are HIV positive is increasing.) Assist in finding support sources for those who are HIV positive.

Evaluation

EXPECTED OUTCOMES
- Reports absence of or decrease in pain
- Complies with measures to prevent bleeding
- Demonstrates effective coping with chronicity and altered lifestyle
- Demonstrates no complications

For more information, see Chapter 30 in Smeltzer and Bare: *Brunner and Suddarth's Textbook of Medical-Surgical Nursing,* 9th edition. Philadelphia: Lippincott Williams & Wilkins, 2000.

HEPATIC ENCEPHALOPATHY AND HEPATIC COMA

Hepatic encephalopathy, a complication of liver disease, occurs with profound liver failure and may result from the accumulation of ammonia and other toxic metabolites in the blood. Hepatic coma represents the most advanced stage of hepatic encephalopathy. Ammonia accumulates because the damaged liver cells fail to detoxify and convert the ammonia to urea. The increased ammonia concentration in the blood causes brain dysfunction and damage, resulting in hepatic encephalopathy and coma. Circumstances that increase serum ammonia levels precipitate or aggravate hepatic encephalopathy, such as digestion of dietary and blood proteins and ingestion of ammonium salts. Other factors that may cause hepatic encephalopathy include excessive diuresis, dehydration, infections, fever, surgery, and some medications. Portal system encephalopathy is the most common type of hepatic encephalopathy.

Clinical Manifestations

- Earliest symptoms of hepatic encephalopathy include minor mental changes and motor disturbances. Slight confusion and alterations in mood occur; the patient becomes unkempt in appearance, experiences altered sleep patterns, and tends to sleep during the day and to experience restlessness and insomnia at night.
- As coma progresses, the patient may be difficult to awaken, and asterixis (flapping tremor of the hands) may occur. Simple tasks, such as handwriting, become difficult.
- In early stages, the patient's reflexes are hyperactive; with worsening encephalopathy, reflexes disappear, and extremities become flaccid.
- Electroencephalogram (EEG) shows slowing and increase in amplitude of brain waves.

- Occasionally, fetor hepaticus, a characteristic breath odor like freshly mowed grass, acetone, or old wine, may be noticed.
- Gross disturbances of consciousness and complete disorientation occur as the disease progresses.
- With further progression, frank coma and seizures occur.

Diagnostic Evaluation
- Serum ammonia
- Symptoms in a susceptible patient; taking a sample handwriting daily or sample drawings (constructional apraxia) reveals progression

Medical Management
- Administer lactulose (Cephulac) to reduce serum ammonia. Observe for watery diarrheal stools, which indicate lactulose overdose.
- Reduce protein intake or eliminate if signs of impending encephalopathy or coma occur.
- Give an enema as prescribed to reduce ammonia absorption from the gastrointestinal tract.
- Administer nonabsorbable antibiotics (neomycin) as an intestinal antiseptic.
- Monitor serum ammonia level daily; monitor electrolyte status, and correct if abnormal.
- Discontinue medications that may precipitate encephalopathy (ie, sedatives, tranquilizers, analgesics).
- Other treatments may include intravenous glucose, vitamins, and oxygen administration.

Nursing Management
- Assess neurologic status frequently. Keep daily record of handwriting and performance in arithmetic to monitor mental status.
- Monitor fluid intake and output and body weight daily; monitor vital signs at least every 4 hours.
- Monitor for peritoneal, pulmonary, or other infection, and report promptly.

Promoting Home and Community-Based Care

- Instruct family to observe the patient for subtle signs of recurrent encephalopathy.
- Instruct in maintenance of low-protein, high-calorie diet.
- Teach administration of lactulose and monitoring for side effects.

H

Continuing Care
- Refer for home care nurse visits.
- Emphasize importance of periodic follow-up.
- The home care nurse assesses the patient's physical and mental status and adherence to the prescribed therapeutic regimen.

For more information, see Chapter 36 in Smeltzer and Bare: *Brunner and Suddarth's Textbook of Medical-Surgical Nursing,* 9th edition. Philadelphia: Lippincott Williams & Wilkins, 2000.

HEPATIC FAILURE, FULMINANT

Fulminant hepatic failure is the clinical syndrome of sudden and severely impaired liver function in a previously healthy person. It is characterized by the development of first symptoms or jaundice within 8 weeks of the onset of disease. Three categories that have been cited are hyperacute, acute, and subacute. There is rapid clinical deterioration caused by massive hepatocellular injury and necrosis. The mortality rate is extremely high. Viral hepatitis is the most common cause; other causes include toxic drugs, chemicals, metabolic disturbances, and structural changes.

Clinical Manifestations
- Jaundice and profound anorexia

- Often accompanied by coagulation defects, renal failure, electrolyte disturbances, infection, hypoglycemia, encephalopathy, and cerebral edema

Medical Management

- Liver transplantation (treatment of choice)
- Blood or plasma exchanges, charcoal hemoperfusion, and corticosteroids
- Liver support systems, such as hepatocytes within synthetic fiber columns, extracorporeal liver-assist devices, and bioartificial liver, until transplantation is possible

---

For more information, see Chapter 36 in Smeltzer and Bare: *Brunner and Suddarth's Textbook of Medical-Surgical Nursing,* 9th edition. Philadelphia: Lippincott Williams & Wilkins, 2000.

HEPATITIS, VIRAL: TYPES A, B, C, D, AND G

HEPATITIS A

Hepatitis A is caused by an RNA virus of the enterovirus family. Mode of transmission of this disease is the fecal–oral route, primarily through ingestion of foods or fluids infected by the virus. The virus is found in the stool of infected patients before the onset of symptoms and during the first few days of illness. The incubation period is estimated to be from 2 to 7 weeks, with an average of 30 days. The course of illness may last from 4 to 8 weeks. The virus is present only briefly in the serum; by the time jaundice appears, the patient is likely to be noninfectious. A person who is immune to hepatitis A may contract other forms of hepatitis. Recovery from hepatitis A is usual; it rarely progresses to acute liver necrosis and fulminant hepatitis. No carrier state exists, and no chronic hepatitis is associated with hepatitis A.

Clinical Manifestations
- Many patients are anicteric (without jaundice) and symptomless.
- When symptoms appear, they are of a mild, flulike, upper respiratory infection, with low-grade fever.
- Anorexia is an early symptom and is often severe.
- Later, jaundice and dark urine may be apparent.
- Indigestion is present in varying degrees.
- Liver and spleen may be moderately enlarged for a few days after onset.
- Adults are more likely to have symptoms than are children.
- Patient may have an aversion to cigarette smoke and strong odors; symptoms tend to clear when jaundice reaches its peak.

Diagnostic Evaluation
- Stool analysis for hepatitis A antigen
- Serum hepatitis A virus antibodies; immunoglobulin

Medical Management
- Bed rest during the acute stage; encourage nutritious diet.
- Give small, frequent feedings supplemented by intravenous glucose if necessary during period of anorexia.
- Promote gradual but progressive ambulation to hasten recovery.

Prevention
- Hepatitis vaccine is recommended for high-risk groups (be cautious of hypersensitivity).
- Administration of immune globulin to prevent hepatitis A if given within 2 weeks of exposure.
- Hepatitis vaccine and immunoglobulin are recommended for those who travel to developing countries and settings with unsatisfactory hygiene or sanitation conditions.
- Immunoglobulin is recommended for household members and sexual contacts of people with hepatitis A.

Promoting Home and Community-Based Care

- The patient is usually managed at home unless symptoms are severe.
- Assist patient and family to cope with the temporary disability and fatigue that are common problems in hepatitis.
- Teach the patient and family the indications to seek additional health care if the symptoms persist or worsen.
- Instruct patient and family regarding guidelines about diet, rest, follow-up blood work, avoidance of alcohol, and sanitation and hygiene measures (hand washing) to prevent spread of disease to other family members.
- Teach patients and families about reducing risk of contracting hepatitis A: good personal hygiene with careful hand washing; environmental sanitation with safe food and water supply and sewage disposal.

HEPATITIS B

Hepatitis B virus is a DNA virus. It is transmitted primarily through blood. The virus has been found in saliva, semen, and vaginal secretions and can be transmitted through mucous membranes and breaks in the skin. Hepatitis B has a long incubation period. It replicates in the liver and remains in the serum for long periods, allowing transmission of the virus. Those at risk include all health care workers, patients in hemodialysis and oncology units, homosexually active and bisexual men, and intravenous drug users. The incubation period is between 1 and 6 months. About 10% of patients progress to a carrier state or develop chronic hepatitis. Hepatitis B is the chief cause of cirrhosis and hepatocellular carcinoma worldwide.

Clinical Manifestations

- Symptoms may be insidious and variable; subclinical episodes frequently occur, fever and respiratory symptoms are rare; some patients have arthralgias and rashes.

- Loss of appetite, dyspepsia, abdominal pain, general aching, malaise, and weakness may occur.
- Jaundice may or may not be evident. With jaundice, there are light-colored stools and dark urine.
- Liver may be tender and enlarged; spleen is enlarged and palpable in a small number of patients. Posterior cervical lymph nodes may also be enlarged.

Diagnostic Evaluation
- Hepatitis B antigen

Medical Management
- Alpha-interferon has shown promising results.
- Bed rest and restriction of activities until hepatic enlargement and elevation of serum bilirubin and liver enzymes have disappeared.
- Maintain adequate nutrition; restrict proteins when the ability of the liver to metabolize protein by-products is impaired.
- Administer antacids, and antiemetics for dyspepsia and general malaise; avoid all medications if vomiting.
- Convalescence may be prolonged, and recovery may take 3 to 4 months; provide hospitalization and fluid therapy if vomiting persists.

Nursing Management
- Encourage gradual activity after complete clearing of jaundice.
- Consider psychological implications of the long disease course and isolation and separation from family and friends.
- Include family in planning patient's care and activities.

Control and Prevention
- Interrupt the chain of transmission.
- Protect those people at high risk with active immunization through use of hepatitis B vaccine.
- Use passive immunization for unprotected people exposed to hepatitis B.

Promoting Home and Community-Based Care

Teaching Patients Self-Care

- Educate patient and family in home care and convalescence.
- Instruct patient and family to provide adequate rest and nutrition before discharge.
- Inform family and intimate friends about risks of contracting hepatitis B.
- Arrange for family and intimate friends to receive hepatitis B vaccine or hepatitis B immune globulin. Hepatitis B vaccine is given in three doses, the second and third doses 1 and 6 months after the first dose.
- Caution against using alcohol.

Continuing Care

- Inform family that follow-up home visits by home care nurse are indicated to assess progress and understanding, reinforce teaching, and answer questions.
- Teach those at risk the early signs of hepatitis B and ways to reduce risk by avoiding all modes of transmission.
- Encourage patient to use strategies, such as avoiding sexual intercourse or use condoms, to prevent exchange of body fluids.

 Gerontologic Considerations

Elderly patients who contract hepatitis B have a serious risk of severe liver cell necrosis or fulminant hepatic failure. The patient is seriously ill, and prognosis is poor.

HEPATITIS C

A significant portion of cases of viral hepatitis are neither A, B, nor D; they are classified as hepatitis C. It is the primary form of hepatitis associated with parenteral means (sharing contaminated needles, needlesticks or injuries by health care workers, blood transfusions) or sexual contact. The incubation period is variable and may range from 15 to 160 days. The clinical course of hepatitis C is similar to that of hepatitis B; symptoms are usually mild. A chronic carrier state occurs frequently. There is increased risk of cirrhosis and liver cancer after hepatitis C. Long-term, low-dose interferon therapy is effective for improvement in patients with hepatitis C and in treating relapses.

HEPATITIS D

Hepatitis D (delta agent) occurs in some cases of hepatitis B. Only patients with hepatitis B are at risk. The virus requires hepatitis B surface antigen for its replication. It is common in people who are intravenous drug users, hemodialysis patients, and recipients of multiple blood transfusions. Sexual contact with those with hepatitis B is an important mode of transmission of hepatitis B and D. Incubation varies between 21 and 140 days. The symptoms are similar to those of hepatitis B except that patients are more likely to have fulminant hepatitis and progress to chronic active hepatitis and cirrhosis. Treatment is similar to that for other forms of hepatitis.

HEPATITIS E

The hepatitis E virus is transmitted by the fecal–oral route, principally through contaminated water and poor sanitation. Incubation is variable and is estimated to range between 15 and 65 days. Onset and symptoms are similar to those of other types of viral hepatitis (resembles hepatitis A). Hepatitis E has a self-limiting course with abrupt onset. Jaundice is nearly always present; chronic forms do not develop. The major method of prevention is avoiding contact with the virus through hygiene (hand washing). Effectiveness of immune globulin in protecting against hepatitis E virus is uncertain.

HEPATITIS G

Hepatitis G (the newest form) is a posttransfusion hepatitis with an incubation period of 14 to 145 days. Autoantibodies are absent. The risk factors are similar to those for hepatitis C.

For more information, see Chapter 36 in Smeltzer and Bare: *Brunner and Suddarth's Textbook of Medical-Surgical Nursing,* 9th edition. Philadelphia: Lippincott Williams & Wilkins, 2000.

HERNIATION OR RUPTURE OF AN INTERVERTEBRAL DISK

In herniation of the intervertebral disk (ruptured disk), the nucleus of the disk protrudes into the annulus (the fibrous ring around the disk), with subsequent nerve compression. Rupture of the disk is usually preceded by degenerative changes that occur with aging. In most patients, the immediate symptoms of trauma are short lived, and those resulting from injury to the disk do not appear for months or years. A herniated disk with accompanying pain may occur in any portion of the spine but usually is cervical (typically the C5-6 and C6-7 interspaces).

Clinical Manifestations
Clinical features depend on location, rate of development (acute or chronic), and effect on surrounding structures.

Pain; stiffness in neck, shoulders, and scapulae; paresthesia and numbness (cervical)

Changes in sensation and reflex action; sensory loss and muscle weakness

Diagnostic Evaluation
• Magnetic resonance imaging (MRI), computed tomography (CT), myelogram

Medical and Nursing Management
For herniation of cervical and lumbar disks, treatment involves conservative management with bed rest and medication. Goals of treatment are to rest and immobilize the spine and to reduce inflammation.

- Bed rest (2 weeks) with proper positioning on a firm mattress
- Spine immobilization with cervical collar, cervical traction, or a brace
- Cervical isometric exercises after patient is pain free

Pharmacologic Therapy
- Analgesics (oxycodone [Tylox], hydrocodone [Vicodin], propoxyphene [Darvon])
- Muscle relaxants and antiinflammatory agents (NSAIDs)
- Hot, moist compresses (10 to 20 minutes)

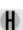

Surgical Interventions
The goal of surgical treatment is to relieve pressure on the nerve root to relieve pain and reverse neurologic deficits.

- Discectomy (with or without fusion)
  - Endoscopic microdiscectomy: removal of herniated or extruded fragments of intervertebral disk
  - With fusion: a bone graft is used to fuse the vertebral spinous process to bridge over the defective disk to stabilize the spine and reduce the rate of recurrence
- Laminectomy: removal of the lamina to expose the neural elements in the spinal canal; allows the surgeon to inspect the spinal canal, identify and remove pathology, and relieve compression of the cord and roots
- Laminotomy: division of the lamina of the vertebra

For more information, see Chapter 59 in Smeltzer and Bare: *Brunner and Suddarth's Textbook of Medical-Surgical Nursing,* 9th edition. Philadelphia: Lippincott Williams & Wilkins, 2000.

HIATAL HERNIA

In a hiatal (hiatus) hernia, the opening in the diaphragm through which the esophagus passes becomes enlarged, and part of the upper stomach tends to move up into the lower portion of the thorax. There are two types of hernias: axial and paraesophageal. With an axial, or sliding, hiatal hernia, the upper stomach and the gastroesophageal junction are displaced upward and slide in and out of the thorax; this occurs in about 90% of patients with esophageal hiatal hernias. The less frequent paraesophageal hernias occur when all or part of the stomach pushes through the diaphragm next to the gastroesophageal junction. Hiatal hernia occurs more often in women than men.

Clinical Manifestations
Axial (Sliding) Hernia
- Heartburn, regurgitation, and dysphagia; at least half of cases are asymptomatic
- Often implicated in reflux

Paraesophageal Hernia
- Sense of fullness after eating or may be asymptomatic
- Reflux does not usually occur
- Complications of hemorrhage, obstruction, and strangulation possible

Diagnostic Evaluation
Diagnosis is confirmed by radiographic studies, barium swallow, and fluoroscopy.

Medical Management
- Frequent, small feedings that easily pass through the esophagus are given.
- Elevate head of bed on 4- to 8-inch blocks to prevent the hernia from sliding upward.
- Surgery is indicated in about 15% of patients; paraesophageal hernias may require emergency surgery.

- Medical and surgical management of paraesophageal hernias is similar to that for gastroesophageal reflux (antacids, histamine blockers, gastric acid pump inhibitors, or prokinetic agents (metoclopramide [Reglan], cisapride [Propulcid]).

Nursing Management: The Patient With an Esophageal Condition and Reflux

Assessment
- Take a complete health history, including pain assessment and nutrition assessment.
- Determine if patient appears emaciated.
- Auscultate chest to determine presence of pulmonary complications.

Major Nursing Diagnoses
- Altered nutrition: less than body requirements related to difficulty swallowing
- Risk for aspiration due to difficulty swallowing or tube feeding
- Pain related to difficulty swallowing, ingestion of abrasive agent, a tumor, or reflux
- Knowledge deficit about the esophageal disorder, diagnostic studies, treatments, and rehabilitation

Planning and Goals
The major goals of the patient may include attainment of adequate nutritional intake, avoidance of respiratory compromise from aspiration, relief of pain, and increased knowledge level.

Nursing Interventions
ENCOURAGING ADEQUATE NUTRITIONAL INTAKE
- Instruct patient to eat a low-fat, high-fiber diet.
- Encourage patient to eat slowly and chew all food thoroughly.
- Small frequent feedings of nonirritating foods are recommended; sometimes, liquids with food help passage.

- Prepare food in an appealing manner to help stimulate appetite; avoid irritants (tobacco, alcohol).
- Obtain a baseline weight, and record daily weights; assess nutrient intake.

DECREASING RISK OF ASPIRATION
- Keep patients with difficulty swallowing or handling secretions in at least a semi-Fowler's position.
- Instruct patient in the use of oral suction to decrease risk of aspiration.

RELIEVING PAIN
- Teach patient to eat small, frequent meals, at least 2 hours before bedtime.
- Instruct patient to avoid caffeine, tobacco, carbonated beverages, very hot or very cold beverages, and spicy foods.
- Advise not to recline for 1 to 4 hours after eating to prevent reflux or movement of the hernia.
- Advise to avoid any activities that put strain on the thoracic region and increase pain.
- Elevate the head of the bed on 4- to 8-inch blocks; avoid tight clothes.
- Advise patient not to use over-the-counter antacids because of possible rebound acidity.
- Instruct in use of prescribed antacids or histamine antagonists.

Promoting Home and Community-Based Care

Teaching Patients Self-Care
- Reassure the patient and discuss all procedures and their purposes.
- Give sufficient information for participation in care and diagnostic effort.
- Prepare patient for surgery if required.
- Help patient to plan for needed physical and psychological adjustments and follow-up care if condition is chronic. Help in planning meals, using medications as prescribed, and resuming activity.

- Teach patient and family to use special equipment (enteral or parenteral feeding devices, suction).
- Educate about nutritional requirements and how to measure the adequacy of nutrition (particularly in elderly and debilitated patients).

See Nursing Management under the Preoperative and Postoperative Patient for additional information.

Continuing Care

- Arrange for home health care nursing support and assessment when indicated.
- Teach patient to prepare food in specialized way if indicated (blenderized or soft food).
- Assist patient to adjust medication schedule to daily activities when possible (analgesics, antacids).
- Arrange for nutritionist, social worker, and family member team approach or hospice care when indicated.

For more information, see Chapter 32 in Smeltzer and Bare: *Brunner and Suddarth's Textbook of Medical-Surgical Nursing,* 9th edition. Philadelphia: Lippincott Williams & Wilkins, 2000.

HODGKIN'S DISEASE

Hodgkin's disease is a rare malignancy of unknown cause that is unicentric in origin and spreads along the lymphatic system. There is a familial pattern associated with Hodgkin's as well as an association with the Epstein-Barr virus (20% of patients also infected). It is more common in men and tends to peak in the early 20s and after 50 years of age. The Reed-Sternberg cell, a gigantic atypical tumor cell, is the pathologic hallmark and essential diagnostic criterion for Hodgkin's disease.

Clinical Manifestations

- Painless enlargement of the lymph nodes on one side of the neck. Individual nodes are firm and painless;

common sites are the cervical, supraclavicular, and mediastinal nodes.

- Mediastinal lymph nodes may be large enough to cause severe pressure symptom (eg, dyspnea from pressure against the trachea; dysphagia from pressure against the esophagus).

- Symptoms may result from the tumor compressing other organs, such as cough and pulmonary effusion (from pulmonary infiltrates); jaundice (from hepatic involvement or bile duct obstruction); abdominal pain (from splenomegaly or retroperitoneal adenopathy); or bone pain (due to skeletal involvement).

- Pruritus is common, can be distressing and of unclear etiology. Herpes zoster infection is common.

- Some patients may experience brief but severe pain after drinking alcohol, usually at the site of the tumor.

- A mild anemia develops; the white blood cell count may be elevated or decreased; and anergy, an absence of or decreased response to skin sensitivity tests (eg, candidal infection, mumps), may be noted.

- Constitutional symptoms for prognostic purposes, referred to as *B symptoms,* include fever (without chills), drenching sweats (particularly at night), and unintentional weight loss of more than 10% of body weight.

Diagnostic Evaluation

Diagnosis depends on identification of characteristic histologic features in an excised lymph node. After the diagnosis is confirmed, the total extent of tumor involvement is assessed, and its distribution is defined.

- Laboratory studies: complete blood count; platelet count, sedimentation rate, liver and renal function studies

- Excisional lymph node biopsy, bone marrow biopsy, characteristic presence of Reed-Sternberg cell; staging of node

- Chest radiograph and computed tomography (CT) scan of the chest, abdomen, and pelvis

Medical Management

Treatment is determined by the stage of the disease instead of the histologic type.

- Chemotherapy followed by radiation therapy is used in early-stage disease.
- Combination chemotherapy alone is now the standard treatment for more advanced disease.
- When Hodgkin's does recur, the use of high doses of chemotherapeutic medications, followed by autologous bone marrow or stem-cell transplantation, can be very effective.

Nursing Management

See Nursing Management under Cancer for additional information about nursing interventions for patients undergoing radiation and chemotherapy treatments.

 Promoting Home and Community-Based Care

- Help the patient to cope with undesirable effects of radiation therapy, including esophagitis, anorexia, loss of taste, dry mouth, nausea and vomiting, diarrhea, skin reactions, and lethargy.
- Serve bland, soft foods at mild temperatures.
- Instruct in proper dental hygiene.
- Administer antiemetics during peak times of nausea.
- Teach patient that skin reactions and the appearance of sunburned or tanned skin are common; rubbing the area and applying heat, cold, or lotion should be avoided.
- Encourage the patient to rest and sleep to maintain a reasonable energy level; lethargy accompanies radiation.
- Help patients to prepare for alopecia by encouraging them to purchase a wig before the time of hair loss.
- Encourage the patient to report any sign of infection for immediate treatment.
- Instruct the patient to use contraception during chemotherapy to prevent cytotoxic effects on the fetus.
- Encourage the patient to keep all follow-up appointments.

For more information, see Chapter 30 in Smeltzer and Bare: *Brunner and Suddarth's Textbook of Medical-Surgical Nursing,* 9th edition. Philadelphia: Lippincott Williams & Wilkins, 2000.

HUNTINGTON'S DISEASE

Huntington's disease is a chronic, hereditary disease of the nervous system that results in progressive involuntary choreiform (dancelike) movements and dementia. Researchers believe that glutamine abnormally collects in certain brain cell nuclei, causing cell death. Huntington's disease affects men and women of all races. It is transmitted as an autosomal dominant genetic disorder. Each child of a parent with Huntington's has a 50% risk of inheriting the illness. Onset usually occurs between 35 and 45 years of age.

Clinical Manifestations
- The most prominent clinical features are abnormal involuntary movements (chorea), intellectual decline, and emotional disturbance.
- Constant writhing, twisting, and uncontrollable movements of the entire body occur as the disease progresses.
- Facial movements produce ticks and grimaces; speech becomes slurred, hesitant, often explosive, and then eventually unintelligible.
- Chewing and swallowing are difficult, and aspiration and choking are a danger.
- Gait becomes disorganized, and ambulation is eventually impossible; patient is eventually confined to a wheelchair.
- Bowel and bladder control is lost.
- Progressive intellectual impairment occurs with eventual dementia.
- Uncontrollable emotional changes occur but become less acute as the disease progresses. Patient may be nervous, irritable, or impatient. During the early stages of illness: uncontrollable fits of anger; profound, often suicidal depression; apathy; or euphoria.

- Hallucinations, delusions, and paranoid thinking may precede appearance of disjointed movements.
- Patient succumbs in 10 to 15 years from heart failure, pneumonia, or infection or dies as a result of a fall or choking.

Diagnostic Evaluation

- Diagnosis is made on the basis of clinical presentation, positive family history, and exclusion of other causes.
- Imaging studies, such as computed tomography (CT) and magnetic resonance imaging (MRI), may show atrophy of the striatum.
- A genetic marker for Huntington's disease has been located. It offers no hope of cure or even specific determination of onset.

Medical Management

No treatment stops or reverses the process; palliative care is given.

- Medications such as phenylthiazines, butyrophenones, and thioxanthenes, which block dopamine receptors, and reserpine, tetrabenazine, and antiparkinsonism therapy (L-dopa) may improve chorea and temporarily decrease rigidity in many patients.
- Patient's motor signs are continually assessed and evaluated.
- Psychotherapy aimed at allaying anxiety and reducing stress may be beneficial; antidepressants are given for depression or suicidal ideation.
- The patient's needs and capabilities are the focus of treatment.

Nursing Management

Promoting Home and Community-Based Care

- Reinforce understanding that Huntington's disease takes emotional, physical, social, and financial tolls on every member of the patient's family.

- Encourage crucial genetic counseling, access to long-term psychological counseling, marriage counseling, and financial and legal support.

Teaching Patients Self-Care
- Teach patient and family about medications, including signs indicating need for change in dosage or medication.
- Address strategies to manage symptoms (chorea, swallowing problems, ambulation problems, or altered bowel or bladder function).
- Arrange for consultation with a speech therapist, if needed.

Continuing Care
- Emphasize the need for regular follow-up.
- Refer for home care nursing assistance, respite care, day care centers, and eventually skilled long-term care to assist patient and family to cope.
- Provide information about the Huntington's Disease Foundation of America, which gives information, referrals, education, and support for research.

For more information, see Chapter 59 in Smeltzer and Bare: *Brunner and Suddarth's Textbook of Medical-Surgical Nursing*, 9th edition. Philadelphia: Lippincott Williams & Wilkins, 2000.

HYPERGLYCEMIC HYPEROSMOLAR NONKETOTIC SYNDROME

Hyperglycemic hyperosmolar nonketotic syndrome (HHNKS) is a serious condition in which hyperglycemia and hyperosmolarity predominate with alterations of the sensorium (sense of awareness). Ketosis is minimal or absent. The basic biochemical defect is lack of effective insulin (insulin resistance). The persistent hyperglycemia causes osmotic diuresis, resulting in water and electrolyte losses. Although there is not enough insulin to prevent hyperglycemia, the small amount of insulin present is enough to prevent fat breakdown. This condition occurs most frequently in older people (50 to 70 years of age) who have had no previous history of diabetes or only mild type 2 diabetes. The acute development of the condition can be traced to some precipitating event, such as acute illness (pneumonia, myocardial infarction, stroke), ingestion of medications known to provoke insulin insufficiency (thiazide diuretics, propranolol), or therapeutic procedures (peritoneal dialysis or hemodialysis, hyperalimentation).

Clinical Manifestations
- History of days to weeks of polyuria and polydipsia
- Hypotension, tachycardia
- Profound dehydration (dry mucous membranes, poor skin turgor)
- Variable neurologic signs (alterations of sensorium, seizures, hemiparesis)

Diagnostic Evaluation
- Blood work, including blood glucose, electrolytes, blood urea nitrogen (BUN), complete blood count, serum osmolality, and arterial blood gases
- Clinical picture of severe dehydration

Medical Management
The overall treatment of HHNKS is similar to that of diabetic ketoacidosis (DKA): fluids, electrolytes, and insulin.

- Start fluid treatment with 0.9% or 0.45% normal saline, depending on sodium level and severity of volume depletion.
- Central venous or arterial pressure monitoring may be necessary to guide fluid replacement.
- Add potassium to replacement fluids when urinary output is adequate and is guided by continuous electrocardiogram (ECG) monitoring and laboratory determinations of potassium.

- Insulin is usually given at a continuous low rate to treat hyperglycemia.
- Dextrose is added to replacement fluids when the glucose level decreases to 250 to 300 mg/dL.
- Other treatment modalities are determined by the underlying illness of the patient and results of continuing clinical and laboratory evaluation.
- Treatment is continued until metabolic abnormalities are corrected and neurologic symptoms clear (may take 3 to 5 days for neurologic symptoms to resolve).

Nursing Management

See Nursing Management under Diabetes Mellitus and Diabetic Ketoacidosis for additional information.

Nursing Interventions

- Monitor fluid volume and electrolyte status for prevention of congestive heart failure and cardiac dysrhythmias (because of increased age of typical patient).
- Reinforce that after recovery from HHNKS, many patients can control diabetes with diet alone or diet and oral hypoglycemic agents. Insulin may not be needed after the acute hyperglycemic complication is resolved.

For more information, see Chapter 37 in Smeltzer and Bare: *Brunner and Suddarth's Textbook of Medical-Surgical Nursing,* 9th edition. Philadelphia: Lippincott Williams & Wilkins, 2000.

HYPERPARATHYROIDISM

Hyperparathyroidism is due to overproduction of parathyroid hormone by the parathyroid glands and is characterized by bone calcification and development of renal stones containing calcium. Primary hyperparathyroidism occurs two to four times more often in women than in men and is most frequently seen in patients between 60 and 70 years of age. Secondary hyperparathyroidism with similar manifestations occurs in patients with chronic renal failure and renal rickets.

Clinical Manifestations

The patient may have no symptoms or may experience signs and symptoms resulting from involvement of several body systems.

- Apathy, fatigue, muscular weakness, nausea, vomiting, constipation, hypertension, and cardiac dysrhythmias may occur.
- Psychological manifestations vary from emotional irritability and neuroses to psychoses due to the effect of calcium on the brain and nervous system.
- Stones in one or both kidneys may occur, causing obstruction, polynephritis, and renal failure.
- Musculoskeletal symptoms result from demineralization of the bones or bone tumors. Skeletal pain and tenderness in the back and joints; pain on weight bearing; pathologic fractures; deformities; and shortening of body stature.
- Incidence of peptic ulcer and pancreatitis is increased.

Diagnostic Evaluation

- Persistent increased serum calcium levels and elevated level of parahormone; double antibody parathyroid hormone test.
- Radioimmunoassays for parathormone, radiographs, or bone scan.
- Ultrasound, magnetic resonance imaging (MRI), thallium scan, or fine-needle biopsy

Medical Management

- Surgical removal of abnormal parathyroid tissue for primary hyperparathyroidism: in the preoperative period, encourage the patient to have a fluid intake of 2000 mL or more to prevent calculus formation; cranberry juice is suggested.

- Thiazide diuretics should be avoided because they decrease renal excretion of calcium.
- Mobility is encouraged because bones subjected to normal stress give up less calcium.
- Oral phosphates are administered to lower serum calcium levels (not for long-term use).
- Foods high in calcium and phosphorus are limited; if patient has coexisting peptic ulcer, antacids and protein feedings are added.

Nursing Management
- Initiate efforts to improve patient's appetite.
- Suggest prune juice, stool softeners, and increased fluid intake and physical activity to offset constipation postoperatively.
- Nursing management of the patient undergoing parathyroidectomy is essentially the same as that for a thyroidectomy patient, with emphasis on diet, avoiding dehydration, and increasing mobility.
- Monitor closely to detect symptoms of tetany, an early postoperative complication.
- Remind patient and family of importance of follow-up to ensure normal serum calcium levels.

Hypercalcemic Crisis
Acute hypercalcemic crisis can occur when serum calcium levels exceed 15 mg/dL. This results in neurologic, cardiovascular, and renal symptoms that can be life-threatening.

- Treatment includes rehydration with large volume of intravenous fluids, diuretic agents for renal excretion of excess calcium, and phosphate therapy to correct hypophosphatemia and decrease serum calcium levels.
- Cytotoxic agents, calcitonin, and dialysis may be used in emergency situations to decrease serum calcium quickly.
- Monitor patients in hypercalcemic crisis closely for complications, deterioration of condition, and reversal of serum calcium levels.

- Assess and care for patient to minimize complications and reverse the life-threatening hypercalcemia.
- Administer medications, such as calcitonin, corticosteroids, and bisphosphonates, with care to promote fluid and electrolyte balance.

For more information, see Chapter 38 in Smeltzer and Bare: *Brunner and Suddarth's Textbook of Medical-Surgical Nursing,* 9th edition. Philadelphia: Lippincott Williams & Wilkins, 2000.

H

HYPERTENSION

Hypertension is defined as a systolic blood pressure above 140 mm Hg and a diastolic pressure above 90 mm Hg, based on two or more blood pressure measurements. Hypertension can be classified as follows:

- *Stage 1:* systolic blood pressure, 140 to 159 mm Hg; diastolic pressure, 90 to 99 mm Hg
- *Stage 2:* systolic blood pressure, 160 to 179 mm Hg; diastolic pressure, 100 to 109 mm Hg
- *Stage 3:* systolic blood pressure, 180 mm Hg or higher; diastolic pressure, 110 mm Hg or higher

Hypertension is a major risk factor for atherosclerotic cardiovascular disease, heart failure, stroke, and kidney failure. Hypertension carries the risk of premature morbidity or mortality, which increases as systolic and diastolic pressure rises. Prolonged blood pressure elevation damages blood vessels in target organs (heart, kidneys, brain, and eyes).

ESSENTIAL (PRIMARY) HYPERTENSION
- In the adult population with hypertension, more than 90% have essential (primary) hypertension, which has no identifiable medical cause.
- On occasion, hypertension appears abruptly and severely and takes a "malignant" course that causes rapid deterioration in condition.

- Emotional disturbances, obesity, excessive alcohol intake, and overstimulation with coffee, tobacco, and stimulatory drugs play a role.
- Hypertension is strongly familial.
- Hypertension affects more women than men, but African American men are less able to tolerate the disease.

SECONDARY HYPERTENSION

- Elevations in blood pressure with specific cause, such as arterial disease, renal disease, certain medications, tumors, and pregnancy.
- Hypertension can also be acute, a sign of an underlying condition that causes a change in peripheral resistance or cardiac output.

Clinical Manifestations

- Physical examination may reveal no abnormality other than high blood pressure.
- Changes in the retinae with hemorrhages (small infarcts), exudates, narrowed arterioles, and papilledema may be seen in severe hypertension.
- Symptoms usually indicate vascular damage related to organ systems served by involved vessels.
- Coronary artery disease with angina or myocardial infarction is the most common sequela.
- Left ventricular hypertrophy may occur; left heart failure ensues.
- Pathologic changes may occur in the kidney (nocturia and increased blood urea nitrogen [BUN] and creatinine levels).
- Cerebral vascular involvement may occur (stroke or transient ischemic attack [TIA, ie, temporary hemiplegia, sudden falls, dizziness, weakness, or alterations in vision or speech]).

Diagnostic Evaluation

- History and physical examination, including retinae examination; laboratory studies for organ damage,

including urinalysis, blood chemistry; electrocardiogram (ECG) for left ventricular hypertrophy
- Special studies: intravenous pyelograms, renal arteriograms, split renal function studies, renin levels, 24-hour urine protein, creatinine clearance

Medical Management

The goal of any treatment program is to prevent associated morbidity and mortality by achieving and maintaining an arterial blood pressure below 140/90 mm Hg, whenever possible.

- Nonpharmacologic approaches include weight reduction; restriction of alcohol, sodium, tobacco; exercise and relaxation.
- Select a drug class that has the greatest effectiveness, fewest side effects, and best chance of acceptance by the patient. Promote compliance by avoiding complicated drug schedules.
- Two classes of drugs are available as first-line therapy: diuretics and beta-blockers.

Nursing Management
Assessment

Assess blood pressure at frequent intervals; know baseline level. Note changes in pressure that would require a change in medication. Include the following in the physical examination:

- Apical and peripheral pulse rate, rhythm, and character.
- Symptoms such as nosebleeds; anginal pain; shortness of breath; alterations in vision, speech, or balance (vertigo); headaches; or nocturia.

Major Nursing Diagnoses
- Knowledge deficit regarding the relationship between the treatment regimen and control of the disease process
- Noncompliance related to side effects of prescribed therapy

Collaborative Problems/Potential Complications
- Retinal hemorrhage
- Congestive heart failure
- Renal insufficiency
- Cerebrovascular accident (CVA)
- TIA
- Myocardial infarction
- Left ventricular hypertrophy

Planning and Goals
The major goals of the patient include understanding of the disease process and its treatment and compliance with self-care program.

Nursing Interventions
INCREASING KNOWLEDGE
- Emphasize the concept of controlling hypertension rather than curing it.
- Facilitate consultation with a dietitian to help patient plan weight loss.
- Obtain patient education materials from the American Heart Association.

MONITORING AND MANAGING POTENTIAL COMPLICATIONS
- Assess all body systems when patient returns for follow-up care.
- Question patient about blurred vision, spots, or diminished visual acuity.
- Report any significant findings promptly to determine whether additional studies or changes in medications are required.

🏠 Promoting Home and Community-Based Care

Teaching Patients Self-Care
- Support patient and promote adherence to therapy in a cost-effective manner; collaborate with patients for shared goal setting.

- Reinforce the importance of taking medications as prescribed, scheduling regular follow-up appointments, maintaining dietary restrictions of sodium and fat, increasing fruits and vegetables, and controlling weight control.
- Support the patient in planning lifestyle changes, including an exercise program with regular physical activity.
- Encourage counseling, education, and weight control; cessation of smoking; and stress self-help groups for family and patient.

H

Promoting Compliance With the Self-Care Program
- Encourage active participation of the patient in the program, including self-monitoring of blood pressure and diet for increased compliance.
- Encourage patient to abstain from alcohol because alcohol may have a synergistic effect with medication.
- Discourage use of tobacco and nicotine products.
- Give patient written information regarding expected effects and side effects of medication.
- Teach patient how to take own blood pressure.

Continuing Care
- Reinforce the importance of regular follow-up care.
- Obtain a patient history and perform a physical examination at each clinic visit.
- Assess for presence of medication-related problems (orthostatic hypotension).

Gerontologic Considerations

Isolated systolic hypertension is common in older adults as a result of changes of aging. Compliance with the therapeutic program is even more difficult for elderly people because medication therapy must be continuous, may be complicated, and may be expensive for a person on a fixed income.

- Promote monotherapy, treatment with a single agent, if appropriate for simplifying the medication regimen and making it less expensive.
- Make sure that the patient understands the medication regimen, is able to read the instructions, and is prepared to adjust to postural hypotensive effects of antihypertensive medications (change position slowly, use supportive devices).
- Include the family in the teaching program so that they understand the patient's needs, support adherence to the therapeutic program, and know when to seek guidance from health professionals.
- Encourage return to the outpatient setting for follow-up care.
- Assess all body systems to detect evidence of vascular damage to vital organs, such as eyes (blurred vision, spots in front of eyes, diminished visual acuity), heart, nervous system, and kidney function.

Evaluation

EXPECTED OUTCOMES
- Maintains adequate tissue perfusion
- Complies with the self-care program
- Experiences no complications

 NURSING ALERT: HYPERTENSIVE CRISIS

Hypertensive *emergency* exists when an elevated blood pressure must be lowered within 1 hour. Hypertensive *urgency* exists when blood pressure must be lowered within a few hours. Hypertensive crisis requires prompt treatment in an intensive care setting because of serious organ damage. The medication regimen (eg, nitroprusside, nicardipine hydrochloride) requires extremely close hemodynamic monitoring.

For more information, see Chapter 29 in Smeltzer and Bare: *Brunner and Suddarth's Textbook of Medical-Surgical Nursing,* 9th edition. Philadelphia: Lippincott Williams & Wilkins, 2000.

HYPERTHYROIDISM (GRAVES' DISEASE)

Hyperthyroidism is the second most common endocrine disorder. Graves' disease is the most common type. It results from an excessive output of thyroid hormones due to abnormal stimulation of the thyroid gland by circulating immunoglobulins. Long-acting thyroid stimulator (LATS) is found in significant concentration in the serum of many of these patients. The disorder affects women eight times more frequently than men and peaks in incidence in the third and fifth decades of life. It may appear after an emotional shock, stress, or infection, but the exact significance of these relationships is not understood. Other common causes include thyroiditis and excessive ingestion of thyroid hormone (eg, from the treatment of hypothyroidism).

Clinical Manifestations

Hyperthyroidism presents a characteristic group of signs and symptoms (thyrotoxicosis).

- Nervousness (emotionally hyperexcitable), irritability, apprehensiveness; inability to sit quietly; palpitations; rapid pulse on rest and exertion
- Poor tolerance of heat; excessive perspiration; skin that is flushed and likely to be warm, soft, and moist
- Dry skin and diffuse pruritus in the elderly
- Fine tremor of the hands
- Exophthalmos (bulging eyes)
- Increased appetite and dietary intake, progressive loss of weight, abnormal muscle fatigability, weakness, amenorrhea, and changes in bowel function (constipation or diarrhea)
- Pulse ranges between 90 and 160 beats/min with sinus tachycardia or dysrhythmias; systolic (but not diastolic) blood pressure elevation (increased pulse pressure)
- Atrial fibrillation; cardiac decompensation in the form of congestive heart failure, especially in the elderly
- Osteoporosis and fracture

- May include remissions and exacerbations, terminating with spontaneous recovery in a few months or years
- May progress relentlessly, causing emaciation, intense nervousness, delirium, disorientation, and eventually myocardial hypertrophy and heart failure

Diagnostic Evaluation

- Thyroid gland is enlarged; it is soft and may pulsate; a thrill may be felt and a bruit heard over thyroid arteries.
- Laboratory tests include an increase in serum thyroxine (T_4) and increase in ^{123}I or ^{125}I uptake.

Medical Management

Treatment is directed toward reducing thyroid hyperactivity for symptomatic relief and removing the cause of complications. Three forms of treatment are available:

- Pharmacotherapy with antithyroid medications
- Irradiation involving the administration of ^{131}I or ^{123}I for destructive effects on the thyroid gland
- Surgery with the removal of most of the thyroid gland

Radioactive Iodine (^{131}I)

- ^{131}I is given to destroy the overactive thyroid cells (most common treatment in the elderly).
- ^{131}I is contraindicated in pregnancy and nursing mothers because radioiodine crosses the placenta and is secreted in breast milk.

Pharmacotherapy

- The objective of pharmacotherapy is to inhibit hormone synthesis or release and reduce the amount of thyroid tissue.
- The most commonly used medications are propylthiouracil (Propacil, PTU) and methimazole (Tapazole) until patient is euthyroid.
- Maintenance dose is established, followed by gradual withdrawal of the medication over the next several months.

- Antithyroid drugs are contraindicated in late pregnancy because of a risk for goiter and cretinism in the fetus.
- Thyroid hormone may be administered to put the thyroid to rest.

Adjunctive Therapy
- Potassium iodide, Lugol's solution, and saturated solution of potassium iodide (SSKI) may be added.
- Beta-adrenergic agents may be used to control the sympathetic nervous system effects that occur in hyperthyroidism; for example, propranolol is used for nervousness, tachycardia, tremor, anxiety, and heat intolerance.

Surgical Intervention
- Surgical intervention (reserved for special circumstances) removes about five sixths of the thyroid tissue.
- Before surgery, the patient is given propylthiouracil until signs of hyperthyroidism have disappeared.
- Iodine is prescribed to reduce thyroid size and vascularity and blood loss. The patient is monitored carefully for evidence of iodine toxicity (swelling buccal mucosa, excessive salivation, skin eruptions).
- Risk for relapse and complications necessitates long-term follow-up of patient undergoing treatment of hyperthyroidism.
- Surgery to treat hyperthyroidism is performed after thyroid function has returned to normal (4 to 6 weeks).

Nursing Management
Assessment
- Obtain a health history, including family history of hyperthyroidism, and note reports on irritability or increased emotional reaction and the impact of these changes on the patient's interaction with family, friends, and coworkers.
- Assess stressors and the patient's ability to cope with stress.

- Evaluate nutritional status and presence of symptoms; note excessive nervousness and changes in vision and appearance of eyes.
- Assess and monitor cardiac status periodically (heart rate, blood pressure, heart sounds, and peripheral pulses).
- Assess emotional state and psychological status.

Major Nursing Diagnoses
- Altered nutrition related to exaggerated metabolic rate, excessive appetite, and increased gastrointestinal activity
- Ineffective coping related to irritability, hyperexcitability, apprehension, and emotional instability
- Disturbance in self-esteem related to changes in appearance, excessive appetite, and weight loss
- Altered body temperature

Collaborative Problems/Potential Complications
- Thyrotoxicosis or thyroid storm
- Hypothyroidism

Planning and Goals
The patient's goals may be improved nutritional status, improved coping ability, improved self-esteem, maintenance of normal body temperature, and absence of complications.

Nursing Interventions
IMPROVING NUTRITIONAL STATUS
- Provide several small, well-balanced meals (up to six meals a day) to satisfy patient's increased appetite.
- Replace food and fluids lost through diarrhea and diaphoresis, and control diarrhea that results from increased peristalsis.
- Reduce diarrhea by avoiding highly seasoned foods and stimulants such as coffee, tea, cola, and alcohol; encourage high-calorie, high-protein foods.
- Provide quiet atmosphere during mealtime to aid digestion.
- Record patient's weight and dietary intake daily.

ENHANCING COPING MEASURES

- Reassure family and friends that symptoms are expected to disappear with treatment.
- Maintain a calm, unhurried approach, and minimize stressful experiences.
- Keep the environment quiet and uncluttered.
- Provide information regarding thyroidectomy, and preparatory pharmacotherapy, to alleviate patient anxiety.
- Assist patient to take medications as prescribed and encourage adherence to the therapeutic regimen.
- Repeat information often, and provide written instructions as indicated due to short attention span.

IMPROVING SELF-ESTEEM

- Convey to the patient an understanding of concern regarding problems in appearance, appetite, and weight, and assist in developing coping strategies.
- Provide eye protection if experiencing eye changes secondary to hyperthyroidism; instruct regarding correct installation of eyedrops or ointment to soothe the eyes and protect the exposed cornea.
- Arrange for the patient to eat alone, if desired and if embarrassed by the large meals consumed due to increased metabolic rate. Avoid commenting on intake.

MAINTAINING NORMAL BODY TEMPERATURE

- Provide a cool, comfortable environment and fresh bedding and gown as needed.
- Give cool baths and provide cool fluids; monitor body temperature.
- Explain to patient and family the importance of providing a cool environment.

MONITORING AND MANAGING POTENTIAL COMPLICATIONS

- Monitor closely for signs and symptoms indicative of thyroid storm.
- Assess cardiac and respiratory function: vital signs, cardiac output, electrocardiogram (ECG) monitoring, arterial blood gases, pulse oximetry.

- Administer oxygen to prevent hypoxia.
- Give intravenous fluids to maintain blood glucose levels and replace lost fluids.
- Administer antithyroid medications to reduce thyroid hormone levels.
- Administer propranolol and digitalis to treat cardiac symptoms.
- Implement strategies to treat shock if needed.
- Monitor for hypothyroidism; encourage continued therapy.

 Promoting Home and Community-Based Care

Teaching Patients Self-Care

- Instruct how and when to take prescribed medications.
- Teach patient how the medication regimen fits in with the broader therapeutic plan, and the consequences of failing to take medications.
- Provide an individualized written plan of care for use at home.
- Teach patient and family members about the desired effects and side effects of medications.
- Instruct patient and family about which adverse effects should be reported to the physician.
- Teach patient about what to expect from a thyroidectomy if this is to be performed.
- Teach patient to avoid situations that have the potential of stimulating thyroid storm.

Continuing Care

- Stress long-term follow-up care because of the possibility of hypothyroidism after thyroidectomy or treatment with antithyroid drugs or [131]I.
- Refer to home care for assessment of the home and family environment.
- Assess patient's and family's understanding of the importance of the therapeutic regimen and compliance with it; recommend follow-up monitoring.

- Assess for changes indicating return to normal thyroid function; assess for physical signs of hyperthyroidism and hypothyroidism.

Evaluation

EXPECTED OUTCOMES
- Improved nutritional status
- Demonstrates effective coping methods in dealing with family, friends, and coworkers
- Achieves increased self-esteem
- Maintains normal body temperature
- Absence of complications

 Gerontologic Considerations

The major symptoms of the elderly patient may be depression and apathy, accompanied by significant weight loss and constipation in some. The patient may report cardiovascular symptoms and difficulty climbing stairs or rising from a chair because of muscle weakness; congestive failure may be noted.

Elderly patients may experience a single manifestation, such as atrial fibrillation, anorexia, or weight loss. These general symptoms may mask underlying thyroid disease. Spontaneous remission of hyperthyroidism is rare in the elderly. Measurement of thyroid-stimulating hormone (TSH) uptake is indicated in elderly patients with unexplained physical or mental deterioration.

Use of ^{131}I is generally recommended for treatment of thyrotoxicosis rather than surgery unless an enlarged thyroid gland is pressing on the airway. Thyrotoxicosis must be controlled by antithyroid drugs before ^{131}I is used because radiation may precipitate thyroid storm, which has a high mortality rate in the elderly.

Use of beta-blockers may be indicated to decrease cardiovascular and neurologic signs; use these agents with extreme caution and monitor closely for granulocytopenia. Modify dosages of other medications because of the altered rate of metabolism in hyperthyroidism.

For more information, see Chapter 38 in Smeltzer and Bare: *Brunner and Suddarth's Textbook of Medical-Surgical Nursing,* 9th edition. Philadelphia: Lippincott Williams & Wilkins, 2000.

HYPOGLYCEMIA (INSULIN REACTION)

Hypoglycemia (abnormally low blood glucose level) occurs when the blood glucose falls below 50 to 60 mg/dL. It can be caused by too much insulin or oral hypoglycemic agents, too little food, or excessive physical activity. Hypoglycemia may occur at any time. It often occurs before meals, especially if delayed or if snacks are omitted. Middle-of-the-night hypoglycemia may occur because of peaking evening NPH or Lente insulins, especially in patients who have not eaten a bedtime snack.

Clinical Manifestations
- The symptoms of hypoglycemia may be grouped into two categories: adrenergic symptoms and central nervous system symptoms.
- Hypoglycemic symptoms may occur suddenly and unexpectedly and vary from person to person.
- Patients who have blood glucose in the hyperglycemic range (200 mg/dL or greater) may feel hypoglycemic with adrenergic symptoms when blood glucose quickly drops to 120 mg/dL or less.
- Patients with usual blood glucose levels of low range of normal may not experience symptoms when blood glucose slowly falls under 50 mg/dL.
- Decreased hormonal (adrenergic) response to hypoglycemia may occur in patients who have diabetes for many years.
- As the glucose falls, the normal surge of adrenaline does not occur, and the patient does not feel the usual adrenergic symptoms: sweating and shakiness.

Mild Hypoglycemia
The sympathetic nervous system is stimulated, producing sweating, tremor, tachycardia, palpitations, nervousness, and hunger.

Moderate Hypoglycemia
Moderate hypoglycemia produces impaired function of the central nervous system, including inability to concentrate, headache, lightheadedness, confusion, and memory lapses. Additional symptoms include numbness of the lips and tongue, slurred speech, impaired coordination, emotional changes, irrational or combative behavior, double vision, and drowsiness or any combination of these symptoms.

Severe Hypoglycemia
In severe hypoglycemia, central nervous system function is further impaired. The patient needs the assistance of another for treatment. Symptoms may include disoriented behavior, seizures, difficulty arousing from sleep, or loss of consciousness.

Diagnostic Evaluation
• Measurement of serum glucose levels

Medical Management
• The usual recommendation is 10 to 15 g of a fast-acting sugar orally: (a) three or four commercially prepared glucose tablets; (b) 4 to 6 ounces of fruit juice or regular soda; (c) 6 to 10 Lifesavers or other hard candies; (d) 2 to 3 teaspoons of sugar or honey.
• The patient should avoid adding table sugar to juice, even "unsweetened" juice, which may cause a sharp increase in glucose, resulting in hyperglycemia hours later.
• Treatment is repeated if the symptoms persist more than 10 to 15 minutes; the patient is retested in 15 minutes and retreated if blood glucose level is less than 70 to 75 mg/dL.

- The patient should eat a snack containing protein and starch (milk, or cheese and crackers) after the symptoms resolve or should eat a meal or snack within 30 to 60 minutes.
- Diabetic patients should carry a form of simple sugar with them at all times.
- The patient is discouraged from eating high-calorie, high-fat dessert foods to treat hypoglycemia because high-fat snacks may slow absorption of the glucose.

Management of Hypoglycemia in the Unconscious Patient

- Glucagon, 1 mg subcutaneously or intramuscularly for patients who are unable to swallow, or refuse treatment; the patient may take up to 20 minutes to regain consciousness. Give a simple sugar followed by snack when awake.
- From 25 to 50 mL of 50% dextrose in water (D-50) is administered intravenously to patients who are unconscious or unable to swallow (in a hospital setting).

Nursing Management

🏠 Promoting Home and Community-Based Care

Teaching Patients Self-Care

- Teach patient to prevent hypoglycemia by following a consistent, regular pattern for eating, administering insulin, and exercising. Consume between-meal and bedtime snacks to counteract the maximum insulin effect.
- Reinforce that routine blood glucose tests are performed so that changing insulin requirements may be anticipated and adjusted.
- Encourage patients taking insulin to wear identification bracelet or tag indicating they have diabetes.
- Instruct patient to notify physician after severe hypoglycemia has occurred.

- Instruct patients and family members about symptoms of hypoglycemia and use of glucagon.
- Teach family members that hypoglycemia can cause irrational and unintentional behavior.
- Teach patients the importance of performing blood glucose tests on a frequent and regular basis.
- Teach patients with type 2 diabetes who take oral hypoglycemic agents that symptoms of hypoglycemia may also develop.

 Gerontologic Considerations

Elderly people frequently live alone and may not recognize symptoms of hypoglycemia. With decreasing renal function, it takes longer for oral hypoglycemic agents to be excreted by the kidneys. Teach the patient to avoid skipping meals because of decreased appetite or financial limitations on meal planning. Decreased visual acuity may lead to errors in insulin administration.

For more information, see Chapter 37 in Smeltzer and Bare: *Brunner and Suddarth's Textbook of Medical-Surgical Nursing,* 9th edition. Philadelphia: Lippincott Williams & Wilkins, 2000.

HYPOPARATHYROIDISM

The most common cause of hypoparathyroidism is inadequate secretion of parathyroid hormone after interruption of the blood supply or surgical removal of parathyroid gland tissue during thyroidectomy, parathyroidectomy, or radical neck dissection. Atrophy of the parathyroid glands of unknown etiology is a less common cause. Symptoms are due to deficiency of parathormone that results in an elevation of blood phosphate and decrease in blood calcium levels.

Clinical Manifestations
Tetany is the chief symptom.

- Latent tetany: numbness, tingling, and cramps in the extremities; stiffness in the hands and feet.
- Overt tetany: bronchospasm, laryngeal spasm, carpopedal spasm, dysphagia, photophobia, cardiac dysrhythmias, and seizures.
- Other symptoms: anxiety, irritability, depression, and delirium. Electrocardiogram (ECG) changes and hypotension may also occur.

Diagnostic Evaluation
- Latent tetany is suggested by positive Trousseau's sign or positive Chvostek's sign.
- Diagnosis is difficult because of vague symptoms; laboratory studies show decreased serum calcium, increased serum phosphate; increased bone density and brain calcification on radiograph.

Medical Management
- The patient's serum calcium level is raised to 9 to 10 mg/dL.
- When hypocalcemia and tetany occur after thyroidectomy, intravenous calcium gluconate is given immediately. Sedatives (pentobarbital) may be administered. Parenteral parathormone may be given, watching for an allergic reaction.
- Neuromuscular irritability is reduced by providing an environment that is free of noise, sudden drafts, bright lights, or sudden movement.
- Emergency management with bronchodilating medications, tracheostomy, or mechanical ventilation for respiratory distress.
- Chronic hypoparathyroidism is treated with a diet high in calcium and low in phosphorus. The patient should avoid milk, milk products, egg yolk, and spinach.
- Oral calcium tablets and vitamin D preparation and aluminum hydroxide or aluminum carbonate may be given.

Nursing Management
Nursing Interventions
- Anticipate signs of tetany, convulsions, and respiratory difficulty.
- Keep calcium gluconate at bedside and observe for cardiac problems, such as dysrhythmias. If receiving digitalis, then calcium gluconate must be administered slowly and cautiously.
- Provide continuous cardiac monitoring and careful assessment; calcium and digitalis increase systolic contraction and potentiate each other and the risk for fatal dysrhythmias.
- Provide oral tablets of calcium salts (calcium gluconate); give aluminum hydroxide gel after meals to bind phosphate.
- Provide vitamin D preparations to enhance calcium absorption from the gastrointestinal tract.

H

🏠 Promoting Home and Community-Based Care

Teaching Patients Self-Care
- Teach patient about medications and diet therapy and reason for high calcium and low phosphate intake; teach patient to contact physician if symptoms occur.
- Teach the importance of maintaining a diet high in calcium and low in phosphorus for patients with chronic hypoparathyroidism.
- Caution patient to restrict milk, milk products, and egg yolk because they contain high levels of phosphorus and to eliminate spinach because it contains oxalate, which forms insoluble calcium substances.

For more information, see Chapter 38 in Smeltzer and Bare: *Brunner and Suddarth's Textbook of Medical-Surgical Nursing,* 9th edition. Philadelphia: Lippincott Williams & Wilkins, 2000.

HYPOPITUITARISM

Hypopituitarism is pituitary insufficiency from destruction of the anterior lobe of the pituitary gland or hypofunction of the hypothalamus. Panhypopituitarism (Simmonds' disease) is total absence of all pituitary secretions and is rare. Postpartum pituitary necrosis (Sheehan's syndrome) is another uncommon cause of failure of the anterior pituitary. It is more likely to occur in women with severe blood loss, hypovolemia, and hypotension at the time of delivery. Hypopituitarism is also a complication of radiation therapy to the head and neck. Total destruction of the pituitary gland by trauma, tumor, or vascular lesion removes all stimuli that are normally received by the thyroid, gonads, and adrenal glands. The result is extreme weight loss, emaciation, atrophy of all endocrine glands and organs, hair loss, impotence, amenorrhea, hypometabolism, and hypoglycemia. Coma and death occur without replacement of missing hormones.

For more information, see Chapter 38 in Smeltzer and Bare: *Brunner and Suddarth's Textbook of Medical-Surgical Nursing,* 9th edition. Philadelphia: Lippincott Williams & Wilkins, 2000.

HYPOTHYROIDISM AND MYXEDEMA

Hypothyroidism is a condition of thyroid deficiency (suboptimal levels of thyroid hormone). Types of hypothyroidism include primary, which refers to dysfunction of the thyroid gland (more than 95% of cases); central, due to failure of the pituitary gland, hypothalamus, or both; secondary or pituitary, which is due entirely to a pituitary disorder; and hypothalamic or tertiary, due to a disorder of the hypothalamus resulting in inadequate secretion of thyroid-stimulating hormone (TSH) from decreased stimulation by thyrotropin-releasing hormone (TRH). Hypothyroidism occurs more often in older women. Its causes include autoimmune thyroiditis (Hashimoto's thyroiditis, most common type in adults); therapy for hyperthyroidism (radioiodine, surgery, or antithyroid drugs); radiation therapy for head and neck cancer; infiltrative diseases of the thyroid (amyloidosis and scleroderma); iodine deficiency; and iodine excess. When thyroid deficiency is present at birth, the condition is known as *cretinism.* The term *myxedema* refers to the accumulation of mucopolysaccharides in subcutaneous and other interstitial tissue and is used only to describe the extreme symptoms of severe hypothyroidism.

H

Clinical Manifestations
- Nonspecific early symptoms
- Extreme fatigue
- Hair loss, brittle nails, dry skin, and numbness and tingling of the fingers
- Husky voice and hoarseness
- Menstrual disturbances; menorrhagia or amenorrhea; loss of libido
- Severe hypothyroidism: subnormal temperature and pulse rate; weight gain without corresponding increase of food intake; cachexia
- Sensation of cold in a warm environment
- Subdued emotional responses as the condition progresses; dulled mental processes and apathy
- Slowed speech; enlarged tongue, hands, and feet; constipation; possibly deafness
- Hypothyroidism (affects women five times more frequently than men); associated tendency toward atherosclerosis with all consequences
- Advanced hypothyroidism: personality and cognitive changes, pleural effusion, pericardial effusion, and respiratory muscle weakness
- Myxedema: thickened skin, thinning hair or alopecia; expressionless and masklike facial features
- Advanced hypothyroidism with hypothermia: abnormal sensitivity to sedatives, opiates, and anesthetic agents (these drugs are given with extreme caution)

Medical Management

The primary objective is to restore a normal metabolic state by replacing thyroid hormone.

- Synthetic levothyroxine (Synthroid or Levothroid) is the preferred preparation.
- Additional treatment consists of maintaining vital functions, monitoring arterial blood gas (ABG) values, and administering fluids cautiously because of danger of water intoxication.
- External heat application is avoided because it increases oxygen requirements and may lead to vascular collapse.
- Concentrated glucose may be given if hypoglycemia is evident.
- If myxedema coma is present, thyroid hormone is given intravenously until consciousness is restored.

Interaction of Thyroid Hormones With Other Drugs

- Thyroid hormones increase blood glucose levels, which may necessitate adjustment in doses of insulin or oral hypoglycemic agents.
- The effects of thyroid hormone may be increased by phenytoin and tricyclic antidepressants.
- Thyroid hormone may increase the pharmacologic effect of digitalis, glycosides, anticoagulants, and indomethacin, requiring careful observation and assessment for side effects of these drugs.

 NURSING ALERT

Severe untreated hypothyroidism increases susceptibility to all hypnotic and sedative drugs.

Nursing Management

Assessment

- Monitor and record vital signs for baseline.
- Monitor respiratory rate, depth, pattern, pulse oximetry, and ABG values.

- Assess all body systems; note any abnormal functions.
- Explore the impact of condition on patient and family members and coping skills.

Major Nursing Diagnoses
- Activity intolerance related to fatigue and depressed cognitive process
- Altered body temperature
- Ineffective breathing pattern related to depressed ventilation
- Constipation related to depressed gastrointestinal function
- Knowledge deficit about the therapeutic regimen for lifelong thyroid replacement therapy
- Altered thought processes related to depressed metabolism and altered cardiovascular and respiratory status

Planning and Goals
The major goals of the patient may include ability to tolerate moderate activity, maintenance of normal body temperature and effective breathing pattern, prevention of constipation, understanding of therapeutic regimen, and maintenance of effective thought processes.

Nursing Interventions
IMPROVING RESPIRATORY STATUS
- Encourage deep breathing and coughing.
- Administer medications with caution (hypnotics and sedatives).
- Maintain patent airway through suction and ventilatory support if indicated.

INCREASED PARTICIPATION IN ACTIVITIES
- Support the patient by assisting with care and hygiene while encouraging to participate in activities within tolerance to prevent complications of immobility (major role of nurse).
- Space activities to promote rest and exercise as tolerated.

- Monitor vital signs and cognitive level closely during diagnostic workup and initiation of treatment to detect (1) deterioration of physical and mental status, (2) symptoms indicating that an increased metabolic rate exceeds the ability of the cardiovascular and pulmonary systems to respond, and (3) continued limitations and complications of myxedema.

MAINTAINING NORMAL BODY TEMPERATURE AND PROMOTING COMFORT
- Provide extra clothing and blankets for chilling and extreme intolerance to cold.
- Avoid heating pads and electric blankets; patient could be burned because of delayed responses and decreased mental status.
- Monitor patient's body temperature, and report decreases from baseline.
- Protect from exposure to cold and drafts.

PROMOTING RETURN OF BOWEL FUNCTION
- Encourage increased fluid intake within limits of fluid restriction.
- Provide foods high in fiber.
- Instruct patient about foods with high water content.
- Monitor bowel function.
- Encourage increased mobility within exercise tolerance.
- Encourage patient to use laxatives and enemas sparingly.

PROVIDING EMOTIONAL SUPPORT
- Assist patient and family in dealing with emotional reactions to changes in appearance and body image.
- Inform patient that symptoms subside when hypothyroidism is treated successfully.
- Provide assistance and counseling to deal with the emotional concerns and reactions that result.

IMPROVING THOUGHT PROCESSES
- Orient patient to time, place, date, and events.
- Provide stimulation through conversation and nonthreatening activities.

- Explain to patient and family that change in cognitive and mental functioning is a result of disease process.
- Monitor cognitive and mental processes and response of these to medication and other therapy.

MONITORING AND PREVENTING COMPLICATIONS
- Monitor increasing severity of signs and symptoms of hypothyroidism.
- Assist in ventilatory support if needed.
- Administer medications (thyroxine) with caution.
- Turn and reposition patient at intervals.
- Avoid use of hypnotic, sedative, and analgesic agents in myxedema.
- Document and report subtle signs and symptoms that indicate inadequate thyroxine hormone.

🏠 Promoting Home and Community-Based Care

Teaching Patients Self-Care
- Provide follow-up, teaching, and health care before hospital discharge.
- Provide dietary instruction to promote weight loss after medication has been initiated and to promote return of normal bowel pattern.
- Inform and instruct family members about treatment goals, medication schedules, and signs of overdose or underdose or side effects to be reported.

Continuing Care
- Give encouragement and assistance in the daily administration of medications; encourage development of schedule and administration checklist.
- Reinforce knowledge that continued thyroid hormone replacement is necessary, with periodic follow-up testing.
- If indicated, arrange a weekly visit from the home care nurse to assess the patient's physical and cognitive status and ability to cope with recent changes.

Gerontologic Considerations

The higher prevalence of hypothyroidism in the elderly population may be related to alterations in immune function with age. Depression, apathy, or decreased mobility or activity may be the major initial symptom.

The effects of analgesics, sedatives, and anesthetic agents are prolonged in all patients with hypothyroidism, and these agents should be administered with caution. Thyroid hormone replacement must be started with low doses and gradually increased to prevent serious cardiovascular and neurologic side effects, such as angina. Testing of serum TSH is recommended every 5 years. Myxedema and myxedema coma generally occur exclusively in patients older than 50 years of age.

NURSING ALERT

Patients with unrecognized hypothyroidism undergoing surgery are at increased risk for intraoperative hypotension, postoperative congestive heart failure, and altered mental status. Myocardial ischemia or infarction may occur in response to therapy in patients with severe, long-standing hypothyroidism or myxedema coma. Nurses must be alert for signs of angina, especially during the early phase of treatment and should discontinue administration of thyroid hormone immediately if symptoms occur.

For more information, see Chapter 38 in Smeltzer and Bare: *Brunner and Suddarth's Textbook of Medical-Surgical Nursing,* 9th edition. Philadelphia: Lippincott Williams & Wilkins, 2000.

IDIOPATHIC THROMBOCYTOPENIA PURPURA

Idiopathic thrombocytopenia purpura (ITP) is a disease affecting all ages but is more common in children and young women. Although the precise cause remains unknown, viral infection sometimes precedes the disease in children. Other conditions (eg, systemic lupus erythematosus, pregnancy) or medications (eg, sulfa drugs) can also produce ITP. Antiplatelet autoantibodies are produced, which attack platelets; platelet life-span is markedly shortened. Usually the diagnosis is made from decreased platelet count, survival time, and increased bleeding time. There are two forms: acute (primarily in children) and chronic.

Clinical Manifestations
- Petechiae and easy bruising (dry purpura)
- Heavy menses in women and mucosal bleeding (wet purpura, high risk of intracranial bleeding)
- Platelet count generally below 20,000 mm^3
- Acute form self-limiting, possibly with spontaneous remissions

Diagnostic Evaluation
- Exclusion of other causes of thrombocytopenia
- Platelet count, complete blood count
- Bone marrow aspiration

Medical Management

- Immunosuppressive medications: corticosteroids are the treatment of choice.
- Intravenous gamma globulin (very expensive) and vincristine are effective.
- Splenectomy is sometimes performed.
- A new approach involves using anti-D for patients who are Rh(D) positive.
- Platelet use is avoided except to stop catastrophic bleeding.
- Instruct to avoid all drugs that interfere with platelet function (eg, quinine, sulfa-containing medication, aspirin, nonsteroidal antiinflammatory drugs [NSAIDs]).

Nursing Management

Assessment

- Obtain history of medication use, including over-the-counter medications, recent viral illness, or complaints of headache or visual disturbances (intracranial bleed).
- Physical assessment should include thorough search for signs of bleeding, including neurologic assessment, along with vital sign measurement.

Nursing Interventions

MINIMIZE BLEEDING

- Avoid medications that alter platelet function (drugs containing aspirin, sulfa-containing medications, NSAIDs).
- Avoid injections and rectal medications.

🏠 Promoting Home and Community-Based Care

Teaching Patients Self-Care

- Address signs of exacerbation of disease (petechiae, ecchymoses); how to contact health care personnel, and the names of medications that induce ITP.

- Include information about current medication treatment (tapering schedule, if relevant), frequency of platelet count monitoring, and medications to avoid.
- Instruct patient to avoid constipation, the Valsalva maneuver, tooth flossing, and razors (nonelectric) for shaving.
- Instruct patient to use soft-bristled toothbrushes instead of stiff-bristled brushes; patient should refrain from vigorous sexual intercourse when platelet count is less than 10,000/mm^3.

For more information, see Chapter 30 in Smeltzer and Bare: *Brunner and Suddarth's Textbook of Medical-Surgical Nursing,* 9th edition. Philadelphia: Lippincott Williams & Wilkins, 2000.

IMPETIGO

Impetigo is a superficial infection of the skin caused by staphylococci, streptococci, or multiple bacteria. Exposed areas of the body, face, hands, neck, and extremities are most frequently involved. Impetigo is contagious and may spread to other parts of the patient's skin or to other members of the family who touch the patient or who use towels or combs that are soiled with the exudate of the lesion. Impetigo is particularly common among children living in poor hygienic conditions. In adults, chronic health problems, poor hygiene, and malnutrition may predispose to impetigo.

Clinical Manifestations

- Lesions begin as small, red macules that become discrete, thin-walled vesicles that rupture and become covered with a honey-yellow crust.
- These crusts, when removed, reveal smooth, red, moist surfaces on which new crusts develop.
- If the scalp is involved, the hair is matted, distinguishing the condition from ringworm.

- Bullous impetigo, a deep-seated infection of the skin caused by *Staphylococcus aureus*, is characterized by the formation of bullae from original vesicles. The bullae rupture, leaving a raw, red area.

Medical Management
Systemic Antibiotic Therapy
- Usual treatment for impetigo
- Reduces contagious spread and prevents possible aftermath of glomerulonephritis
- Nonbullous impetigo: benzathine penicillin, or oral penicillin or erythromycin
- Bullous impetigo: penicillinase-resistant penicillin or erythromycin

Topical Antibacterial Therapy
- Usual treatment for disease that is limited to a small area
- Applied to lesions several times daily for 1 week
- Lesions soaked or washed with soap solution to remove central site of bacterial growth and to give the topical antibiotic opportunity to reach the infected site
- Gloves worn when giving care to these patients
- Antiseptic solutions (chlorhexidine [Hibiclens]) to cleanse the skin and reduce bacterial content and prevent spread

🏠 Promoting Home and Community-Based Care

- Instruct patient and family to bathe at least once daily with bactericidal soap.
- Encourage cleanliness and good hygienic practices to prevent spread of lesion from one skin area to another and from one person to another. Provide each person with separate towel and washcloth. Avoid physical contact between the infected person and other people.

For more information, see Chapter 52 in Smeltzer and Bare: *Brunner and Suddarth's Textbook of Medical-Surgical Nursing,* 9th edition. Philadelphia: Lippincott Williams & Wilkins, 2000.

INCREASED INTRACRANIAL PRESSURE

Increased intracranial pressure (ICP) is the result of the amount of brain tissue, intracranial blood volume, and cerebrospinal fluid (CSF) within the skull at any one time. The volume and pressure of these three components are usually in a state of equilibrium. Because there is limited space for expansion within the skull, an increase in any of these components causes a change in the volume of the other by either displacing or shifting CSF, increasing the absorption of CSF, or decreasing cerebral blood volume. The normal ICP is 10 to 20 mm Hg. Although elevated ICP is most commonly associated with head injury, an elevated pressure may be seen secondary to brain tumors, subarachnoid hemorrhage, and toxic and viral encephalopathies. Increased ICP from any cause affects cerebral perfusion and produces distortion and shifts of brain tissue.

Clinical Manifestations

- When ICP increases to where the brain's ability to adjust has reached its limits, neural function is impaired. Increased ICP is manifested by changes in level of consciousness and abnormal respiratory and vasomotor responses.
- The patient's level of responsiveness and consciousness is the most important indicator of his or her condition.
- Lethargy is the earliest sign of increasing ICP. Slowing of speech and delay in response to verbal suggestions are early indicators.
- Sudden change in condition, such as becoming restless (without apparent cause), appearing confused, or displaying increasing drowsiness, has neurologic significance.
- As pressure increases, patient becomes stuporous and may react only to loud auditory or painful stimuli. This indicates serious impairment of brain circulation, and immediate surgical intervention may be required. With further deterioration, coma and abnormal motor

responses in the form of decortication, decerebration, or flaccidity may occur.

- When coma is profound, pupils dilate and fix, respirations are impaired, and death is usually inevitable.

Diagnostic Evaluation

- Cerebral angiography, computed tomography (CT), magnetic resonance imaging (MRI), positron emission tomography (PET), transcranial Doppler studies, or electrophysiologic monitoring may be done. Lumbar puncture is avoided owing to risk of herniation.
- ICP monitoring provides beneficial information.

Medical Management

- Increased ICP constitutes a true emergency and must be treated promptly. The immediate management for relief of ICP is based on decreasing cerebral edema, lowering the volume of CSF, and decreasing blood volume while maintaining cerebral perfusion.
- Osmotic diuretics and corticosteroids are administered, fluid is restricted, CSF is drained, the patient is hyperventilated, fever is controlled (using antipyretics, hypothermia blanket with chlorpromazine [Thorazine] to control shivering), and cellular metabolic demands are reduced (with barbiturates, paralyzing agents).
- If patient is not responsive to conventional treatment, reduction of cellular metabolic demands may be accomplished through administration of high doses of barbiturates or administration of pharmacologic paralyzing agents, such as pancuronium (Pavulon). The patient requires care in a critical care unit.

Nursing Management

Assessment

- Obtain a patient history with subjective data including events leading to present illness.
- Complete a neurologic examination as patient's condition allows.

- Use the Glasgow Coma Scale to assess three types of behavior: verbal response, motor response, and eye opening.
- Note subtle changes, such as restlessness, headache, forced breathing, mental cloudiness, and purposeless movements, which may be early indications of rising ICP.
- Assess headache (usually is constant, increasing in intensity, and aggravated by movement or straining).
- Note recurrent or projectile vomiting, which indicates increased pressure.
- Monitor ICP closely as an essential part of management.

CHANGES IN VITAL SIGNS
- Alterations in vital signs may be a late sign of increased ICP.
- As ICP increases, pulse rate and respiratory rate decrease, and blood pressure and temperature rise.
- Observe for widening pulse pressure, bradycardia, and respiratory irregularity: Cheyne-Stokes breathing and ataxic breathing (Cushing's triad). Widened pulse pressure is a serious development.
- Immediate surgical intervention is indicated if the major circulation begins to decrease as a result of brain compression.

PUPILLARY CHANGES
- Inspect pupils for size, configuration, and reaction to light.
- Evaluate gaze as to whether it is conjugate (paired, working together) or disconjugate.
- Assess ability of eyes to abduct or adduct.
- Inspect retina and optic nerve for hemorrhage and papilledema.

Major Nursing Diagnoses
- Altered cerebral tissue perfusion related to the effects of increased ICP
- Ineffective breathing patterns related to neurologic dysfunction (brain-stem compression, structural displacement)

- Ineffective airway clearance related to accumulation of secretions secondary to depression of level of responsiveness
- Risk for fluid volume deficit related to dehydration procedures
- Risk for infection related to ICP monitoring system (fiberoptic or intraventricular catheter)

Collaborative Problems/Potential Complications
- Brain-stem herniation
- Diabetes insipidus
- Syndrome of inappropriate antidiuretic hormone (SIADH)

Planning and Goals
The major goals of the patient may include adequate cerebral tissue perfusion through reduction of ICP, normalization of respiration, maintenance of a patent airway, restoration of fluid balance, normal urine and bowel elimination, absence of infection, and absence of complications.

Nursing Interventions
PRESERVING AND IMPROVING
CEREBRAL TISSUE PERFUSION
- Monitor for bradycardia, bradypnea, and a rising blood pressure (Cushing's reflex or response).
- Avoid raising jugular venous pressure and ICP by keeping patient's head in a neutral (midline) position and maintaining slight elevation of the head to aid in venous drainage.
- Avoid extreme rotation and flexion of the neck because compression or distortion of the jugular veins increases the ICP.
- Avoid extreme hip flexion because this position causes an increase in intraabdominal and intrathoracic pressures, which produce a rise in ICP.
- Avoid the Valsalva maneuver or even moving in bed; provide stool softeners and a high-fiber diet if patient is able to eat; note any abdominal distention.

- Avoid isometric muscle contractions.
- Avoid suctioning longer than 15 seconds; hyperventilate on ventilator with 100% oxygen before suctioning.
- Maintain a calm atmosphere, and reduce environmental stimuli.
- Avoid enemas and cathartics.
- During nursing care, the ICP should not rise above 25 mm Hg and should return to baseline levels within 5 minutes. Space interventions to prevent transient increases in ICP.
- When moving or turning in bed, instruct patient to exhale to avoid the Valsalva maneuver.

ATTAINING NORMAL RESPIRATORY PATTERN
- Monitor patient constantly for respiratory irregularities.
- Collaborate with respiratory therapist in monitoring arterial carbon dioxide pressure ($PaCO_2$), which is usually maintained between 30 and 35 mm Hg when hyperventilation therapy is used.
- Maintain continuous neurologic observation record with repeated assessments.

MAINTAINING A PATENT AIRWAY
- Maintain patency of the airway; oxygenate patient before and after suctioning.
- Auscultate lung fields for presence of adventitious sounds every 8 hours.
- Elevate head of bed to aid in clearing secretions and improve venous drainage of the brain.
- Discourage coughing and straining.

ATTAINING FLUID BALANCE
- Assess patient's skin turgor, mucous membranes, and serum and urine osmolality for signs of dehydration.
- Monitor vital signs to assess fluid volume status.
- Give oral hygiene for mouth dryness.
- Insert indwelling catheter to assess renal and fluid status.
- Monitor urine output every hour in the acute phase.

- Administer intravenous fluids by pump at a slow to moderate rate; monitor patients receiving mannitol for congestive failure.
- Administer corticosteroids and dehydrating agents as ordered.
- Test stools for blood if patient is on high doses of corticosteroids (gastrointestinal bleeding is a complication).

PREVENTING INFECTION
- Strictly adhere to the written protocols for managing ICP monitoring systems in the health care facility.
- Keep dressings over ventricular catheters dry because wet dressings are conducive to bacterial growth.
- Use aseptic technique at all times when managing the ventricular drainage system and changing drainage bag.
- Check carefully for any loose connections that cause leaking and contamination of the ventricular system and contamination of CSF as well as inaccurate ICP readings.
- Monitor for signs and symptoms of meningitis: fever, chills, nuchal (neck) rigidity, and increasing or persistent headache.

MONITORING AND MANAGING
POTENTIAL COMPLICATIONS
- ICP elevation: monitor ICP closely for continuous elevation or significant increase over baseline; assess vital signs at time of ICP increase. Assess for and immediately report manifestations of increasing ICP.
- Impending brain herniation: monitor for increase in blood pressure, decrease in pulse, and change in pupillary response.
- Patients not on paralyzing agents may change from decerebrate to decorticate posturing to a flaccid or rag doll appearance; this requires rapid intervention using mannitol or drainage of CSF. Monitor urine output closely.
- Diabetes insipidus requires fluid and electrolyte replacement and administration of vasopressin; monitor serum electrolytes for replacement.

- SIADH requires fluid restriction and serum electrolyte monitoring.

Evaluation

EXPECTED OUTCOMES

- Remains free of excessive airway secretions; airway is patent
- Attains normal respirations
- Demonstrates improved cerebral tissue perfusion
- Attains improved fluid balance
- Has no sign of infection
- Remains free of complications

For more information, see Chapter 57 in Smeltzer and Bare: *Brunner and Suddarth's Textbook of Medical-Surgical Nursing,* 9th edition. Philadelphia: Lippincott Williams & Wilkins, 2000.

INFLUENZA

Influenza is an acute viral disease that occurs in epidemic proportions every 2-3 years with a highly variable degree of severity. The virus is easily spread from host to host through droplet exposure. Previous infection with influenza does not guarantee protection from future exposure. Mortality rate is probably attributable to influenza and its accompanying pneumonia (viral or superimposed bacterial pneumonia) and other chronic cardiopulmonary sequelae. Transmission is most likely to occur in the first 3 days of illness.

Nursing and Medical Management

Goals of management are to relieve symptoms, treat complications, and prevent transmission to others. See Nursing and Medical Management under Pharyngitis and Pneumonia for additional information.

Prevention

Annual influenza vaccinations are recommended for those at high risk for complications of influenza: those over 65 years of age; residents of extended care facilities; those with chronic pulmonary or cardiovascular diseases, diabetes, immunosuppression, or renal dysfunction; children who require long-term aspirin therapy, which puts them at increased risk of developing Reye's syndrome; and health care personnel.

For more information, see Chapter 21 in Smeltzer and Bare: *Brunner and Suddarth's Textbook of Medical-Surgical Nursing,* 9th edition. Philadelphia: Lippincott Williams & Wilkins, 2000.

INTERSTITIAL CYSTITIS

Interstitial cystitis, sometimes called *urethral* or *painful bladder syndrome*, is chronic inflammation of the bladder wall that eventually causes disintegration of the lining and loss of bladder elasticity. It occurs most often in women aged 40 to 50 years but can affect people of any age, race, or sex. Its cause is unknown, but there is some suggestion of an inflammatory or autoimmune basis. Suggested causes include penetration of urinary irritants into the urothelium or suburothelial tissues due to a defect in the barrier between the urine and bladder wall mucosa. Interstitial cystitis may progress to contraction of the bladder with diminished bladder volume. It is a physical disorder with psychological consequences.

Clinical Manifestations

- Severe irritable voiding symptoms (urinary frequency, nocturia, urgency, suprapubic pressure, and pain with bladder filling) and markedly diminished bladder capacity occur. Some patients (60%) report painful intercourse.

• Urine contains both red and white blood cells even though it is sterile, and cytology is benign.

Diagnostic Evaluation
• Elimination of other causes
• Health history, symptoms, signs, cystoscopy, urodynamic studies, histology and laboratory test findings
• Micturition chart or diary of frequent voidings, biopsy, and radiographic studies such as radiographs, ultrasound, and computed tomography (CT) scans
• Presence of Hunner's ulcers (superficial erosions of the bladder wall; diagnostic)

Medical Management
• Tricyclic antidepressants (amitriptyline and doxepin) may decrease excitability of smooth muscle in the bladder.
• Bladder instillation of silver nitrate, dimethyl sulfoxide, or oxychlorosene (Clorpactin) or intravesical heparin (self-catheterization) may be effective.
• Antispasmodics, such as oxybutynin (Ditropan) and mucosal anesthetics (phenazopyridine [Pyridium]), may be useful.
• A bladder protectant (pentosan polysulfate sodium [Elmiron]) has been approved for use.
• Destruction of ulcers with laser photoirradiation and bladder removal and urinary diversion (severe cases) may be used.
• Transcutaneous electrical nerve stimulation (TENS) may relieve symptoms.

Nursing Management
Nursing Interventions
• Assess the effectiveness of the patient's ability to cope with the disorder.

- Convey to patient the belief that symptoms exist, and appreciate their severity and effects on lifestyle.
- Provide explanations about diagnostic tests and treatment regimens.
- Provide psychological support.

For more information, see Chapter 41 in Smeltzer and Bare: *Brunner and Suddarth's Textbook of Medical-Surgical Nursing,* 9th edition. Philadelphia: Lippincott Williams & Wilkins, 2000.

KAPOSI'S SARCOMA

Kaposi's sarcoma (KS) is the most common malignancy related to the human immunodeficiency virus (HIV) and involves the endothelial layer of blood and lymphatic vessels. It is subdivided into three categories: classic KS, African (endemic) KS, and KS associated with immunosuppressant therapy. Classic KS occurs predominantly in men between the ages of 40 and 70 years who are of Eastern European ancestry. This type of KS is chronic, relatively benign, and rarely fatal. The endemic form, found most often in young men and also in children in equatorial Africa, may infiltrate and progress to lymphadenopathic forms. Immunosuppressive therapy–associated KS occurs when patients are treated with immunosuppressive agents. The greater the immunosuppression, the higher the incidence of KS. Although the histopathologic features of all forms of KS are virtually identical, the clinical manifestations differ with AIDS-related KS, which exhibits a more variable and aggressive course, ranging from localized cutaneous lesions to disseminated disease involving multiple organ systems.

Clinical Manifestations
- Cutaneous lesions can occur anywhere on the body and are brownish pink to deep purple in color.
- AIDS-related KS has a more variable and aggressive disease course.

- KS is characteristically presented as lower-extremity skin lesions.
- AIDS-related KS lesions may be flat or raised and surrounded by ecchymosis and edema; they develop rapidly and cause extensive disfigurement.
- The location and size of the lesions can lead to venous stasis, lymphedema, and pain. Common sites of visceral involvement include the lymph nodes, gastrointestinal tract, and lungs.
- KS associated with immunosuppressive therapy, as in transplant recipients, is characterized by local skin lesions and disseminated visceral and mucocutaneous diseases.
- Internal organ involvement leads to organ failure, hemorrhage, infection, and death.

Diagnostic Evaluation

- Diagnosis is confirmed by biopsy of suspected lesions.
- Prognosis depends on extent of tumor, presence of constitutional symptoms, and the $CD4^+$ count.
- Death occurs from tumor progression, but more often from other complications of AIDS.

Medical Management

The treatment goal is reduction of symptoms by decreasing the size of the skin lesions, reducing discomfort associated with edema and ulcerations, and controlling symptoms associated with mucosal or visceral involvement.

- Localized treatment includes surgical excision of the lesions or application of liquid nitrogen to lesions and injection of intraoral lesions with dilute vinblastine.
- Chemotherapy regimen with ABV (doxorubicin [Adriamycin], bleomycin, and vincristine) has been effective; however, significant myelosuppression occurs in some patients.
- Radiation therapy is effective as a palliative measure to relieve localized pain from KS lesions that are in sites

such as the oral mucosa, conjunctiva, face, and soles of the feet.

- Patients with cutaneous KS treated with alpha-interferon have experienced tumor regression.
- Pain management may include nonsteroidal anti-inflammatory drugs (NSAIDs) and opioids.

Nursing Management

- Provide thorough and meticulous skin care involving regular turning, cleansing, and application of medicated ointments and dressings.
- Provide analgesics given at regular intervals around the clock. Teach patient relaxation and guided imagery, which may be helpful in reducing pain and anxiety.

K

🏠 Promoting Home and Community-Based Care

- Teach patients to self-administer alpha-interferon at home or arrange for patient to receive it in an outpatient setting.
- Support patient in coping with disfigurement of condition; stress that lesions are temporary, when applicable (after immunotherapy is discontinued).
- Provide supportive care and treatment as ordered to minimize pain and edema, address complications, and promote healing.

For more information, see Chapters 48 and 52 in Smeltzer and Bare: *Brunner and Suddarth's Textbook of Medical-Surgical Nursing,* 9th edition. Philadelphia: Lippincott Williams & Wilkins, 2000.

L

LEUKEMIA

The common feature of the leukemias is an unregulated proliferation or accumulation of white blood cells in the bone marrow, replacing normal marrow elements. There is also proliferation in the liver and spleen and invasion of nonhematologic organs, such as meninges, lymph nodes, gums, and skin. The leukemias are often classified as either lymphocytic or myelocytic and according to the stem cell line involved. Leukemia is also classified as acute (abrupt onset) or chronic (evolves over months to years). Its cause is unknown. There is some evidence that genetic influence and viral pathogenesis may be involved. Bone marrow damage from radiation exposure or chemicals (benzine) and alkylating agents can cause leukemia.

Nursing Management
Assessment
- Identify range of signs and symptoms reported by patient in nursing history and physical examination.
- Be alert for key symptoms of leukemia: weakness and fatigue, bleeding tendencies, petechiae and ecchymosis, pain, headache, vomiting, fever, and infection.
- Assess blood studies, and report alterations of white blood cells, hematocrit, platelets, electrolytes, absolute neutrophil count (ANC), hepatic function tests and creatinine findings, and culture results.

Major Nursing Diagnoses
- Risk for infection and bleeding

- Alterations in mucous membranes due to changes in epithelial lining of the gastrointestinal tract from chemotherapy or antimicrobial medications
- Pain and discomfort related to mucositis, leukocytic infiltration of systemic tissues, fever, and infection
- Altered nutrition: less than body requirements related to hypermetabolic state, anorexia, mucositis, pain, and nausea.
- Diarrhea due to altered gastrointestinal flora, mucosal denudation
- Fluid imbalance due to potential for bleeding and renal dysfunction
- Fatigue and activity intolerance related to anemia and infection
- Impaired skin integrity and alopecia related to toxic effects of chemotherapy
- Grieving related to anticipatory loss and altered role functioning
- Disturbance in body image related to change in appearance, function, and roles
- Self-care deficit due to fatigue and malaise
- Potential for diminished spiritual well-being
- Knowledge deficit about disease process, treatment, complication management, and self-care measures
- Anxiety due to knowledge deficit and uncertain future

Collaborative Problems/Potential Complications
- Infection
- Bleeding
- Renal dysfunction
- Tumor lysis syndrome
- Nutritional depletion
- Mucositis

Planning and Goals
The major goals of the patient may include self-care, activity tolerance, attainment or maintenance of comfort,

attainment or maintenance of adequate nutrition, promotion of positive body image, understanding of the disease process and its treatment, ability to cope with the diagnosis and prognosis, and absence of complications.

Nursing Interventions

PREVENTING BLEEDING
- Assess for thrombocytopenia, granulocytopenia, and anemia.
- Report any increase in petechiae, melena, hematuria, or nosebleeds.
- Avoid trauma and injections; use small-gauge needles when analgesics are administered parenterally, and apply pressure after injections to avoid bleeding.
- Use acetaminophen instead of aspirin for analgesia.
- Give prescribed hormonal therapy to prevent menses.
- Treat hemorrhage with bed rest and transfusions of red blood cells and platelets.

PREVENTING INFECTION
Infection is a major cause of death in leukemia patients.

- Assess temperature elevation, flushed appearance, chills, tachycardia and appearance of white patches in the mouth.
- Observe for redness, swelling, heat, or pain in eyes, ears, throat, skin, joints, abdomen, and rectal and perineal areas.
- Assess for cough and changes in character or color of sputum.
- Give frequent oral hygiene.
- Wear sterile gloves to start infusions.
- Provide daily intravenous site care; observe for signs of infection.
- Ensure normal elimination; avoid rectal thermometers, enemas, and rectal trauma; avoid vaginal tampons.
- Avoid catheterization unless essential. Practice scrupulous asepsis if catheterization necessary.

MANAGING MUCOSITIS
- Assess the oral mucosa thoroughly; identify and describe lesions; note color and moisture (remove dentures first).
- Assist patient with oral hygiene with soft-bristled toothbrush.
- Avoid lemon-glycerin swabs and commercial mouthwashes.
- Emphasize the importance of medications to prevent yeast infections.
- Instruct patient to cleanse the perirectal area after each bowel movement; monitor frequency of stools, and stop stool softener with loose stool.

EASING PAIN AND COMFORT
- Prevent undue pain in the abdomen, lymph node areas, bones, and joints with careful positioning of patient.
- Avoid sudden movements, and promote comfort with soft supports such as pillows; back and shoulder massage may provide comfort.
- Administer acetaminophen rather than aspirin for analgesia.
- Sponge patient with cool water for fever; avoid cold water or ice packs.
- Provide oral hygiene, and assist the patient with use of patient-controlled analgesia (PCA) for pain.
- Use creative strategies to permit uninterrupted sleep (a few hours).
- Provide active listening to patients enduring pain.

ATTAINING AND MAINTAINING ADEQUATE NUTRITION
- Supply good nutrition by careful timing of chemotherapeutic drug administration and prophylactic use of antiemetics.
- Give frequent oral hygiene to prevent oral lesions and promote appetite; with oral anesthetics, be cautious to prevent self-injury.
- Maintain nutrition with palatable, small, frequent feedings of soft nonirritating foods and fluids that are high in protein and vitamins.

L

- Maintain calorie counts and formal nutritional assessment; monitor daily body weights.
- Encourage intake of low-microbial diet. Administer total parenteral nutrition (TPN) as ordered.

MAINTAINING FLUID AND ELECTROLYTE BALANCE
- Measure intake and output accurately; weigh the patient daily.
- Assess for signs of fluid overload or dehydration
- Monitor laboratory tests (electrolytes, blood urea nitrogen [BUN], creatinine), and replace as ordered and indicated.

DECREASING FATIGUE AND DECONDITIONING
- Assist in choosing activity priorities; help patient balance activity and rest; suggest a stationary bicycle and sitting up in chair.
- Assist patient in using a high-efficiency particulate air (HEPA) filter mask to ambulate outside room.
- Assess for dyspnea, tachycardia, and other evidence of inadequate oxygen supply to vital organs.
- Arrange for physical therapy when indicated.

IMPROVING SELF-CARE
- Encourage the patient to do as much as possible.
- Listen empathetically to the patient.
- Assist patient to resume more self-care during recovery from treatment.

MANAGING ANXIETY AND GRIEF
- Provide emotional support, and discuss the impact of uncertain future.
- Assess patient's understanding of illness, treatment, and potential complications.
- Assist patient to identify the source of grief, and encourage patient to allow time to adjust to the major life changes rendered by the illness.
- Arrange to have communication with nurses across care settings to reassure patient that he or she has not been abandoned.

PROMOTING POSITIVE BODY IMAGE
- Prepare patient for the occurrence of alopecia, and help patient to express and resolve feelings.
- Help patient adjust to body image problems by encouraging involvement and support of family or support system.

ENCOURAGING SPIRITUAL WELL-BEING
- Assess the patient's spiritual and religious practices, and offer relevant services.
- Assist the patient to maintain realistic hope over the course of the illness (initially for a cure, in later stage for a quiet, dignified death).

 NURSING ALERT

The usual manifestations of infection are altered in patients with leukemia. Corticosteroid therapy may blunt the normal febrile and inflammatory responses to infection.

 Promoting Home and Community-Based Care

Teaching Patients Self-Care
- Ensure that patients and their families have a clear understanding of disease and complications (risk for infection and bleeding).
- Teach family members about home care while patient is still in the hospital, particularly vascular access device management if applicable.

Continuing Care
- Maintain communications between patient and nurses across care settings.
- Provide specific instructions regarding when and how to seek care from the physician.

Terminal Care
- Respect patient's choices about treatment, including measures to prolong life, when they no longer respond

to therapy. Provide for advance directives and living wills to give patient control during terminal phase.

- Support families and coordinate home care services to alleviate anxiety about managing patient's care in the home.
- Provide respite for caregivers and patient with hospice volunteers.
- Give patient and caregivers assistance to cope with changes in their roles and responsibilities, that is, anticipatory grieving.
- Provide information on hospital-based hospice programs for patients to receive palliative care in the hospital when care at home is no longer possible.

Evaluation

EXPECTED OUTCOMES
- Demonstrates absence of infection
- Demonstrates absence of bleeding
- Exhibits intact oral mucous membranes
- Attains optimal level of nutrition
- Reports less pain and discomfort
- Experiences less fatigue and increases activity
- Maintains fluid and electrolyte balance
- Participates in self-care
- Copes with anxiety and grief
- Experiences absence of complications

🍁 Gerontologic Considerations

Aging is accompanied by a gradual decline of physiologic processes, among which is a reduction in the immune function, resulting in increased susceptibility to infections.

Older patients often delay reporting symptoms because of lack of knowledge, financial resources, or support systems. The complications of leukemia can be devastating to the already decreased reserves of the elderly patient. Comprehensive nursing care is crucial in assisting the older patient to tolerate the side effects and treatment of the disease and to cope with the psychological and financial aspects.

For more information, see Chapter 30 in Smeltzer and Bare: *Brunner and Suddarth's Textbook of Medical-Surgical Nursing,* 9th edition. Philadelphia: Lippincott Williams & Wilkins, 2000.

LEUKEMIA, LYMPHOCYTIC, ACUTE

Acute lymphocytic leukemia (ALL) results from an uncontrolled proliferation of immature cells (lymphoblasts). It is most common in young children; boys are affected more frequently than girls, with a peak incidence at 4 years of age. After 15 years of age, ALL is uncommon. Therapy for this childhood leukemia has improved to the extent that about 80% of children survive at least 5 years.

Clinical Manifestations
Skeletal
- Immature lymphocytes proliferate in marrow and crowd development of normal cells.
- Normal hematopoiesis is inhibited, and leukopenia, anemia, and thrombocytopenia develop.
- Pain results from enlarged liver or spleen and bone, headache and vomiting are due to leukemic cell infiltration into other organs (more common with ALL than with other forms of leukemia).
- Erythrocyte and platelet counts are low.
- Leukocyte counts are low or high but always include immature cells.

Medical Management
The major form of treatment is chemotherapy with vinca alkaloids and glucocorticoids.

- Combinations of vincristine, prednisone, daunorubicin, and asparaginase are used for initial induction therapy.
- Combinations of medications are used for maintenance (maintenance doses of medications for up to 3 years).

- Irradiation of the cerebrospinal region and intrathecal injection of chemotherapeutic drugs help prevent central nervous system recurrence.

For more information, see Chapter 30 in Smeltzer and Bare: *Brunner and Suddarth's Textbook of Medical-Surgical Nursing,* 9th edition. Philadelphia: Lippincott Williams & Wilkins, 2000.

LEUKEMIA, LYMPHOCYTIC, CHRONIC

Chronic lymphocytic leukemia (CLL) is a common malignancy of older adults (two thirds of patients are older than 60 years of age). It derives from a malignant clone of B lymphocytes. There are more mature leukemia cells than immature cells, so it tends to be a mild disorder compared with the acute form. It is diagnosed during physical examination or treatment for another disease.

Clinical Manifestations
- Many cases are asymptomatic.
- CLL patients can develop *B symptoms*: fevers, sweats (especially night), unintentional weight loss, and infections are common.
- Anergy (decreased or absent reaction to skin sensitivity tests) reveals the defect in cellular immunity.
- Lymphadenopathy (enlargement of lymph nodes), which is sometimes severe and painful, and splenomegaly may be noted.
- Erythrocyte and platelet counts may be normal or decreased.
- Lymphocytosis is always present.

Medical Management
- In its early stages, CLL may require no treatment. When symptoms are severe, chemotherapy with steroids and chlorambucil (Leukeran) is often used. Agents may include cyclophosphamide, vincristine, and doxorubicin.

- Patients who do not respond to ordinary therapy may achieve remission by, for example, fludarabine monophosphate.
- Intravenous immunoglobulin may prevent recurrent bacterial infections in selected patients.

Nursing Management
See Nursing Management under Leukemia for additional information.

For more information, see Chapter 30 in Smeltzer and Bare: *Brunner and Suddarth's Textbook of Medical-Surgical Nursing,* 9th edition. Philadelphia: Lippincott Williams & Wilkins, 2000.

L

LEUKEMIA, MYELOID, ACUTE

Acute myeloid leukemia (AML) results from a defect in the hematopoietic stem cell that differentiates into all myeloid cells: monocytes, granulocytes (basophils, neutrophils, eosinophils), erythrocytes, and platelets. All age groups are affected; incidence rises with age and peaks at 60 years of age. It is the most common nonlymphocytic leukemia. Death usually occurs secondary to infection or hemorrhage.

Clinical Manifestations
- Most signs and symptoms evolve from insufficient production of normal blood cells: fever and infection result from neutropenia, weakness and fatigue are due to anemia, bleeding tendencies are a result of thrombocytopenia. Major hemorrhage occurs with platelet count of less than 10,000/mm^3.
- Proliferation of leukemic cells within organs leads to a variety of additional symptoms: pain from enlarged liver or spleen, lymphadenopathy, headache or vomiting secondary to meningeal leukemia, and bone pain from expansion of marrow.

- AML has its onset without warning; symptoms develop over 1 to 6 weeks or over months.
- Peripheral blood shows decreased erythrocyte and platelet counts.
- The leukocyte count is low, normal, or high; the percentage of normal cells is usually vastly decreased.

Diagnostic Evaluation
- Bone marrow specimen (excess of immature blast cells)
- Platelet count, complete blood count

Medical Management
- Objective is to achieve complete remission.
- Chemotherapy is the major form of therapy and in some instances results in remissions lasting a year or longer.

Chemotherapy
- Daunorubicin (Cerubidine), cytarabine (Cytosar-U)
- Mercaptopurine (Purinethol), mitoxantrone, or idarubicin
- Consolidation therapy (postremission therapy with chemotherapy agents)

Supportive Care
- Administration of blood products
- Prompt treatment of infections
- Granulocyte colony-stimulting factor (G-CSF: filgrastim) or granulocyte-macrophage colony-stimulating factor (GM-CSF: sargamastim) to decrease neutropenia

Bone Marrow Transplantation
- Used when a tissue match of a close relative can be obtained
- Transplantation follows destruction of leukemic marrow by chemotherapy

Nursing Management
See Nursing Management under Leukemia for additional information.

For more information, see Chapter 30 in Smeltzer and Bare: *Brunner and Suddarth's Textbook of Medical-Surgical Nursing,* 9th edition. Philadelphia: Lippincott Williams & Wilkins, 2000.

LEUKEMIA, MYELOGENOUS, CHRONIC

Chronic myelogenous leukemia (CML) arises from a mutation in the myeloid stem cells. More normal cells are present than in the acute form, however, and the disease is milder. A cytogenetic abnormality termed the *Philadelphia chromosome* is found in 90% to 95% of patients. Uncommon before 20 years of age, the incidence of CML rises with age (median age, 40 to 50 years).

CML has three stages: chronic, transformation, and accelerated or blast crisis. Marrow expands into cavities of the long bones, and cells are formed in the liver and spleen, with resultant painful enlargement problems. Infection and bleeding are rare until the disease transforms to the acute phase.

Clinical Manifestations

The clinical picture of CML is similar to that of acute myeloid leukemia, but signs and symptoms are less severe. Many patients are without symptoms for years.

- Onset is insidious; patients demonstrate malaise, anorexia, weight loss.
- Leukocytosis is always present, sometimes at extraordinary levels. Patient may be short of breath or slightly confused from leukostasis.
- Splenomegaly with tenderness and hepatomegaly are common.
- In the transforming phase, bone pain, fever, weight loss, anemia, and thrombocytopenia are noted.

Medical Management

- Therapies of choice are busulfan (Myleran) and hydroxyurea, or chlorambucil (Leukeran) alone or with steroids. An anthracycline chemotherapeutic agent (eg, daunomycin) may be used.

- Bone marrow transplantation increases survival significantly and best if done in chronic phase.
- Other drug choices are alpha-interferon, fludarabine (Fludara), and cytosine, or oral chemotherapy (hydroxyurea or busulfan) in the chronic phase.
- Leukapheresis may be needed if the white blood cell count exceeds 300,000/mm^3.
- In the transformation phase, treatment is chemotherapy used in ALL.

Nursing Management

Nursing management is similar to that for chronic lymphocytic leukemia. See Nursing Management under Leukemia for additional information.

For more information, see Chapter 30 in Smeltzer and Bare: *Brunner and Suddarth's Textbook of Medical-Surgical Nursing,* 9th edition. Philadelphia: Lippincott Williams & Wilkins, 2000.

LUNG ABSCESS

A lung abscess is a localized necrotic lesion of the lung parenchyma containing purulent materials; the lesion collapses and forms a cavity. Most lung abscesses occur because of aspiration of nasopharyngeal or oral anaerobes into the lung.

Abscesses may also occur secondary to mechanical or functional obstruction of the bronchi. At-risk patients include those with impaired cough reflexes, loss of glottal closures, or swallowing difficulties, which may cause aspiration of foreign material. Other at-risk patients include those with central nervous system disorders (seizure, stroke, altered mental status, drug or alcohol addiction), esophageal disease, and those fed by nasogastric tube.

The site of lung abscess is related to gravity and is determined by the patient's position. For patients in recumbent position, the posterior segment of the upper right lobe is the most common site. The organisms most frequently associated with lung abscess are *Klebsiella* species and *Staphylococcus aureus.*

Clinical Manifestations
- The clinical features vary from a mild productive cough to acute illness.
- Fever is accompanied by a productive cough of moderate to copious amounts of foul-smelling sputum, often bloody.
- Pleurisy, or dull chest pain, dyspnea, weakness, anorexia, and weight loss are common.
- Dullness on percussion and decreased or absent breath sounds are found, with an intermittent pleural friction rub and possibly crackles on auscultation.

Diagnostic Evaluation
Chest radiograph, sputum culture, and fiberoptic bronchoscopy. A computed tomography (CT) scan of the chest may be required.

Medical Management
Prevention
To reduce the risk for lung abscess: give appropriate antibiotic therapy before dental procedures and maintain adequate dental and oral hygiene. Give appropriate antimicrobial therapy for pneumonia.

Treatment
Findings of the history, physical examination, chest radiograph, and sputum culture indicate type of organism and treatment.

- Coughing, postural drainage (chest physiotherapy), and possibly percutaneous catheter placement or,

infrequently, bronchoscopy for abscess drainage
are used.

- Intravenous antimicrobial therapy: clindamycin (Cleocin)
  is the medication of choice, followed by penicillin with
  metronidazole (Flagyl); ceftazidime plus aminoglycoside,
  or cefoperazone is used to treat *Pseudomonas aeruginosa*
  infection; *S. aureus* infection is treated with oxacillin, naf-
  cillin, or a first-generation cephalosporin (cefuroxime).
  Large intravenous doses are required because the antibiotic must penetrate necrotic tissue and abscess fluid.
- The patient is advised to eat a high-protein, high-calorie
  diet.
- Antibiotics are administered orally instead of intravenously after signs of improvement: normal temperature,
  lowering of white blood cell count, and improvement seen
  on chest radiograph (reduction in size of cavity).
- Antibiotic therapy may last 6 to 16 weeks.
- Surgical intervention is rare. Pulmonary resection
  (lobectomy) is performed when there is massive
  hemoptysis or no response to medical management.

Nursing Management
Nursing Interventions

- Administer antibiotic and intravenous therapy as
  prescribed, and monitor for any adverse effects.
- Initiate chest physiotherapy as prescribed to drain
  abscess.
- Teach patient deep breathing and coughing exercises.
- Encourage diet high in protein and calories.
- Provide emotional support; abscess may take a long time
  to resolve.

Promoting Home and Community-Based Care

Teaching Patients Self-Care

- Teach patient or caregiver how to change dressings to
  prevent skin excoriation and offensive odor.

- Perform deep breathing and coughing exercises every 2 hours during the day.
- Teach postural drainage and percussion techniques to caregiver.
- Provide counseling for attaining and maintaining an optimal state of nutrition.
- Emphasize importance of completing antibiotic regimen, rest, and appropriate activity levels to prevent relapse.
- Arrange home visits by an intravenous therapy nurse to administer intravenous antibiotic therapy.

For more information, see Chapter 21 in Smeltzer and Bare: *Brunner and Suddarth's Textbook of Medical-Surgical Nursing,* 9th edition. Philadelphia: Lippincott Williams & Wilkins, 2000.

L

LYMPHEDEMA AND ELEPHANTIASIS

Lymphedemas are classified as primary (congenital malformations) or secondary (acquired obstruction). A swelling of tissues in the extremities occurs because of an increased quantity of lymph that results from an obstruction of the lymphatic vessels. It is especially marked when the extremity is in a dependent position. The most common type is congenital lymphedema (lymphedema praecox), caused by hypoplasia of the lymphatic system of the lower extremity. It is usually seen in women and appears first between the ages of 15 and 25 years. The obstruction may be in both the lymph nodes and the lymphatic vessels. At times, it is seen in the arm after a radical mastectomy and in the leg in association with varicose veins or a chronic thrombophlebitis (from lymphangitis). Lymphatic obstruction caused by a parasite (filaria) is seen frequently in the tropics. When chronic swelling is present, there may be frequent bouts of infection (high fever and chills) and increased residual edema after inflammation has resolved. These lead to chronic fibrosis, thickening of the subcutaneous tissues, and hypertrophy of the skin. This condition, in which chronic swelling of the extremity recedes only slightly with elevation, is referred to as *elephantiasis*.

Medical Management

The goals of medical therapy are to reduce and control the edema and prevent infection.

Rest, Activity, and Comfort

- Strict bed rest with leg elevation to aid in mobilizing fluids
- Active and passive exercises to assist in movement of lymphatic fluid into the bloodstream
- External compression devices
- Custom-fitted elastic stockings, when patient is ambulatory

Pharmacologic Treatment

- Furosemide (Lasix) initially to prevent fluid overload
- Diuretics, palliatively for lymphedema
- Antibiotic therapy, if lymphangitis or cellulitis is present

Surgical Treatment

- Surgery (excision of affected tissue and fascia with skin grafting, relocation of lymphatic vessels) is performed if edema is severe and uncontrolled by medical therapy, or if infection is present.
- Surgery is also performed if mobility is severely compromised.

Nursing Management

Nursing Interventions

- Teach the patient to inspect the skin for evidence of infection.

- Instruct the patient to elevate extremities.
- Teach passive and active exercises.

POSTOPERATIVE
- Provide standard care of skin grafts and flaps.
- Instruct patient to take antibiotics as prescribed (the total 5 to 7 days).
- Elevate affected extremity, and observe for complications constantly (eg, flap necrosis, hematoma or abscess under the flap, cellulitis).

For more information, see Chapter 28 in Smeltzer and Bare: *Brunner and Suddarth's Textbook of Medical-Surgical Nursing,* 9th edition. Philadelphia: Lippincott Williams & Wilkins, 2000.

L

M

MALIGNANT MELANOMA

A malignant melanoma is a malignant neoplasm in which atypical melanocytes (pigment cells) are present in both the epidermis and the dermis (and sometimes the subcutaneous cells). It is the most lethal of all skin cancers. It can occur in one of several forms: superficial spreading melanoma, lentigo-maligna melanoma, nodular melanoma, and acral-lentiginous melanoma. Most melanomas derive from cutaneous epidermal melanocytes; some appear in preexisting nevi (moles) in the skin or develop in the uveal tract of the eye. Melanomas frequently appear simultaneously with cancer of other organs. The incidence and mortality rate of malignant melanoma are increasing, probably related to increased recreational sun exposure. Its prognosis is related to the depth of dermal invasion and the thickness of lesion. Malignant melanoma can spread through both the bloodstream and lymphatic system and can metastasize to the bones, liver, lungs, spleen, central nervous system, and lymph nodes.

Causes and Risk Factors

The etiology of malignant melanoma is unknown; ultraviolet rays are strongly suspected. Risk factors include the following:

- Fair complexion, blue eyes, red or blond hair, and freckles
- Celtic or Scandinavian origin.
- Tendency to burn and not tan
- Older age; residence in the southwestern United States

- Family history of melanoma, presence of giant congenital nevi, or significant history of severe sunburn
- Dysplastic nevus syndrome

Clinical Manifestations
Superficial Spreading Melanoma
- Most common form, usually affects middle-aged people, occurs most frequently on trunk and lower extremities
- Circular lesions with irregular outer portions
- Margins of lesion flat or elevated and palpable
- May appear in combination of colors, with hues of tan, brown, and black mixed with gray, bluish-black, or white; sometimes, a dull, pink-rose color noted in a small area within the lesion

Nodular Melanoma

M

- Second most common type, spherical, blueberry-like nodule with relatively smooth surface and uniform blue-black color
- May have other shadings of red, gray, or purple
- May appear as irregularly shaped plaques
- May be described as a blood blister that fails to resolve
- Invades directly into adjacent dermis (vertical growth); poor prognosis

Lentigo-Maligna Melanoma
- Slowly evolving pigmented lesion
- Occurs on exposed skin areas; head and neck in elderly people
- First appears as tan, flat lesions; in time, undergo changes in size and color

Acral-Lentiginous Melanoma
- Occurs in areas not excessively exposed to sunlight
- Found on the palms of the hands, soles, in nail beds, and mucous membranes in dark-skinned people
- Appear as irregular pigmented macules that develop nodules
- Become invasive early

Diagnostic Evaluation
- Excisional biopsy specimen
- Chest radiograph, complete blood count, liver function tests, radionuclide or computed tomography (CT) scans ordered for staging once melanoma is confirmed

Medical Management
- The therapeutic approach to malignant melanoma depends on the level of invasion and the depth of the lesion. Chemotherapy may be used.
- Immunotherapy (interferon, monoclonal antibodies) may be used.
- Laboratory assay of tyrosinase is under investigation for treatment.

Surgery
- Surgical excision is the treatment of choice for small superficial lesions.
- Deeper lesions require wide local excision and skin graft.
- A regional lymph node dissection may be performed to rule out metastasis.
- Debulking the tumor or other palliative care may be done.

Nursing Management
Assessment
Assessment is based on history and symptoms.
- Question specifically about pruritus, tenderness, and pain, which are not features of a benign nevus.
- Question about changes in preexisting moles or development of new pigmented lesions.
- Assess people at risk carefully.

ASSESS SKIN
- Use a magnifying lens to examine for irregularity and changes in the mole.
- Signs that suggest malignant changes include variegated color, irregular border, asymmetry (irregular surface) and large diameter.

- Pay attention to common sites of melanoma occurrence.
- Measure diameter of mole; melanomas are often larger than 6 mm.

Major Nursing Diagnoses
- Pain related to surgical incision and grafting.
- Anxiety and depression related to possible life-threatening consequences of melanoma and disfigurement.
- Knowledge deficit about early signs of melanoma.

Collaborative Problems/Potential Complications
- Metastasis
- Infection of the surgical site

Planning and Goals
The major goals of the patient may include relief of pain and discomfort, reduction of anxiety, knowledge of early signs of melanoma, and absence of complications.

Nursing Interventions
RELIEVING PAIN AND DISCOMFORT
- Anticipate need for and administer appropriate analgesic.

REDUCING ANXIETY
- Give support, and allow patient to express feelings.
- Convey understanding of anger and depression.
- Answer questions, and clarify information during the diagnostic workup and staging of the tumor.
- Point out patient resources, past effective coping mechanisms, and support systems to help the patient cope with diagnosis and treatment.
- Include immediate family in all discussions to clarify information and provide emotional support.

MONITORING AND MANAGING POTENTIAL
COMPLICATIONS: METASTASIS
- Educate patient about treatment:
  ○ Present treatment is largely unsuccessful, and cure is generally not possible.

M

○ Surgical intervention may be performed to debulk the tumor or to remove part of the organ involved.
○ More extensive surgery is for relief of symptoms, not for cure.
○ Chemotherapy may be effective in controlling the metastasis.
• Provide time for patient to express fears and concerns about the future; arrange for hospice and palliative care services.
• Encourage patient to have hope in the therapy while being realistic.
• Offer information about support groups and contact people.

🏠 Promoting Home and Community-Based Care

Teaching Patients Self-Care
• Teach patient to recognize the early signs of melanoma.
• Instruct patient to examine the skin and scalp monthly in an orderly manner.
  ○ Use a full-length mirror and a small hand mirror to aid in examination.
  ○ Learn where moles and birthmarks are located.
  ○ Inspect moles and other pigmented lesions; immediately report to physician or clinic moles that change colors, enlarge, become raised or thicker, itch, or bleed.
• Inform person who has had a malignant melanoma to have lifelong follow-up; these people are at higher risk of developing a second one.
• Avoid exposure to sunlight.
• Arrange palliative and hospice care.

Evaluation
EXPECTED OUTCOMES
• Experiences relief of pain and discomfort
• Achieves reduction of anxiety

- Demonstrates understanding of disease
- Experiences absence of metastasis

For more information, see Chapter 52 in Smeltzer and Bare: *Brunner and Suddarth's Textbook of Medical-Surgical Nursing*, 9th edition. Philadelphia: Lippincott Williams & Wilkins, 2000.

MASTOIDITIS

Mastoiditis is an inflammation of the mastoid resulting from an infection of the middle ear (otitis media). Since the discovery of antibiotics, acute mastoiditis is rare. Chronic otitis media may cause chronic mastoiditis. If it is untreated, osteomyelitis may occur.

M

Clinical Manifestations
- Pain and tenderness behind the ear (postauricular)
- Discharge from the middle ear (otorrhea)
- Mastoid area that becomes erythematous and edematous
- Otoscopic evaluation of the tympanic membrane revealing cholesteatoma (an in-growth of the skin of the external layer of the eardrum into the middle ear)

Medical Management
- General symptoms are usually successfully treated with antibiotics; occasionally, myringotomy is required.
- If recurrent or persistent tenderness, fever, headache, and discharge from the ear, mastoidectomy may be necessary to remove the cholesteatoma and gain access to diseased structures.

Nursing Management: The Patient Undergoing Mastoid Surgery
Assessment
- During the health history, collect data about the ear problem, including hearing loss and vertigo, duration

and intensity, causation, prior treatments, health problems, current medications, family history, and drug allergies.
- During the physical assessment, observe for erythema, edema, otorrhea, lesions, and odor of discharge.
- Review results of audiogram.

Major Nursing Diagnoses
- Pain related to mastoid surgery
- Risk for infection related to mastoidectomy, placement of grafts, prostheses, or electrodes; surgical trauma to surrounding tissues and structures
- Anxiety related to surgical procedure, potential loss of hearing, potential taste disturbance, and potential loss of facial movement
- Auditory sensory perception alterations related to ear disorder, surgery, or packing
- Risk for trauma related to balance difficulties or vertigo
- Knowledge deficit about mastoid disease, surgical procedure, and postoperative care and expectations

Planning and Goals
The major goals for mastoidectomy include reduction of anxiety; freedom from discomfort; prevention of infection; stable or improved hearing and communication; absence of injury or vertigo; absence of, or adjustment to, altered sensory perceptual alterations; return of skin integrity; and increased knowledge regarding disease, surgical procedure, and postoperative care.

Nursing Interventions
REDUCING ANXIETY
- Reinforce information the otologic surgeon has discussed.
- Encourage patient to discuss any anxiety or concerns.

RELIEVING PAIN
- Give prescribed analgesic for the first 24 hours postoperatively and then only as needed.

- Instruct patient in use of and side effects of medication.
- If a tympanoplasty is also performed, inform patient that he or she may have packing or a wick in the external auditory canal and may experience sharp shooting pains in the ear for 2 to 3 weeks postoperatively.

PREVENTING INFECTION
- Give prescribed prophylactic antibiotics; instruct to prevent water from entering the ear for 6 weeks.
- Keep postauricular incision dry for 2 days.
- Observe for and report signs of infection, inform patient that some serous drainage is normal postoperatively.

IMPROVING HEARING AND COMMUNICATION
- Initiate measures to improve hearing and communication: reduce environmental noise, face patient when speaking, and speak clearly and distinctly without shouting, providing good lighting if patient must speech read and using nonverbal clues.
- Instruct family members that patient will have temporarily reduced hearing from surgery as a result of edema, packing, and fluid in middle ear; instruct family in effective ways to improve communication with patient.

INCREASING KNOWLEDGE
- Inform the patient about the surgery and operating room environment.
- Discuss postoperative expectations to decrease anxiety about the unknown.
- Provide postoperative instructions for mastoid surgery as appropriate for particular otologic surgeon's preferences.

🏠 Promoting Home and Community-Based Care
Teaching Patients Self-Care
- Provide patient with instruction about prescribed medications: analgesics, antivertiginous agents, and antihistamines for balance disturbance.

- Inform patient about the expected effects and potential side effects of the medication.
- Instruct patient about any activity restrictions.
- Teach patient to monitor for possible complications, such as infection, facial nerve weakness, or taste disturbances, including the signs and symptoms to report immediately.

Continuing Care

- Refer patients, particularly elderly patients, for home care nursing.
- Caution the caregiver and patient that the patient may experience some vertigo and will therefore require help with ambulation to avoid falling.
- Instruct patient that any symptoms of complications are to be promptly reported to the surgeon.
- Stress the importance of scheduling and keeping follow-up appointments.

Evaluation

EXPECTED OUTCOMES
- Demonstrates reduced anxiety about surgical procedure
- Remains free of discomfort or pain
- Demonstrates no signs or symptoms of infection
- Exhibits signs that hearing has stabilized or improved
- Remains free of injury and trauma secondary to vertigo
- Experiences adjustment to or remains free of altered sensory perception
- Demonstrates no skin breakdown
- Demonstrates understanding (as confirmed by conversation) about the reasons for and methods of care and treatment

---

For more information, see Chapter 55 in Smeltzer and Bare: *Brunner and Suddarth's Textbook of Medical-Surgical Nursing*, 9th edition. Philadelphia: Lippincott Williams & Wilkins, 2000.

MÉNIÈRE'S DISEASE

Ménière's disease is an inner ear fluid balance problem (too much circulatory fluid) caused by malabsorption in the endolymphatic sac or blockage in the duct. Its cause is unknown. Some attribute the impairment of the microvasculature of the inner ear to abnormally high levels of metabolites (glucose, insulin, triglycerides, and cholesterol) in the blood. Ménière's disease is more common in adults, with the average age of onset in the fourth decade of life. There is no cure for this disease. There are two possible subsets of the disease: cochlear and vestibular.

Clinical Manifestations
- Cochlear Ménière's disease presents with four major symptoms: (1) episodic incapacitating vertigo (lasting minutes to hours, with nausea and vomiting), (2) tinnitus or a roaring sound, (3) fluctuating progressive sensorineural hearing loss, and (4) feeling of pressure or fullness in the ear.
- At the onset, only one or two symptoms are manifested.
- Attacks occur with increasing frequency.
- Diaphoresis and a persistent feeling of disequilibrium may last for days.
- Usually only one ear is involved.
- Vestibular Ménière's disease reveals episodic vertigo associated with aural pressure with no cochlear symptoms; eventually, all symptoms are noted.

Diagnostic Evaluation
- Disease is not diagnosed until the four major symptoms are present; careful history of vertigo and nausea and vomiting contributes to diagnosis.
- There is no absolute diagnostic test for this disease.
- Audiovestibular diagnostic procedures, including Weber's test, are used.
- Other laboratory and radiographic tests are performed to rule out other causes for symptoms.

M

Medical Management

The goals of treatment may include recommendations for changes in lifestyle and habits or surgical treatment. The treatment is designed to eliminate vertigo or to stop the progression of or stabilize the disease.

- Treatment approaches include rehabilitative, dietary, medical, and surgical treatment.
- Psychological evaluation may be indicated if patient is anxious, uncertain, fearful, or depressed.

Pharmacologic Treatment

- Tranquilizers and antihistamines to suppress the vestibular system; antiemetics for nausea and vomiting
- Diuretics to lower pressure in the endolymphatic system; vasodilators
- Middle and inner ear perfusion or systemic injections of ototoxic medications: streptomycin, gentamicin to eliminate vertigo; procedure accompanied by a significant risk for hearing loss

Dietary Management

- Low sodium (2000 mg/day)
- Avoidance of alcohol, nicotine, and caffeine

Surgical Management

- Endolymphatic sac decompression or shunt
- Labyrinthectomy (destruction of the inner ear)
- Vestibular nerve section (eighth cranial nerve)

Nursing Management: The Patient With Vertigo
Assessment

- Obtain a history of symptoms, causative factors, and alleviating factors.
- Determine extent of disability related to activities of daily living as well as emotional response to symptoms.
- Elicit medications being taken, including over-the-counter drugs.

Major Nursing Diagnoses
- Risk for injury related to altered mobility because of gait disturbance and vertigo
- Impaired adjustment related to disability requiring change in lifestyle because of unpredictability of vertigo
- Risk for fluid volume imbalance and deficit related to increased fluid output, altered intake, and medications
- Anxiety related to threat of, or change in, health status and disability effects of vertigo
- Ineffective individual coping related to personal vulnerability and unmet expectations stemming from vertigo
- Self-care deficit: feeding, bathing/hygiene, dressing/grooming, and toileting related to labyrinth dysfunction and episodes of vertigo

Planning and Goals
Patient goals include remaining free of injuries associated with imbalance or falls; adjusting to or modifying lifestyle to decrease disability and exert maximum control and independence; maintaining a normal fluid and electrolyte balance; experiencing less or no anxiety; maintaining ability to care for self; and maintaining freedom from complications.

Nursing Interventions
PREVENTING INJURY
- Assess for vertigo.
- Assist patient in identifying aura that suggests an impending attack.
- Encourage patient to sit down when dizzy.
- Recommend that patient keep eyes open and stare straight ahead when lying down and experiencing vertigo; place pillows on side of head to restrict movement.
- Reinforce vestibular and balance therapy as prescribed.
- Administer and teach administration of antivertiginous medication and vestibular sedation; instruct in side effects.

ADJUSTING TO DISABILITY

- Encourage patient to identify personal strengths and roles that can be fulfilled.
- Provide information about vertigo and what to expect.
- Include family and significant others in rehabilitative process.
- Encourage patient in making decisions and assuming more responsibility for care.

MAINTAINING FLUID VOLUME

- Assess intake and output; monitor laboratory values.
- Assess indicators of dehydration.
- Encourage oral fluids as tolerated; avoid caffeine (a vestibular stimulant).
- Teach administration of antiemetics and antidiarrheal medications.

RELIEVING ANXIETY

- Assess level of anxiety; help identify successful coping skills.
- Encourage patient to discuss anxieties and explore concerns about vertigo attacks.
- Teach stress management; provide comfort measures.

MONITORING AND MANAGING COMPLICATIONS

- Assist patient in preparing for diagnostic tests.
- Prepare patient for surgery if indicated.
- Observe for potential complications.
- Assist unsteady patient as required; expect vertigo and nausea after labyrinthectomy.
- Arrange for psychosocial and family support as necessary.
- Provide patient and family with the appropriate hearing aid service information.

🏠 Promoting Home and Community-Based Care

Teaching Patients Self-Care

- Teach patient to administer antiemetic and other prescribed medications to relieve nausea and vomiting.

- Encourage patient to care for bodily needs when free of vertigo.
- Review diet with patient and caregivers; offer fluids as necessary.

For more information, see Chapter 55 in Smeltzer and Bare: *Brunner and Suddarth's Textbook of Medical-Surgical Nursing*, 9th edition. Philadelphia: Lippincott Williams & Wilkins, 2000.

MENINGITIS

Meningitis is an inflammation of the meninges (membranes surrounding the brain and spinal cord) and is caused by a viral, bacterial, or fungal organism. Types of meningitis include aseptic, septic, and tuberculous. Aseptic refers to viral meningitis or meningeal irritation, such as encephalitis. Septic refers to a bacterial cause, such as influenza bacillus. Tuberculosis meningitis is caused by the tubercle bacillus. Meningeal infections generally originate in one of two ways: either through the bloodstream from other infections (cellulitis) or by direct extension (after a traumatic injury to the facial bones). In a small number of cases, the cause is iatrogenic or secondary to invasive procedures (lumbar puncture) or devices (intracranial pressure [ICP] monitoring devices) or to opportunistic infections, such as acquired immunodeficiency syndrome (AIDS) or Lyme disease.

Bacterial meningitis is the most significant form. The common bacteria are *Neisseria meningitidis* (meningococcal meningitis), *Streptococcus pneumoniae* (in adults), and *Haemophilus influenzae* (in children and young adults). These three organisms account for about 75% of the cases. Mode of transmission is direct contact, including droplets and discharges from nose and throat of carriers or infected people. Bacterial meningitis starts as an infection of the oropharynx and is followed by septicemia, which extends to the meninges of the brain and upper region of the spinal cord.

Clinical Manifestations

Bacterial Meningitis

- Symptoms result from infection and increased ICP.
- Headache and fever are frequently initial symptoms.
- Changes in level of consciousness are associated with bacterial type.
- Disorientation and memory impairment are common early in the illness.
- Lethargy, unresponsiveness, and coma may develop as illness progresses.
- Signs of meningeal irritation include the following:
  - Early sign: nuchal rigidity (stiff neck)
  - Positive Kernig's sign: when lying with thigh flexed on abdomen, cannot completely extend leg
  - Positive Brudzinski's sign: when neck is flexed, flexion of the knees and hips is produced; when passive flexion of lower extremity of one side is made, similar movement is seen for opposite extremity
  - Photophobia
- Seizures and increased ICP
  - Seizures secondary to focal areas of cortical irritability
  - Signs of increasing ICP: widened pulse pressure and bradycardia, respiratory irregularity, headache, vomiting, and depressed levels of consciousness
- Rash (*Neisseria meningitidis*): ranges from petechial rash with purpuric lesions to large areas of ecchymosis

Meningococcal Meningitis

Ten percent of patients present with a fulminating infection, with signs of overwhelming septicemia.

- Abrupt onset of high fever
- Extensive purpuric lesions (over face and extremities)
- Shock and signs of disseminated intravascular coagulopathy (DIC)
- Death possible within a few hours of onset of infection
- In AIDS patients: few if any symptoms because of blunted inflammatory response occurring in the immunocompromised patient

Diagnostic Evaluation

Infecting organisms are usually identified through culture of cerebrospinal fluid and blood.

Medical Management

- Antimicrobial therapy: penicillin, ampicillin, or chloramphenicol, or cephalosporins. Cryptococcal meningitis treatment is intravenous administration of amphotericin B; may be used with or without 5-flucytosine.
- Dehydration and shock are treated with fluid volume expanders.
- Seizures are controlled with diazepam or phenytoin.
- Cerebral edema is treated with an osmotic diuretic (mannitol).

Prevention

- People who have close contact with patient should be considered candidates for antimicrobial prophylaxis (Rifampin).
- Close contacts should be observed and examined immediately if fever or other signs and symptoms of meningitis develop.
- Group C meningococcal vaccination may be of benefit for some travelers visiting countries that are experiencing epidemic meningococcal disease.
- Vaccination should be considered as an adjunct to antibiotic chemoprophylaxis for anyone living with a patient who has meningococcal disease.
- Polysaccharide vaccine (hemophilia B polysaccharide vaccine) against invasive *Haemophilus influenzae* type B infection is used routinely in children for prevention of meningitis.

Nursing Management

Prognosis depends on supportive care given.

Nursing Interventions

- Monitor vital signs constantly, determine arterial blood gases, insert cuffed endotracheal tube (or tracheostomy), and place on mechanical ventilation as prescribed.

- Give oxygen to maintain arterial partial pressure of oxygen (pO_2).
- Monitor central venous pressure (CVP) for incipient shock, which precedes cardiac or respiratory failure.
- Note generalized vasoconstriction, circumoral cyanosis, and cold extremities.
- Reduce high fever to decrease load on heart and brain oxygen demands.
- Rapid intravenous fluid replacement may be prescribed, but take care not to overhydrate patient because of risk of cerebral edema.
- If syndrome of inappropriate antidiuretic hormone (SIADH) secretion is suspected, monitor closely for body weight, serum electrolytes, urine volume, specific gravity, and osmolality.
- Assess continuously for clinical status; evaluate skin and oral hygiene; promote comfort, and protect during seizures and while comatose.
- Advise respiratory isolation for 24 hours after start of antibiotic therapy.

For more information, see Chapter 59 in Smeltzer and Bare: *Brunner and Suddarth's Textbook of Medical-Surgical Nursing*, 9th edition. Philadelphia: Lippincott Williams & Wilkins, 2000.

MITRAL REGURGITATION (INSUFFICIENCY)

Mitral regurgitation results when the margins of the mitral valve are unable to close during systole. There is a problem with one or more of the leaflets, the annulus, or the papillary muscles, preventing closure of the leaflets. At each beat, the left ventricle forces some blood back into the left atrium, causing dilation and hypertrophy. This backward flow of blood from the ventricle eventually causes the lungs to become congested, which adds strain to the right ventricle, resulting in heart failure.

Clinical Manifestations

- Chronic mitral regurgitation is often asymptomatic; acute regurgitation usually presents as heart failure.
- Symptoms include dyspnea on exertion, fatigue, weakness, palpitation of the heart, and cough due to chronic passive pulmonary congestion.
- Irregular pulse as a result of either extra systoles or atrial fibrillation may persist indefinitely.

Medical Management

Management is the same as that for congestive heart failure. Surgical intervention consists of mitral valve replacement or valvuloplasty.

For more information, see Chapter 26 in Smeltzer and Bare: *Brunner and Suddarth's Textbook of Medical-Surgical Nursing*, 9th edition. Philadelphia: Lippincott Williams & Wilkins, 2000.

M

MITRAL STENOSIS

Mitral stenosis is the progressive thickening and contracture of the mitral valve cusps, which causes narrowing of the orifice and progressive obstruction to blood flow. Normally, the mitral valve opening is as wide as three fingers. In cases of marked stenosis, the opening narrows to the width of a lead pencil.

Clinical Manifestations

- Progressive fatigue (result of low cardiac output), hemoptysis and dyspnea (due to pulmonary venous hypertension), cough, and repeated respiratory infections
- Weak and often irregular pulse (because of atrial fibrillation)

Diagnostic Evaluation

- Electrocardiography (ECG)
- Echocardiography
- Cardiac catheterization with angiography

Medical and Nursing Management

See Medical Management and Nursing Management under Cardiac Failure for additional information.

- Antibiotic therapy to prevent recurrence of infections
- Cardiotonics and diuretics for treatment of congestive heart failure
- Surgical intervention (valvuloplasty, commissurotomy, or replacement of the mitral valve)
- Percutaneous transluminal valvuloplasty, for palliation of symptoms

---

For more information, see Chapter 26 in Smeltzer and Bare: *Brunner and Suddarth's Textbook of Medical-Surgical Nursing*, 9th edition. Philadelphia: Lippincott Williams & Wilkins, 2000.

MITRAL VALVE PROLAPSE

Mitral valve prolapse is a dysfunction of the mitral valve leaflets that prevents the mitral valve from closing completely and results in valvular regurgitation. It occurs more frequently in women. Blood regurgitates from the left ventricle back into the left atrium.

Clinical Manifestations

- The syndrome may produce no symptoms or may progress rapidly and result in sudden death.
- Patients may experience symptoms of fatigue, shortness of breath, lightheadedness, dizziness, syncope, palpitations, chest pain, and anxiety.
- During the physical examination, a mitral click is identified. Presence of a click indicates early valvular incompetence.
- The mitral click may deteriorate into a murmur over time as the valve leaflets become more dysfunctional.
- As the murmur progresses, there may be signs and symptoms of heart failure.

Medical Management
Medical management is directed at controlling symptoms.
- Antidysrhythmic agents are prescribed.
- In advanced stages, mitral valve replacement may be necessary.

Nursing Management
- Teach the patient to read product labels to avoid caffeine and alcohol (eg, in cough medicine).
- Explain that alcohol, ephedrine, and epinephrine, which may be in over-the-counter preparations, may stimulate dysrhythmias.
- Educate patient about the need for prophylactic antibiotic therapy before undergoing invasive procedures (eg, dental work, genitourinary procedures, or gastrointestinal procedures).
- Advise patient to consult physician if in doubt about need for antibiotics before a procedure.

For more information, see Chapter 26 in Smeltzer and Bare: *Brunner and Suddarth's Textbook of Medical-Surgical Nursing*, 9th edition. Philadelphia: Lippincott Williams & Wilkins, 2000.

MULTIPLE MYELOMA

Multiple myeloma is a malignant disease of plasma cells that infiltrates bone, lymph nodes, liver, spleen, and kidneys. It is not classified as a lymphoma. The malignant cell is the plasma cell, the neoplastic proliferation taking place mainly in the bone marrow. Median survival is 3 to 5 years, with death resulting from infection or renal failure.

Clinical Manifestations
- Normochromic, normocytic anemia, back pain, and sometimes leukopenia or thrombocytopenia due to bone marrow infiltration by malignant plasma cells

- Constant bone pain that may be incapacitating
- Hypercalcemia and bone fractures common, especially in the vertebrae or ribs

Diagnostic Evaluation
- Aspiration or biopsy of the bone marrow
- Bence Jones proteins (fragments of abnormal globulins) excreted in urine

Medical Management
- Melphalan (Alkeran), cyclophosphamide, and steroids to decrease tumor mass and relieve bone pain
- Radiation for relieving bone pain
- Good hydration to prevent renal damage resulting from Bence Jones proteins in the renal tubules, hypercalcemia, and hyperuricemia
- Narcotic analgesics and local radiation for severe pain

Nursing Management
- Assess patients for signs and symptoms of renal insufficiency.
- Keep patients as active as possible to prevent pathologic fractures.
- Observe for bacterial infections (pneumonia).
- Avoid fasting regimens for diagnostic tests because dehydrating procedures can precipitate acute renal failure.
- Instruct patients in appropriate infection prevention measures.

🍁 Gerontologic Considerations

The incidence of multiple myeloma increases with age, rarely occurring before 40 years of age. Closely investigate any back pain, which is often presented as a complaint.

For more information, see Chapter 30 in Smeltzer.and Bare: *Brunner and Suddarth's Textbook of Medical-Surgical Nursing,* 9th edition. Philadelphia: Lippincott Williams & Wilkins, 2000.

MULTIPLE SCLEROSIS

Multiple sclerosis (MS) is a chronic, degenerative, progressive disease of the central nervous system characterized by small patches of demyelination in the brain and spinal cord. Demyelinization refers to the destruction of myelin and results in impaired transmission of nerve impulses. The cause of MS is not known but a defective immune response probably plays a major role. MS is more common in people living in northern temperate climate zones. It is one of the most disabling neurologic diseases of young adults (20 to 40 years), affecting twice as many women as men.

Clinical Manifestations

COURSE TYPES

- Relapsing-remitting course with complete recovery between relapses
- Chronic progressive course from the onset with a progressive decline in function
- Benign course with a normal life-span; symptoms so mild that patients do not seek health care and treatment
- Signs and symptoms varied and multiple, reflecting the location of the lesion or combination of lesions
- Primary symptoms: fatigue, weakness, numbness, difficulty in coordination, and loss of balance
- Visual disturbances: blurring of vision, patchy blindness (scotoma), or total blindness
- Spastic weakness of the extremities and loss of abdominal reflexes; ataxia and tremor
- Sensory dysfunction
- Cognitive and psychosocial problems; emotional lability and euphoria
- Bladder, bowel, and sexual problems possible

Secondary Manifestations Related to Complications

- Urinary tract infections, constipation
- Pressure ulcers, contracture deformities, dependent pedal edema

M

- Pneumonia
- Reactive depressions
- Emotional, social, marital, economic, and vocational problems

Exacerbations and Remissions
- Relapses may be associated with periods of emotional and physical stress.
- There is evidence that remyelinization occurs in some patients.

Diagnostic Evaluation
- Magnetic resonance imaging (MRI) (primary diagnostic tool) to visualize small plaques, evaluate course and effect of treatment
- Electrophoresis study of the cerebrospinal fluid (CSF); abnormal immunoglobulin G antibody appears in the CSF in up to 95% of patients
- Neuropsychological testing as indicated to assess cognitive impairment
- Urodynamic studies
- Sexual history to identify changes in sexual function

Medical Management
- No cure exists for MS.
- An individualized treatment program is indicated to relieve symptoms and provide support.

Pharmacotherapy
- Immunotherapeutic medications to modulate the immune response and reduce the rate at which the disease progresses, its frequency, and the severity of exacerbations (azathioprine, interferon, cyclophosphamide)
- Corticosteroids and adrenocorticotrophic hormone (ACTH) as antiinflammatory agents and to improve nerve conduction
- Baclofen: treatment of choice for spasticity
- Interferon-beta (Betaseron) for relapsing-remitting MS

Radiation
- May be used for immunosuppression

Bowel and Bladder Management
- Medications and intermittent self-catheterization
- Assessment of urinary tract infections; ascorbic acid to acidify urine; antibiotics when appropriate

Nursing Management
Assessment
- Assess actual and potential problems associated with the disease: neurologic problems, secondary complications, and impact of the disease on patient and family.
- Assess patient's function when well rested and when fatigued; look for weakness, spasticity, visual impairment, and incontinence.
- Assess sexual history for specific areas of concern.

Major Nursing Diagnoses
- Impaired physical mobility related to weakness, muscle paresis, spasticity
- Risk for injury related to sensory and visual impairment
- Altered urinary and bowel elimination related to spinal cord dysfunction
- Altered thought processes (loss of memory, dementia, euphoria) related to cerebral dysfunction
- Ineffective coping
- Impaired home maintenance management related to physical, psychological, and social limits imposed by MS
- Impaired speech and swallowing related to cranial nerve involvement
- Potential for sexual dysfunction related to spinal cord involvement or psychological reactions to condition

Planning and Goals
The major goals of the patient may include promotion of physical mobility, avoidance of injury, achievement of bladder and bowel continence, improvement of cognitive func-

M

tion, development of coping strengths, improved self-care, and adaptation to sexual dysfunction, promotion of speech and swallowing mechanism.

Nursing Interventions

PROMOTING PHYSICAL MOBILITY

- Encourage progressive resistance exercises to strengthen weak muscles.
- Encourage patient to work up to the point just short of fatigue.
- Advise patient to take frequent short rest periods, preferably lying down, to prevent extreme fatigue.
- Encourage walking exercises to improve gait.
- Provide warm packs to spastic muscles.
- Encourage daily exercises for muscle stretching to minimize joint contractures.
- Encourage swimming, stationary bicycling, and progressive weight bearing to relieve spasticity in legs.
- Avoid hurrying the patient in any activity because hurrying increases spasticity.
- Prevent complications of immobility by assessment and maintenance of skin integrity and through coughing and deep breathing exercises.

PREVENTING INJURY

- Teach patient to walk with feet wide apart to increase walking stability if motor dysfunction causes incoordination.
- Teach patient to watch the feet while walking if there is a loss of position sense.
- Provide a wheelchair if gait remains insufficient after gait training (walker, cane, braces, crutches, parallel bars, and physical therapy).
- Assess skin for pressure ulcers when patient is confined to wheelchair.

ENHANCING BLADDER AND BOWEL CONTROL

- Keep bedpan or urinal readily available because the need to void must be heeded immediately.

- Set up a voiding schedule, with gradual lengthening of time intervals.
- Instruct patient to drink a measured amount of fluid every 2 hours and to attempt to void 30 minutes after drinking.
- Encourage patient to take prescribed medications for bladder spasticity.
- Teach intermittent self-catheterization, if necessary.
- Provide adequate fluids, dietary fiber, and a bowel-training program for bowel problems, including constipation, fecal impaction, and incontinence.

IMPROVING SENSORY AND COGNITIVE FUNCTION

- Provide an eye patch or eyeglass occluder to block visual impulses of one eye when diplopia (double vision) occurs.
- Advise patient about free talking-book services from the library.
- Refer patient and family to a speech-language pathologist when mechanisms of speech are involved.
- Provide compassion and emotional support to patients and family to adapt to new self-image and to cope with life disruption.
- Keep a structured environment; use lists and other memory aids to help patient maintain a daily routine.

STRENGTHENING COPING MECHANISMS

- Alleviate stress, and make referrals for counseling and support to minimize adverse effects of dealing with chronic illness.
- Provide information on the illness to patient and family.
- Help patient define problems and develop alternatives for management.

IMPROVING SELF-CARE ABILITIES

- Suggest modifications that allow independence in self-care activities at home (raised toilet seat, bathing aids, telephone modifications, long-handled comb, tongs, modified clothing).

M

- Avoid physical and emotional stress when possible.
- Maintain moderate environmental temperature; heat increases fatigue and muscle weakness; extreme cold may increase spasticity.

PROMOTING SEXUAL FUNCTIONING
- Suggest a sexual counselor to assist patient and partner with sexual dysfunction (ie, erectile and ejaculatory disorders in men; orgasmic dysfunction and adductor spasms of the thigh muscles in women; bladder and bowel incontinence; urinary tract infections).

Promoting Home and Community-Based Care

Teaching Patients Self-Care
- Teach patient and family about use of assistive devices, self-catheterization, and administration of medications.
- Assist patient and family to deal with new disabilities and changes as disease progresses.

Continuing Care
- Refer for home health care nursing assistance as indicated.
- Encourage patient to contact the local chapter of the National Multiple Sclerosis Society for services, publications, and contact with other MS patients.
- Teach and reinforce new self-care techniques.
- Assess changes in patient's health status and coping strategies.
- Reinforce the importance of follow-up care.

Evaluation
EXPECTED OUTCOMES
- Adapts to impaired mobility and spasticity
- Avoids injury
- Attains or maintains improved bladder and bowel control
- Participates in strategies to improve speech and swallowing

- Compensates for cognitive dysfunction
- Demonstrates improved coping strategies
- Adapts to changes in sexual function

For more information, see Chapter 59 in Smeltzer and Bare: *Brunner and Suddarth's Textbook of Medical-Surgical Nursing,* 9th edition. Philadelphia: Lippincott Williams & Wilkins, 2000.

MUSCULAR DYSTROPHIES

Muscular dystrophies are a group of chronic muscle disorders characterized by a progressive weakening and wasting of the skeletal or voluntary muscles. Most are inherited. The pathologic features include degeneration and loss of muscle fibers, variation in muscle fiber size, phagocytosis and regeneration, and replacement of muscle tissue by connective tissue. Types of symptoms are affected by patterns of inheritance, muscles involved, age of onset, and rate of progression.

Clinical Manifestations and Diagnostic Evaluation

- Muscle wasting and weakness
- Abnormal elevation in serum creatinine phosphokinase (CPK)
- Myopathic electromyography (EMG) pattern
- Myopathic findings on muscle biopsy

Medical Management

Treatment focuses on supportive care and prevention of complications. Supportive management is intended to keep the patient active and functioning as normally as possible and to minimize functional deterioration.

- A therapeutic exercise program is individualized to prevent muscle tightness, contractures, and disuse atrophy. Use night splints and stretching exercises to delay joint contractures (especially ankles, knees, and hips). Braces may be used to compensate for muscle weakness.

- Fit patient with orthotic jacket to improve sitting stability, reduce trunk deformity, and support cardiovascular status. Spinal fusion may be performed to maintain spinal stability.
- Treat vigorously all upper respiratory infections and fractures from falls to minimize immobilization and to prevent joint contractures.
- Advise genetic counseling because of the genetic nature of this disease.

Other Difficulties That Should Be Treated Symptomatically

- Dental and speech problems
- Gastrointestinal tract problem resulting in gastric dilation, rectal prolapse, and fecal impaction
- Cardiomyopathy (common complication in all forms of muscular dystrophy)

Nursing Management

Nursing Interventions

The goals of the patient and the nurse are to maintain function at optimal levels and enhance the quality of life.

- Attend to patient's physical requirements and emotional and developmental needs.
- Actively involve patient and family in decision making, include end-of-life decisions.
- During hospitalization for treatment of complications, assess the knowledge and expertise of the patient and family members responsible for caregiving in the home.
- Assist patient and family to maintain coping strategies used at home while in hospital.

🏠 Promoting Home and Community-Based Care

Teaching Patients Self-Care

- Provide the patient and family with information and instruction about the disorder, its anticipated course, and care and management strategies that will optimize

the patient's growth and development and physical and psychological status.
- Communicate recommendations to all members of the health care team so that they may work toward common goals.

Continuing Care
- Encourage use of self-help devices to achieve a greater degree of independence; refer for home care nursing as appropriate.
- Encourage range-of-motion exercises to prevent disabling contractures.
- In teaching family to monitor patient for respiratory problems, give specific information regarding appropriate respiratory support, such as negative-pressure devices and positive-pressure ventilators.
- Assist family in adjusting home environment to maximize functional independence; patient may require manual or electric wheelchair, gait aids, seating systems, bathroom equipment, lifts, ramps, and additional activity of daily living aids.
- Assess for signs of depression, prolonged anger, bargaining, or denial and help patient to cope and adapt to chronic disease. Arrange for referral to a psychiatric nurse clinician or other mental health professional if indicated to assist the patient to cope and adapt to the disease.
- Provide a hopeful, supportive, and nurturing environment.

M

For more information, see Chapter 59 in Smeltzer and Bare: *Brunner and Suddarth's Textbook of Medical-Surgical Nursing,* 9th edition. Philadelphia: Lippincott Williams & Wilkins, 2000.

MUSCULOSKELETAL TRAUMA

Injury to one part of the musculoskeletal system usually results in injury or dysfunction of adjacent structures and of structures enclosed or supported by them. If the bone is broken, the muscles cannot function, and blood vessels and nerves in the vicinity of the fracture may be injured. If the nerves do not send impulses to the muscles, as in paralysis, the bones cannot move. If the joint surfaces do not articulate normally, neither the bones nor the muscles can function properly.

Contusions, Strains, and Sprains

A *contusion* is a soft tissue injury produced by blunt force (eg, a blow, kick, or fall). Many small blood vessels rupture into soft tissues (ecchymosis, or bruising). A hematoma develops when the bleeding is sufficient to cause an appreciable collection of blood. Most contusions resolve in 1 to 2 weeks.

A *strain* is a "muscle pull" from overuse, overstretching, or excessive stress. Strains are microscopic, incomplete muscle tears with some bleeding into the tissue.

A *sprain* is an injury to the ligaments surrounding a joint, caused by a wrenching or twisting motion. A torn ligament loses its stabilizing ability. Blood vessels rupture and edema occurs.

Joint Dislocations

A *dislocation* of a joint is a condition in which the articular surfaces of the bones forming the joint are no longer in anatomic contact. The bones are literally "out of joint." Dislocations may be congenital, present at birth (most often the hip); spontaneous or pathologic, due to disease of the articular or the periarticular structures; or traumatic, resulting from injury in which the joint is disrupted by force. A *subluxation* is a partial dislocation of the articulating surfaces. Traumatic dislocations are orthopedic emergencies because the associated joint structures, blood supply, and nerves are distorted and severely stressed. If the dislocation is not treated promptly, avascular necrosis (tissue death due to anoxia and diminished blood supply) and nerve palsy may occur.

Clinical Manifestations

- Contusion: local symptoms (pain, swelling, and discoloration)
- Strain: soreness or sudden pain with local tenderness on muscle use and isometric contraction
- Sprain: tenderness of the joint, painful movement; increased disability and pain the first 2 to 3 hours after injury because of associated swelling and bleeding
- Dislocation or subluxation: pain, change in contour of the joint, change in the length of the extremity, loss of normal mobility, and change in the axis of the dislocated bones

Diagnostic Evaluation

- Radiographic examination to evaluate for bone injury (eg, avulsion fracture, in which a bone fragment is pulled away by a ligament or tendon), which may be associated with a sprain

Medical Management

- Treatment of injury of the musculoskeletal system involves providing support for the injured part until healing is complete.
- Treatment of contusions, strains, and sprains consists of rest, applying ice for cold, applying a compression bandage, and elevating the affected part (*RICE*—rest, ice, compression, elevation).
- Ice or some form of moist or dry cold is applied intermittently for 20 to 30 minutes during the first 24 to 48 hours after injury to produce vasoconstriction, which decreases bleeding, edema, and discomfort.
- An elastic compression bandage controls bleeding, reduces edema, and provides support for the injured tissues.

M

- Elevation controls the swelling. If the sprain is severe (torn muscle fibers and disrupted ligaments), surgical repair or cast immobilization may be necessary, so that the joint will not lose its stability.
- After the acute inflammatory stage (eg, 24 to 48 hours after injury), heat may be applied intermittently (for 15 to 30 minutes, four times a day) to relieve muscle spasm and to promote vasodilation, absorption, and repair.
- Depending on the severity of injury, progressive passive and active exercises may begin in 2 to 5 days.
- Severe sprains may require 1 to 3 weeks of immobilization before protected exercises are initiated.
- Strains and sprains take weeks or months to heal. Splinting may be used to prevent reinjury.
- With a dislocation, the affected joint needs to be immobilized while the patient is transported to the hospital.
- The dislocation is promptly reduced (ie, displaced parts brought into normal position) to preserve joint function. Analgesia, muscle relaxants, and possibly anesthesia are used to facilitate closed reduction.
- The joint is immobilized by bandages, splints, casts, or traction and is maintained in a stable position.
- Several days to weeks after reduction, gentle, progressive, active, and passive movement three or four times a day is begun to preserve range of motion and restore strength.
- The joint is supported between exercise sessions.

Nursing Management
Nursing Interventions
- Administer analgesics and provide measures to promote comfort.
- Evaluate the patient's neurovascular status.
- Protect the joint during healing.
- Teach the patient about pain management, medications (analgesics, antibiotics), cast care, wound care, possible complication (eg, altered neurovascular status, infection, skin breakdown), and self-care.

- Teach the patient proper use of ambulatory devices, the healing process, and activity limitation to promote healing.
- Teach the patient how to manage the immobilizing devices and how to protect the joint from reinjury.

For more information, see Chapter 63 in Smeltzer and Bare: *Brunner and Suddarth's Textbook of Medical-Surgical Nursing,* 9th edition. Philadelphia: Lippincott Williams & Wilkins, 2000.

MYASTHENIA GRAVIS

Myasthenia gravis is a disorder affecting the neuromuscular transmission of the voluntary muscles of the body. Excessive weakness and fatigability occur. It affects women between the ages of 15 and 35 years and men older than 40 years. It is considered an autoimmune disease in which antibodies directed against acetylcholine receptor (AChR) impair neuromuscular transmission.

M

Clinical Manifestations

Symptoms include extreme muscular weakness and easy fatigability, which worsen after effort and are relieved by rest.

Varied Symptoms According to Muscles Affected
- Early symptoms: diplopia and ptosis
- Sleepy, masklike expression because facial muscles are affected
- Dysphonia (voice impairment), with nasal sound or difficulty in articulation
- Problems with chewing and swallowing, which can present danger of choking and aspiration
- Complaints of weakness of arm and hand muscles; less commonly, leg muscles
- Progressive weakness of the diaphragm and intercostal muscles, which may produce respiratory distress (an acute emergency)

Diagnostic Evaluation

- Presumptive diagnosis is based on history and physical examination.
- Injection of edrophonium (Tensilon) is used to confirm diagnosis.
- Improvement in muscle strength represents a positive test and usually confirms diagnosis.
- Tests include serum analysis for AChR and electromyography (EMG) to measure electrical potential of muscle cells.

Medical Management

Management is directed at improving function through the administration of anticholinesterase medications and through reducing and removing circulating antibodies.

Anticholinesterase Medications

- Pyridostigmine bromide (Mestinon), neostigmine bromide (Prostigmin)
- Given to increase response of the muscles to nerve impulses and improve strength; results expected within 1 hour after administration

Immunosuppressive Therapy

- Directed toward reducing production of antireceptor antibody or removing it directly by plasma exchange
- Corticosteroids to suppress the immune response, decreasing the amount of blocking antibody
- Plasma exchange (plasmapheresis) to produce a temporary reduction in the titer of circulating antibodies
- Thymectomy (surgical removal of the thymus), which causes substantial remission, especially in patients with tumor or hyperplasia of the thymus gland

Complications

MYASTHENIC CRISIS

- Sudden onset of muscular weakness that is usually the result of undermedication or no cholinergic medication at all

- May result from progression of the disease, emotional upset, systemic infections, medications, surgery, or trauma
- Manifested by sudden onset of acute respiratory distress and inability to swallow or speak

CHOLINERGIC CRISIS
- Caused by overmedication with cholinergic or anticholinesterase drugs
- Muscle weakness and respiratory depression of myasthenic crisis as well as gastrointestinal symptoms (nausea, vomiting, diarrhea), sweating, increased salivation, and bradycardia

Nursing Management
Assessment

M

- Assess health history, focusing on muscle weakness (respiratory and esophageal muscles), eye and vision changes, and the patient's and family's knowledge about the disease and the drug treatment program.
- Assess patient's functional capability and support system to determine discharge needs for services.
- Patients with myasthenia gravis are usually managed on an outpatient basis unless hospitalization is required for managing symptoms or complications.

Major Nursing Diagnoses
- Ineffective breathing pattern related to respiratory muscle weakness
- Impaired physical mobility due to voluntary muscle weakness
- Risk for aspiration related to weakness of bulbar muscles
- Impaired verbal communication related to weakened speech muscles
- Sensory-perceptual alteration related to impaired vision

Collaborative Problems/Potential Complications
- Myasthenic crisis
- Cholinergic crisis

Planning and Goals

The major goals of the patient may include improved respiratory function, increased physical mobility, improved ability to communicate, avoidance of aspiration, and absence of complications (myasthenic and cholinergic crisis).

Nursing Interventions

IMPROVING RESPIRATORY FUNCTION

- Assess respiratory status frequently to detect pulmonary problems before changes in arterial blood gas levels appear.
- Provide chest physical therapy, including postural drainage, to mobilize secretions and suction to remove secretions.
- Acknowledge patient's fears, and give assurance.

INCREASING PHYSICAL MOBILITY

- Teach patient facts about anticholinesterase drugs: action, timing, dosage, symptoms of overdose, and toxic effects.
- Emphasize taking medication on time to improve strength and endurance.
- Encourage patient to keep a diary to determine fluctuation of symptoms.
- Teach patient to avoid factors that may increase weakness and precipitate myasthenic crisis: emotional upset, infections (respiratory), vigorous physical activity, exposure to heat and cold.
- Advise patient to wear an identification bracelet, such as MedicAlert.
- Educate patient regarding self-help devices, provide as desired.

IMPROVING COMMUNICATION

- Teach patients with weakened speech muscles techniques for improving communication (eg, blink eyes, wiggle fingers or toes).

PROVIDING EYE CARE
- Help patient cope with impaired vision (eg, taping eyes open for short intervals, instilling artificial tears to prevent corneal damage).
- Suggest patient use a patch over one eye for double vision and wear sunglasses to diminish the effects of bright light that increase eye problems.

PREVENTING ASPIRATION
- Assess for drooling, regurgitation through the nose, and choking while attempting to swallow.
- Provide standby suction.
- Encourage rest before meals; place patient in an upright position to facilitate swallowing.
- Provide soft foods that are easily swallowed.
- Schedule meals to coincide with the peak effects of anticholinesterase.
- Assist with gastrostomy feedings if necessary.

MONITORING AND MANAGING POTENTIAL COMPLICATIONS: MYASTHENIC AND CHOLINERGIC CRISES
Respiratory distress combined with varying signs of dysphagia (difficulty swallowing), dysarthria (difficulty speaking), eyelid ptosis, diplopia, and prominent muscle weakness are symptoms of crisis of either type.

- Provide immediate adequate ventilatory assistance.
- Suction patient as needed.
- Monitor arterial blood gases, serum electrolytes, intake and output, and daily weights.
- Assist with endotracheal intubation and mechanical ventilation; place patient in intensive care unit for constant monitoring.
- Assist with administration of intravenous edrophonium to differentiate type of crisis; this agent improves patient in myasthenic crisis; temporarily worsens patient in cholinergic crisis. Neostigmine methylsulfate is given with myasthenic crisis.

M

- Assist with nasogastric tube feedings if patient is unable to swallow.
- Avoid sedatives and tranquilizing drugs because they aggravate hypoxia and hypercapnia and can cause respiratory and cardiac depression.

🏠 Promoting Home and Community-Based Care

Teaching Patients Self-Care

- Teach patient to consult with physician before taking any new medications. Many prescription and nonprescription medications aggravate myasthenia gravis.
- Teach patient the importance of administering medication as prescribed.
- Inform patient and family about crisis intervention, ways to deal with daily needs, and ways to cope with the disease.
- Teach family emergency measures that may be needed; provide opportunity to practice these.

🚦 NURSING ALERT

A nursing priority is to give the prescribed anticholinesterase drug according to an exact time schedule to control patient symptoms; delay in drug administration may result in inability to swallow.

Continuing Care

Inform patient of community and support groups provided by the Myasthenia Gravis Foundation.

Evaluation

EXPECTED OUTCOMES

- Achieves adequate respiratory function
- Adapts to impaired mobility
- Experiences no aspiration
- Uses communication methods

- Reports ability to see objects and people in environment
- Recovers from myasthenic and cholinergic crisis.

For more information, see Chapter 59 in Smeltzer and Bare: *Brunner and Suddarth's Textbook of Medical-Surgical Nursing,* 9th edition. Philadelphia: Lippincott Williams & Wilkins, 2000.

MYOCARDIAL INFARCTION

Myocardial infarction (MI) refers to the process by which myocardial tissue is destroyed in regions of the heart that are deprived of an adequate blood supply because of reduced coronary artery blood flow. The cause is usually a critical narrowing of a coronary artery due to atherosclerosis or complete occlusion of an artery due to embolus or thrombus. Decreased coronary blood flow may also result from vasospasm of a coronary artery, decreased oxygen supply (eg, shock and hemorrhage), or increased demand for oxygen (eg, tachycardia, and thyrotoxicosis). In each case, there is a profound imbalance between myocardial oxygen supply and demand. An MI may be defined by the location of the injury to the heart muscle or by the point in time within the process of infarction (acute, evolving, old).

M

Clinical Manifestations
- Chest pain that occurs suddenly and continues despite rest and medication is the primary presenting symptom.
- In many cases, the signs and symptoms cannot be distinguished from those of unstable angina.
- Pain may radiate to the jaw, neck, shoulders, and arm (usually left).
- Pain may be accompanied by cool skin, pallor, clammy diaphoresis, tachycardia, and tachypnea, if stimulation of the sympathetic nervous system occurs.
- Patients with diabetes mellitus may not experience severe pain because the neuropathy that accompanies diabetes

can interfere with neuroreceptors (dulling the pain experience).

Diagnostic Evaluation
- Patient history
- Electrocardiogram (ECG)
- Serial serum enzymes and isoenzymes, myoglobin, and troponin

Medical Management
The goals of medical management are to minimize myocardial damage, preserve myocardial function, and prevent complications such as lethal dysrhythmias and cardiogenic shock.

- Oxygen administration initiated at the onset of chest pain
- Emergent percutaneous transluminal coronary angioplasty (PTCA)
- Coronary artery bypass or minimally invasive direct coronary artery bypass (MIDCAB)

Pharmacotherapy
- Nitrates to increase oxygen supply (NTG)
- Anticoagulants (heparin)
- Analgesics (morphine sulfate)
- Thrombolytics (streptokinase, tissue-type plasminogen activator [t-PA], and anistreplase); most effective if administered as early as possible after the onset of chest pain, before transmural tissue necrosis occurs

Nursing Management
Assessment
Establish a baseline management to get information on present status of patient so deviations may be noted immediately. Include history of chest pain, dyspnea, palpitations, faintness, or sweating.

COMPLETE PHYSICAL ASSESSMENT

The physical assessment is crucial to detect complications and should include the following:

- Assess level of consciousness.
- Evaluate chest pain (most important clinical finding).
- Assess heart rate and rhythm; dysrhythmias may indicate not enough oxygen to the myocardium.
- Assess heart sounds; S3 can be an early sign of impending left ventricular failure.
- Measure blood pressure to determine response to pain and treatment; note pulse pressure, which may be narrowed after an MI, suggesting ineffective ventricular contraction.
- Assess peripheral pulses: rate, rhythm, and volume.
- Evaluate skin color and temperature.
- Auscultate lung fields at frequent intervals for signs of ventricular failure (crackles in lung bases).
- Assess bowel motility; mesenteric artery thrombosis is a potentially fatal complication.
- Observe urinary output; check for edema; note that early sign of cardiogenic shock is hypotension with oliguria.

Major Nursing Diagnoses

- Decreased myocardial perfusion related to reduced coronary blood flow due to coronary thrombus and atherosclerotic plaque
- Potential impaired gas exchange related to fluid overload due to left ventricular dysfunction
- Potential altered peripheral tissue perfusion related to decreased cardiac output due to left ventricular function
- Anxiety related to fear of death
- Knowledge deficit about post-MI self-care

Collaborative Problems/Potential Complications

- Dysrhythmias and cardiac arrest
- Acute pulmonary edema

M

- Congestive heart failure
- Thromboembolism
- Myocardial rupture
- Pericardial effusion and cardiac tamponade

Planning and Goals

The major goals of the patient include relief of symptoms of ischemia (chest pain, ST segment changes), absence of respiratory difficulties, maintenance or attainment of adequate tissue perfusion, reduction of anxiety, adherence to self-care program, and prevention or early recognition of complications.

Nursing Interventions

RELIEVING CHEST PAIN

- Administer vasodilator (NTG) and anticoagulant (heparin) medications and aspirin to preserve heart muscle.
- Provide thrombolytic therapy if patient clinically qualifies.
- Administer analgesic agents (morphine sulfate).
- Administer oxygen in tandem with analgesia to ensure maximum relief of pain (inhalation of oxygen reduces pain associated with low levels of circulating oxygen).
- Assess vital signs as long as patient is experiencing pain.
- Provide physical rest with back elevated or in cardiac chair to decrease chest discomfort and dyspnea.

IMPROVING RESPIRATORY FUNCTION

- Assess respiratory function to detect early signs of complications.
- Pay attention to fluid volume status to prevent overloading the heart and the lungs.
- Encourage patient to breathe deeply and change position to prevent pooling of fluid in lung bases.

PROMOTING ADEQUATE TISSUE PERFUSION

- Keep patient on bed or chair rest to reduce cardiac workload.

- Check skin temperature and peripheral pulses frequently to determine adequate tissue perfusion.
- Administer oxygen to enrich supply of circulating oxygen.

REDUCING ANXIETY
- Develop a trusting and caring relationship with patient.
- Provide frequent and private opportunities to share concerns and fears.
- Provide an atmosphere of acceptance to help know that his or her feelings are both realistic and normal.

MONITORING AND MANAGING COMPLICATIONS
- Monitor closely for cardinal signs and symptoms that signal onset of complications.

M

Cardiac Rehabilitation
Goals of rehabilitation for the patient with a MI are to extend and improve quality of life. The immediate objectives are to limit the effects and progression of atherosclerosis, return the patient to work and a preillness lifestyle, enhance the psychosocial and vocational status of the patient, and prevent another cardiac event.
- Encourage physical activity and physical conditioning.
- Educate both patient and family.
- Provide counseling and behavioral interventions when necessary.

 Promoting Home and Community-Based Care

Teaching Patients Self-Care
- Educate about the disease process.
- Work with patient to develop a plan to meet specific needs to enhance compliance.

 Gerontologic Considerations

The gerontologic considerations for MI are the same as those for angina (atypical pain sensitivity to cold temperatures). The mortality rate is higher in elderly (older than 65

years of age) patients with an acute MI. Age, other illnesses, and preexisting conditions may prevent the patient from receiving otherwise indicated treatment for acute MI.

NURSING ALERT

The resolution of pain is the primary clinical indicator that myocardial oxygen demand and supply are in equilibrium.

Evaluation

EXPECTED OUTCOMES
- Experiences relief of pain
- Shows no signs of respiratory difficulties
- Maintains adequate tissue perfusion
- Expresses less anxiety
- Complies with self-care program
- Experiences absence of complications

For more information, see Chapter 25 in Smeltzer and Bare: *Brunner and Suddarth's Textbook of Medical-Surgical Nursing,* 9th edition. Philadelphia: Lippincott Williams & Wilkins, 2000.

MYOCARDITIS

Acute myocarditis is an inflammatory process involving the myocardium. When the muscle fibers of the heart are damaged, life is threatened. Myocarditis usually results from an infectious process (eg, viral, bacterial, mycotic, parasitic, protozoal, or spirochetal). It may be produced in systemic infections, such as rheumatic fever, in patients receiving immunosuppressive therapy, or in patients with infective endocarditis. Myocarditis can cause heart dilation, mural thrombi (on the heart wall), infiltration of circulating blood cells around coronary vessels and between muscle fibers, and degeneration of the muscle fibers.

Clinical Manifestations
- Clinical features depend on type of infection, degree of myocardial damage, and capacity of the myocardium to recover.
- Symptoms may be moderate, mild or absent.
- Patient may report fatigue and dyspnea, palpitations, and occasional discomfort in the chest and upper abdomen.
- Patient may develop severe congestive heart failure or sustain sudden cardiac death.
- Pericardial friction rub may be heard if associated with pericarditis.
- Pulsus alternans may be present.
- Fever and tachycardia are frequently seen, and symptoms of congestive heart failure may develop.

M

Diagnostic Evaluation
- Diagnosis is confirmed by endomyocardial biopsy.
- Cardiac enlargement, faint heart sounds, gallop rhythm, and systolic murmur may be found on clinical examination.

Medical Management
Prevention
- Appropriate immunizations and early treatment to decrease the incidence of myocarditis

Treatment
The specific underlying cause is treated.
- Bed rest to decrease cardiac workload and prevent complications
- Continuous cardiac monitoring if dysrhythmia occurs
- Medications to slow the heart rate and augment myocardial contractility (digitalis) when there is evidence of congestive heart failure

Nursing Management

- Because patients with myocarditis are sensitive to digitalis, monitor for digitalis toxicity (dysrhythmia, anorexia, nausea, vomiting, bradycardia, headache, malaise).
- Apply, and instruct patient and family in use of, elastic stockings and passive and active exercises to prevent thrombosis.
- Instruct patient to increase physical activity slowly and to report any symptoms that occur with increased activity, including rapid heart rate.
- Instruct patient to avoid competitive sports and alcohol.

For more information, see Chapter 26 in Smeltzer and Bare: *Brunner and Suddarth's Textbook of Medical-Surgical Nursing,* 9th edition. Philadelphia: Lippincott Williams & Wilkins, 2000.

N

NEPHROTIC SYNDROME

Nephrotic syndrome is a primary glomerular disease characterized by proteinuria, hypoalbuminemia, edema, and hyperlipidemia. It is seen in any condition that seriously damages the glomerular capillary membrane causing increased glomerular permeability with loss of protein in the urine. Generally a disorder of childhood, it does occur in adults, including the elderly. Causes include chronic glomerular nephritis and diabetes mellitus among other conditions.

Clinical Manifestations
- Major manifestation: edema (usually periorbital, in dependent areas [sacrum, ankles, and hands], and ascites)
- Malaise, headache, irritability, and fatigue

Diagnostic Evaluation
- Proteinuria (exceeding 3 to 3.5 g/day)
- Microscopic hematuria, urinary casts
- Needle biopsy of the kidney for histologic examination to confirm diagnosis

Medical Management
The objective of management is to preserve renal function.

- Bed rest for a few days to promote diuresis and reduce edema

- High biologic protein diet to replenish urinary losses
- Low-sodium low saturated fat, liberal potassium
- Diuretics for severe edema, combination with angiotensin-converting enzyme (ACE) inhibitors
- Adrenocorticosteroids to reduce proteinuria
- Antineoplastic agents (Cytoxan) or immunosuppressive agents (Imuran, Leukeran, or cyclosporine)

Nursing Management
Nursing Interventions
- In the early stages, nursing management is similar to that of the patient with acute glomerulonephritis.
- As the disease worsens, management is similar to that of the patient with chronic renal failure.

 # Promoting Home and Community-Based Care

- Instruct patient receiving steroids or cyclosporine regarding medication and signs and symptoms that must be reported to the physician.
- Instruct patient in selecting a high-protein diet while restricting cholesterol and fat intake.
- Monitor intake and output; note signs of low plasma volume and impaired circulation with prerenal acute renal failure.

For more information, see Chapter 41 in Smeltzer and Bare: *Brunner and Suddarth's Textbook of Medical-Surgical Nursing,* 9th edition. Philadelphia: Lippincott Williams & Wilkins, 2000.

O

OSTEOARTHRITIS (DEGENERATIVE JOINT DISEASE)

Osteoarthritis (OA), also known as *degenerative joint disease* or *osteoarthrosis,* is the most common and frequently disabling of the joint disorders. OA is characterized by a progressive loss of joint cartilage. Besides age, risk factors for OA include female gender, genetic predisposition, obesity, mechanical joint stress, joint trauma, congenital and developmental disorders of the hip, previous bone and joint disorders, inflammatory joint diseases, and endocrine and metabolic diseases. OA has been classified as primary (idiopathic) and secondary (related to risk factors). Obese women have been shown to have an incidence of OA of the knee nearly four times that of women of average weight. OA peaks between the fifth and sixth decades of life.

Clinical Manifestations
- Pain, stiffness, and functional impairment are primary clinical manifestations.
- Stiffness is most common in the morning after awakening, usually lasts less than 30 minutes, and decreases with movement.
- Functional impairment is due to pain on movement and limited joint motion when structural changes develop.
- Osteoarthritis occurs most often in weight-bearing joints (hips, knees, cervical, and lumbar spine); finger joints are also involved.
- Bony nodes may be present (painless unless inflamed).

Diagnostic Evaluation

- Radiograph (shows narrowing of joint space and osteophytes (spurs) at the joint margins and on the subchondral bone).
- These two findings together are sensitive and specific.

Medical Management

The goals of management focus on slowing and treating symptoms because there is no treatment available that stops the degenerative joint disease process.

Preventive Measures

- Weight reduction
- Prevention of injuries
- Perinatal screening for congenital hip disease
- Ergonomic approaches to job stress modification

Pharmacotherapy

- Acetaminophen; nonsteroidal antiinflammatory drugs (NSAIDs) if joint symptoms persist
- Intraarticular injections of corticosteroids for acute joint inflammation (short-term only)

Conservative Measures

- Heat, weight reduction, joint rest, and avoidance of joint overuse
- Orthotic devices to support inflamed joints (splints, braces)
- Isometric and postural exercises
- Occupational and physical therapy

Surgical Approaches

Use when pain is intractable and function is lost.

- Tidal irrigation, arthroscopic débridement, drilling of osteochondral defects, or abrasion arthroplasty may be performed.
- Viscosupplementation is a new therapeutic concept being used.

- Joint arthroplasty (replacement) is used in patients with end-stage disease.

Nursing Management

The nursing care of the patient with OA is generally the same as the basic care plan for the patient with rheumatic disease.

For more information, see Chapter 50 in Smeltzer and Bare: *Brunner and Suddarth's Textbook of Medical-Surgical Nursing,* 9th edition. Philadelphia: Lippincott Williams & Wilkins, 2000.

OSTEOMALACIA

Osteomalacia is a metabolic bone disease characterized by inadequate mineralization of bone. (Rickets, a similar condition, afflicts children.) The primary defect is a deficiency in activated vitamin D (calcitriol), which causes an imbalance of calcium and phosphate and faulty bone mineralization. In adults, the condition is chronic, and skeletal deformities are not as severe as in children. Risk factors include dietary deficiencies, malabsorption, gastrectomy, chronic renal failure, prolonged anticonvulsant therapy, and insufficient vitamin D (eg, from inadequate dietary intake or inadequate sunlight exposure).

Clinical Manifestations
- Bone pain and tenderness
- Muscle weakness from calcium deficiency
- Waddling or limping gait; legs bowed in more advanced disease
- Pathologic fractures
- Softened vertebrae compressed, shortening the patient's trunk and deforming the thorax (kyphosis)
- Weakness and unsteadiness, presenting risk of falls and fractures

Diagnostic Evaluation
- Radiograph, bone biopsy
- Laboratory studies, which show low serum calcium and phosphorus levels; moderately elevated alkaline phosphatase level; decreased urine calcium and creatinine excretion

Medical Management
- The underlying cause is corrected when possible (eg, diet modifications, vitamin D and calcium supplements, sunlight).
- Long-term monitoring is undertaken to ensure stabilization or reversal.
- Orthopedic deformities are treated with braces or surgery.
- Physical, psychological, and pharmacologic measures are used to reduce pain and discomfort.

Nursing Management
Assessment
- Assess for generalized bone pain in the low back and extremities, with associated tenderness.
- Assess for fracture.
- Obtain information concerning coexisting diseases (malabsorption syndrome) and dietary habits.
- Note skeletal deformities on physical examination and any muscle weakness.

Major Nursing Diagnoses
- Knowledge deficit about the disease process and the treatment regimen
- Pain related to bone tenderness and possible fracture
- Self-concept disturbance related to bowing legs, waddling gait, spinal deformities

Planning and Goals
The major goals of the patient may include knowledge of the disease process and treatment regimen, relief of pain, and improved self-concept.

Nursing Interventions

RELIEVING PAIN
- Assist patient in reducing discomfort by physical, psychological, and pharmaceutical measures.
- Change positions often to decrease discomfort from immobility.
- Administer prescribed analgesics as needed.

IMPROVING SELF-CONCEPT
- Establish a trusting relationship, and encourage patient to discuss any changes in body image and methods of coping.
- Encourage patient to recognize and use existing strengths.
- Include patient in plan of care to promote self-control and improve feelings of self-worth.

Promoting Home and Community-Based Care

Teaching Patients Self-Care
- Educate patient about the cause of osteomalacia and approaches to controlling it.
- Instruct patient about dietary sources of calcium and vitamin D and safe use of vitamin supplements.
- Inform patient that high doses of vitamin D are toxic and enhance risk of hypercalcemia.
- Note importance of monitoring serum calcium levels.
- Encourage outdoor activities to expose skin to sunshine.

Gerontologic Considerations

Promote adequate intake of calcium and vitamin D and a nutritious diet in disadvantaged elderly patients. Encourage patient to spend time in the sun. Reduce incidence of fractures with prevention, identification, and management of osteomalacia. When osteomalacia is combined with osteoporosis, the incidence of fracture increases.

For more information, see Chapter 62 in Smeltzer and Bare: *Brunner and Suddarth's Textbook of Medical-Surgical Nursing,* 9th edition. Philadelphia: Lippincott Williams & Wilkins, 2000.

OSTEOMYELITIS

Osteomyelitis is an infection of the bone. It may occur by extension of soft tissue infections, direct bone contamination (eg, bone surgery, gunshot wound), or hematogenous (bloodborne) spread from other foci of infection. *Staphylococcus aureus* causes 70% to 80% of bone infections. Other pathogenic organisms frequently found include *Proteus* and *Pseudomonas* species and *Escherichia coli.* Patients at risk include poorly nourished, elderly, and obese patients; those with impaired immune systems and chronic illness (eg, diabetes); and those on long-term corticosteroid therapy. The condition may be prevented by prompt treatment and management of focal and soft tissue infections.

Clinical Manifestations
Hematogenous Infection
- Onset is sudden, occurring with clinical manifestations of septicemia (eg, chills, high fever, rapid pulse, and general malaise).
- The extremity becomes painful, swollen, and tender.
- Patient may describe a constant pulsating pain that intensifies with movement (due to the pressure of collecting pus).
- When osteomyelitis is caused by adjacent infection or direct contamination, there are no symptoms of septicemia.
- The area is swollen, warm, painful, and tender to touch.
- With chronic osteomyelitis, there is continually draining sinus or recurrent periods of pain, inflammation, swelling, and drainage.

Diagnostic Evaluation
- Early radiographs show only soft tissue swelling.
- Bone scans and magnetic resonance imaging (MRI) may be performed.
- Blood studies and blood cultures are taken.
- Chronic osteomyelitis: radiograph shows large, irregular cavities, a raised periosteum, sequestrae, or dense bone formations.

Medical Management
The initial goal is to control and arrest the infective process.
- Affected area is immobilized; warm saline soaks are provided for 20 minutes several times a day.
- Blood and wound cultures are performed to identify organisms and select the antibiotic.
- Intravenous antibiotic therapy is instituted around-the-clock.
- Antibiotic is administered orally when infection appears to be controlled and is continued for 3 months.
- Surgical débridement of bone is performed with irrigation; adjunctive antibiotic therapy is maintained.

Nursing Management
Assessment
- Assess for risk factors (eg, older age, diabetes, long-term steroid therapy) and for previous injury, infection, or orthopedic surgery.
- Observe for guarded movement of infected area and generalized weakness due to systemic infection.
- Observe for swelling and warmth of affected area, purulent drainage, and elevated temperature.
- Note that patients with chronic osteomyelitis may have minimal temperature elevations, occurring in the afternoon or evening.

Major Nursing Diagnoses
- Pain related to inflammation and swelling
- Impaired physical mobility associated with pain, immobilization devices, and weight-bearing limitations

- Risk for extension of infection: bone abscess formation
- Knowledge deficit about the treatment regimen

Planning and Goals
The major goals of the patient may include relief of pain, improved physical mobility within therapeutic limitations, control and eradication of infection, and knowledge of treatment regimen.

Nursing Interventions
RELIEVING PAIN
- Restrict activity and immobilize affected part with splint to decrease pain and muscle spasm.
- Place joints above and below the affected part gently through range of motion.
- Handle wounds with great care and gently to avoid pain.
- Elevate affected part to reduce swelling and discomfort.
- Administer prescribed analgesics and other techniques for reducing pain perception.
- Monitor neurovascular status of the affected extremity.

IMPROVING PHYSICAL MOBILITY
- Teach the rationale for activity restrictions (bone is weakened by the infective process).
- Encourage activities of daily living within the physical limitations.

CONTROLLING INFECTIOUS PROCESS
- Monitor the patient's response to antibiotic therapy, and observe the intravenous sites for evidence of phlebitis or infiltration; monitor for signs of superinfection with long-term, intensive antibiotic therapy (eg, oral or vaginal candidiasis).
- If surgery was necessary, ensure adequate circulation (wound suction, elevation of area, avoidance of pressure on grafted area); maintain needed immobility; comply with weight-bearing restriction if surgery performed. Change dressings using aseptic technique to promote healing and prevent cross-contamination.

- Monitor general health and nutrition of patient.
- Provide a balanced diet high in protein and vitamin C to ensure positive nitrogen balance and promote healing; encourage adequate hydration.

🏠 Promoting Home and Community-Based Care

Teaching Patients Self-Care

- Teach patient and family the importance of strict adherence to the therapeutic regimen of antibiotics and prevention of falls or other injury that could result in bone fracture.
- Teach patients how to maintain and manage the intravenous access and intravenous administration equipment.
- Provide in-depth medication education (eg, drug name, dosage, frequency, administration rate), including laboratory monitoring.
- Instruct the patient to observe and report odor, increased inflammation, elevated temperature, drainage, adverse reactions, and signs of superinfection.
- Teach patient and family how to perform aseptic dressing changes and warm compress techniques.

Continuing Care

- Complete home assessment to determine patient's and family's abilities regarding continuation of the therapeutic regimen.
- Refer for a home care nurse if indicated.
- Monitor the patient for response to treatment, signs and symptoms of superinfections, and adverse drug reactions.
- Stress the importance of follow-up health care appointments.

Evaluation

EXPECTED OUTCOMES
- Experiences pain relief
- Increases physical mobility

- Shows absence of infection
- Complies with therapeutic plan

For more information, see Chapter 62 in Smeltzer and Bare: *Brunner and Suddarth's Textbook of Medical-Surgical Nursing,* 9th edition. Philadelphia: Lippincott Williams & Wilkins, 2000.

OSTEOPOROSIS

Osteoporosis is a disorder in which there is a reduction of total bone mass. The rate of bone resorption is greater than the rate of bone formation. The bones become progressively porous, brittle, and fragile, and they fracture easily. Multiple compression fractures of the vertebrae result in skeletal deformity (kyphosis). This kyphosis is frequently associated with loss of height in some postmenopausal women. Patients at risk include postmenopausal women and small-framed, nonobese white women of European ancestry. Risk factors include nutrition and lifestyle choices (eg, smoking, caffeine, and alcohol consumption); genetics; and lack of physical activity. Age-related bone loss begins soon after peak bone mass is achieved (about 35 years of age). Withdrawal of estrogens at menopause or oophorectomy causes accelerated bone resorption, which continues during menopausal years. Endogenous and exogenous catabolic agents may contribute to osteoporosis: excessive corticosteroids, Cushing's syndrome, hyperthyroidism, and hyperparathyroidism. Further causes include coexisting medical conditions: malabsorption syndromes, lactose intolerance, renal failure, liver failure, and endocrine disorders. Contributing medications may include isoniazid, heparin, tetracycline, aluminum-containing antacids, furosemide, anticonvulsants, and thyroid supplements. Immobility contributes to the development of osteoporosis.

Diagnostic Evaluation

- Osteoporosis is identified on routine radiograph when there has been 25% to 40% demineralization.

- Laboratory studies, including serum calcium and serum phosphate, and radiographs are used to exclude other diagnoses.
- Dual-energy x-ray absorptiometry (DXA) provide information about spine and hip bone mass.
- Ultrasonic heel-density studies are used for diagnosis and to predict risk for fracture.

Medical Management
- Adequate, balanced diet rich in calcium and vitamin D
- May increase calcium intake in adolescence, young adulthood, and the middle years, or prescribe a calcium supplement with meals or high vitamin C beverages
- Hormone replacement therapy (HRT) to retard bone loss
- Regular weight-bearing exercise to promote bone formation
- Other medications: calcitonin, alendronate (Fosamax)

Nursing Management: The Patient With a Spontaneous Vertebral Fracture Related to Osteoporosis
Assessment
- To identify patient's risk for and recognition of problems associated with osteoporosis, interview patient regarding family history, previous fractures, dietary intake of calcium and caffeine, exercise patterns, onset of menopause, and use of steroids, alcohol, or cigarettes.
- Observe for fracture, kyphosis of the thoracic spine, or shortened stature upon physical examination.

Major Nursing Diagnoses
- Knowledge deficit about the osteoporotic process and treatment regimen
- Pain related to fracture and muscle spasm
- Constipation related to immobility or development of ileus
- Risk for injury: fracture related to osteoporotic bone

Planning and Goals

The major goals of the patient may include knowledge about osteoporosis and the treatment regimen, relief of pain, improved bowel elimination, and absence of additional fracture.

Nursing Interventions

UNDERSTANDING OSTEOPOROSIS AND THE TREATMENT REGIMEN

- Focus patient teaching on factors influencing the development of osteoporosis, interventions to slow or arrest the process, and measures to relieve symptoms.
- Inform patient about adequate dietary or supplemental calcium, regular weight-bearing exercise, and modification of lifestyle (ie, reduced use of caffeine, smoking and alcohol cessation).
- Emphasize exercise and physical activity to develop high-density bones.
- Inform patient about foods high in calcium, such as skim or whole milk, swiss cheese, canned salmon with bones.
- Encourage taking calcium supplements with meals and adequate fluids.
- Inform patients that at menopause, HRT may be prescribed, or that aldendronate should be taken on an empty stomach.
- Inform patient that estrogen therapy has been associated with a slightly increased incidence of breast and endometrial cancer; patient must examine her breasts monthly and have regular pelvic examinations.
- Inform elderly patients to continue to take sufficient calcium, vitamin D, sunshine, and exercise to minimize the process.

RELIEVING PAIN

- Teach relief of back pain through bed rest and use of a firm, nonsagging mattress, knee flexion, local heat, and back rubs.

- Instruct patient to move the trunk as a unit and avoid twisting; encourage good posture and good body mechanics.
- Apply lumbosacral corset for immobilization and temporary support when out of bed.

IMPROVING BOWEL ELIMINATION
- Encourage a high-fiber diet, increased fluids, and use of prescribed stool softeners.
- Monitor patient's intake, bowel sounds, and bowel activity; ileus may develop if the vertebral collapse involves T10 to L2 vertebrae.

PREVENTING INJURY
- Promote physical activity to strengthen muscles, prevent disuse atrophy, and retard progressive bone demineralization.
- Encourage isometric exercises to strengthen trunk muscles.
- Encourage walking, good body mechanics, and good posture.
- Avoid sudden bending, jarring, and strenuous lifting.
- Encourage outdoor activity in the sunshine to enhance body's ability to produce vitamin D.

🍁 Gerontologic Considerations

Elderly people fall frequently as a result of environmental hazards, neuromuscular disorders, diminished senses, and cardiovascular responses to medications.

Identify and eliminate harmful environmental hazards that may cause the elderly patient to fall; include the patient and family in planning for continued care and preventive management regimens.

Assess home environment for potential hazards, such as scatter rugs, pets under foot, and cluttered rooms. Create a safe, well-lit environment, including grab-bars in the bathroom and properly fitting footwear.

Evaluation

EXPECTED OUTCOMES

- Acquires knowledge about osteoporosis and the treatment regimen
- Achieves pain relief
- Demonstrates normal bowel elimination
- Experiences no new fractures

For more information, see Chapter 62 in Smeltzer and Bare: *Brunner and Suddarth's Textbook of Medical-Surgical Nursing,* 9th edition. Philadelphia: Lippincott Williams & Wilkins, 2000.

OTITIS MEDIA, ACUTE

Acute otitis media is an acute infection of the middle ear usually lasting less than 6 weeks. The primary cause is the entrance of pathogenic bacteria into the normally sterile middle ear when there is eustachian tube dysfunction, that is, obstruction caused by upper respiratory infections, inflammation of surrounding structures (sinusitis), or allergic reactions (allergic rhinitis). Causative organisms are *Streptococcus pneumoniae, Haemophilus influenzae,* and *Moraxella catarrhalis.* Mode of entry of the bacteria is the eustachian tube from contaminated secretions in the nasopharynx, and middle ear from a tympanic membrane perforation.

Clinical Manifestations

- Vary with the severity of the infection and may be either mild and transient or severe
- Usually unilateral in adults
- Pain in and about the ear (otalgia), which may be intense and relieved only after spontaneous perforation of the eardrum or after myringotomy
- Fever; drainage from the ear
- Tympanic membrane that is erythematous and often bulging or perforated

- Conductive hearing loss due to exudate in the middle ear

Medical and Nursing Management

- The outcome is dependent on (1) the efficiency of antibiotic therapy, (2) the virulence of the bacteria, and (3) the physical status of the patient.
- With early and appropriate broad-spectrum antibiotic therapy, otitis media may clear with no serious sequelae.
- Patient must take prescribed doses of antibiotic and all of the prescribed medication.
- If the condition becomes subacute (3 weeks to 3 months) with purulent discharge, it is rare that it is accompanied by permanent hearing loss.
- Perforation of the tympanic membrane may persist and develop into chronic otitis media.
- Secondary complications involve the mastoid (mastoiditis), meningitis, or brain abscess (rare but can occur).

Myringotomy (Tympanotomy)

- An incision is made into the tympanic membrane to relieve pressure and to drain serous or purulent fluid from the middle ear.
- If mild cases of otitis media are treated effectively, a myringotomy may not be necessary.

For more information, see Chapter 55 in Smeltzer and Bare: *Brunner and Suddarth's Textbook of Medical-Surgical Nursing,* 9th edition. Philadelphia: Lippincott Williams & Wilkins, 2000.

OTITIS MEDIA, CHRONIC

Chronic otitis media results from repeated episodes of acute otitis media, causing irreversible tissue pathology and persistent perforation of the eardrum. Chronic infections of the middle ear cause damage to the tympanic membrane, can destroy the ossicles, and can involve the mastoid.

Clinical Manifestations

- Symptoms may be minimal with varying degrees of hearing loss and presence of a persistent or intermittent foul-smelling discharge.
- Pain may be present if acute mastoiditis occurs.
- When accompanying mastoiditis is present, postauricular area is tender to touch; erythema and edema may be present.
- Cholesteatoma (sac filled with degenerated skin and sebaceous material) may be present as a white mass behind the tympanic membrane.
- If left untreated, cholesteatoma continues to grow and causes facial nerve or horizontal canal damage or destruction of other surrounding structures.

Medical Management

- Careful cleansing of the ear and instillation of antibiotic drops or application of antibiotic powder
- Tympanoplasty procedures to prevent recurrent infection, reestablish middle ear function, close the perforation, and improve hearing
- Mastoidectomy to remove the cholesteatoma
- Ossiculoplasty to reconstruct the middle ear bones to restore hearing

Nursing Management

See Nursing Management under Mastoiditis for additional information.

For more information, see Chapter 55 in Smeltzer and Bare: *Brunner and Suddarth's Textbook of Medical-Surgical Nursing,* 9th edition. Philadelphia: Lippincott Williams & Wilkins, 2000.

P

PANCREATITIS, ACUTE

Pancreatitis (inflammation of the pancreas) is a serious disorder that can range in severity from a relatively mild, self-limiting disorder to a rapidly fatal disease that does not respond to any treatment.

Acute pancreatitis is an autodigestion of this organ by the enzymes it produces, principally trypsin. Common causes of acute episodes are biliary tract disease and long-term alcohol use; 5% of patients with gallstones develop pancreatitis. Other, less common forms include bacterial or viral infection, with pancreatitis as a complication. There are many disease processes and conditions that have been associated with an increased incidence of pancreatitis: surgery on or near the pancreas, medications, hypercalcemia, and hyperlipidemia. Ten to 30% of the cases are idiopathic, and there is a small incidence of hereditary pancreatitis. Mortality is high because of shock, anoxia, hypotension, or fluid and electrolyte imbalances. Complete recovery may occur, or the condition may become chronic.

Clinical Manifestations
Severe abdominal pain is the major symptom.

- Pain in the mid-epigastrium
- Frequently acute in onset (24 to 48 hours after a heavy meal or alcohol ingestion)
- May be more severe after meals and unrelieved by antacids

- May be accompanied by abdominal distention, poorly defined palpable abdominal mass, and decreased peristalsis
- Patient appears acutely ill
- Abdominal guarding; rigid or boardlike abdomen
- Soft abdomen in the absence of peritonitis
- Ecchymosis in the flank or around the umbilicus, which may indicate severe hemorrhagic pancreatitis
- Nausea and vomiting, fever, jaundice, mental confusion, agitation
- Hypotension related to hypovolemia and shock
- Acute renal failure common
- May develop tachycardia, cyanosis, and cold, clammy skin
- Respiratory distress and hypoxia
- Dyspnea
- Tachypnea
- Abnormal blood-gas values
- Diffuse pulmonary infiltrates
- Myocardial depression, hypocalcemia, hyperglycemia, and disseminated intravascular coagulation (DIC)

Diagnostic Evaluation
- Diagnosis is based on history of abdominal pain, known risk factors, and selected diagnostic findings.
- Serum amylase and serum lipase levels are most indicative.

Medical Management
Acute Phase
During the acute phase, management is symptomatic and directed toward preventing or treating complications.

- Oral intake is withheld to inhibit pancreatic stimulation and secretion of pancreatic enzymes.
- Total parenteral nutrition (TPN) is administered to the debilitated patient.
- Nasogastric suction is used to relieve nausea and vomiting, decrease painful abdominal distention and paralytic

ileus, and remove hydrochloric acid so that it does not stimulate the pancreas.

- Cimetidine (Tagamet) is given to decrease hydrochloric acid secretion.
- Adequate pain medication is administered; morphine and morphine derivatives are avoided because they cause spasm of the sphincter of Oddi.
- Adequate correction of fluid, blood loss, and low albumin levels is necessary.
- Antibiotics are administered if infection is present.
- Insulin is necessary if significant hyperglycemia occurs.
- Aggressive respiratory care is provided for pulmonary infiltrates, effusion, and atelectasis.
- Biliary drainage results in decreased pain and increased weight gain.
- Surgical intervention is required for diagnosis, drainage, resection, or débridement.

Postacute Phase

- Antacids are given when the acute episode begins to resolve.
- Oral feedings low in fat and protein are initiated gradually.
- Caffeine and alcohol are eliminated.
- Medications (eg, thiazide diuretics, glucocorticoids, or oral contraceptives) are discontinued.

Nursing Management
Assessment

- Assess presence and character of pain, its relationship to eating and to alcohol consumption; note effect of patient's efforts to obtain pain relief.
- Assess nutritional fluid status and history of gallbladder attacks and alcohol use.
- Elicit history of gastrointestinal problems: fatty stools, diarrhea, nausea, and vomiting.
- Assess respiratory status, including rate, pattern, and breath sounds.

P

- Assess abdomen for pain, tenderness, guarding, and bowel sounds; note boardlike or soft abdomen.

Major Nursing Diagnoses
- Severe pain and discomfort related to edema, distention of the pancreas, and peritoneal irritation.
- Altered nutrition: less than body requirements related to inadequate dietary intake, impaired absorption, reduced food intake, and increased metabolic demands.
- Ineffective breathing pattern related to severe pain, pulmonary infiltrates, pleural fusion, and atelectasis.

Collaborative Problems/Potential Complications
- Fluid and electrolyte disturbances
- Necrosis of the pancreas
- Shock and multiple organ failure

Planning and Goals
The major goals of the patient include relief of pain and discomfort, improved fluid and nutritional status, improved respiratory function, and absence of complications.

Nursing Interventions
RELIEVING PAIN AND DISCOMFORT
- Administer meperidine (Demerol) as ordered (drug of choice).
- Avoid morphine sulfate because it causes spasm of the sphincter of Oddi.
- Withhold oral fluids to decrease formation and secretion of secretin.
- Use nasogastric suctioning to remove gastric secretions and relieve abdominal distention; avoid tension on tube, and use water-soluble lubricant around nares; give frequent oral hygiene.
- Maintain patient on bed rest to decrease metabolic rate and reduce secretion of pancreatic enzymes; report increased pain (may be pancreatic hemorrhage or inadequate analgesic dosage).

• Provide adequate explanations about treatment; patient may have clouded sensorium from pain, fluid imbalances, and hypoxemia.

IMPROVING NUTRITIONAL STATUS
• Monitor laboratory test results, daily weights, and anthropometric measures.
• Assess nutritional status and increased metabolic requirements (note increased body temperature, restlessness, increased physical activity) and fluid lost through diarrhea.
• Provide mouth care; NPO during an attack.
• Administer fluids, electrolytes, and TPN as prescribed.
• Monitor serum glucose level, and give insulin as prescribed.
• Introduce oral feedings gradually as symptoms subside.
• Avoid heavy meals, alcoholic beverages, excessive use of coffee, and spicy foods.

PROMOTING WOUND CARE
• Assess the wound, drainage sites, and skin carefully for signs of infection, inflammation, and breakdown.
• Carry out wound care as prescribed, and take precautions to protect intact skin from contact with drainage; consult with an enterostomal therapist as needed to identify appropriate skin care devices and protocols.
• Turn the patient every 2 hours; use of specialty beds may be indicated to prevent skin breakdown.

IMPROVING RESPIRATORY FUNCTION
• Maintain patient in semi-Fowler's position to decrease pressure on diaphragm.
• Change position frequently to prevent atelectasis and pooling of respiratory secretions.
• Administer anticholinergic medications to decrease gastric and pancreatic secretions; dry respiratory tract secretions.
• Assess respiratory status frequently, and teach patient techniques of coughing and deep breathing.

MONITORING AND MANAGING COMPLICATIONS
Fluid and Electrolyte Disturbances
- Assess fluid and electrolyte status by noting skin turgor and moistness of mucous membranes.
- Weigh daily; measure all fluid intake and output.
- Assess for factors that may affect fluid and electrolyte status: fever, fluid loss through diarrhea, vomiting, nasogastric suctioning, or wound drainage.
- Observe for ascites, and measure abdominal girth.
- Administer intravenous fluids, electrolytes, blood, and albumin to maintain volume and prevent or treat shock.
- Assist patient to turn and change positions every 2 hours.
- Report decreased blood pressure, reduced urine output, and low serum calcium and magnesium.

Pancreatic Necrosis
- Transfer patient to intensive care unit for close monitoring.
- Administer fluids, medications, and blood products.
- Assist with supportive management, such as ventilator.
- Attend to the patient's physical and psychological care.

Shock and Multiple Organ Failure
- Monitor patient closely for early signs of neurologic, cardiovascular, renal, and respiratory dysfunction.
- Prepare for rapid changes in patient status, treatment, and therapies; respond quickly.
- Inform family of status and progress of patient; allow time with patient.

🏠 Promoting Home and Community-Based Care

Teaching Patients Self-Care
- Provide patient and family with facts and explanations of the acute phase of illness; provide necessary repetition and reinforcement.
- Reinforce the need for a low-fat diet, avoidance of heavy meals, and avoidance of alcohol.
- Provide additional explanations on dietary modifications if biliary tract disease is the cause.

Continuing Care

- Refer for home care (often indicated).
- Provide information about resources and support groups, particularly if alcohol is the cause of acute pancreatitis.
- Permit patient and family to discuss their questions and concerns, and provide education and emotional support.

Evaluation

EXPECTED OUTCOMES
- Reports relief of pain and discomfort
- Experiences improved respiratory function
- Achieves nutritional and fluid and electrolyte balance
- Exhibits intact skin
- Remains free of complications

 Gerontologic Considerations

The mortality from acute pancreatitis increases with advancing age. Patterns of complications change with age (eg, the incidence of multiple organ failure increases with age). Close observation of major organ function (lungs and kidneys) is indicated, and aggressive treatment is necessary to reduce mortality in the elderly.

P

For more information, see Chapter 38 in Smeltzer and Bare: *Brunner and Suddarth's Textbook of Medical-Surgical Nursing*, 9th edition. Philadelphia: Lippincott Williams & Wilkins, 2000.

PANCREATITIS, CHRONIC

Chronic pancreatitis is an inflammatory disorder characterized by a progressive anatomic and functional destruction of the pancreas. Cells are replaced by fibrous tissue with repeat attacks of pancreatitis. The end result is mechanical obstruction of the pancreatic and common bile ducts and duodenum. In addition, inflammation and destruction of the secreting cells of the pancreas occur. Alcohol consumption in Western societies and malnutrition worldwide are the major causes. Among alcoholics, the incidence of pancreatitis is 50 times the rate in the nondrinking population. Chronic consumption of alcohol produces hypersecretion of protein in pancreatic secretions. The result is protein plugs and calculi within the pancreatic ducts. Alcohol has a direct toxic effect on the cells of the pancreas. Damage is more severe in patients with diets low in protein and high or low in fat.

Clinical Manifestations
- Recurring attacks of severe upper abdominal and back pain, accompanied by vomiting; narcotics may not provide relief.
- There may be continuous severe pain or dull, nagging, constant pain.
- Risk of addiction to opiates is high because of the severe pain.
- Weight loss is a major problem.
- Altered digestion (malabsorption) of foods (proteins and fats) results in frequent, frothy, and foul-smelling stools with a high fat content (steatorrhea).
- As disease progresses, calcification of the gland may occur, and calcium stones may form within the ducts.

Diagnostic Evaluation
- Endoscopic retrograde cholangiopancreatography (ERCP) is the most useful study.
- A glucose tolerance test evaluates pancreatic islet cell function.

Medical Management
- Treatment is directed toward prevention and management of acute attacks.
- Pain and discomfort are relieved with analgesics.
- The patient should avoid alcohol and other foods that produce abdominal pain and discomfort.

- No other treatment will relieve pain if patient continues to consume alcohol.
- Diabetes mellitus resulting from dysfunction of pancreatic islet cells is treated with diet, insulin, or oral hypoglycemic agents.
- Patient and family members are taught the hazard of severe hypoglycemia related to alcohol use.
- Pancreatic enzyme replacement therapy is instituted for malabsorption and steatorrhea.
- Surgery is done to relieve abdominal pain and discomfort, restore drainage of pancreatic secretions, and reduce frequency of attacks.
- Morbidity and mortality after surgical procedures are high because of the poor physical condition before surgery and concomitant occurrence of cirrhosis.

Nursing Management

See Nursing Management under Pancreatitis, Acute for treatment guidelines.

For more information, see Chapter 38 in Smeltzer and Bare: *Brunner and Suddarth's Textbook of Medical-Surgical Nursing,* 9th edition. Philadelphia: Lippincott Williams & Wilkins, 2000.

P

PARKINSON'S DISEASE

Parkinson's disease is a slowly progressive neurologic disorder affecting the brain centers that are responsible for control and regulation of movement. Dopamine stores are lost in the substantia nigra and the corpus striatum because of a degeneration process. Regional cerebral blood flow is reduced, and there is a high prevalence of dementia. Biochemical and pathologic data suggest that demented patients with Parkinson's may have coexistent Alzheimer's disease. The cause of the disease is mostly unknown. The disease usually first appears in the fifth decade of life and is the fourth most common neurodegenerative disease.

Clinical Manifestations
Chief Manifestations
- Impaired movement: bradykinesia (slowness of movement); difficulty in initiating, maintaining, and performing motor activities; muscular stiffness or rigidity
- Resting tremors: a slow, unilateral turning of the forearm and hand and a pill-rolling motion of the thumb against the fingers; tremor at rest and increasing with concentration and anxiety
- Muscle weakness
- Hypokinesia, flexed posture, loss of postural reflexes, and the freezing phenomenon

Other Characteristics
- Masklike facial expression
- Loss of postural reflexes: patient stands with head bent forward and walks with propulsive gait (shuffling gait); difficulty pivoting and loss of balance, resulting in risk for falls
- Depression and psychiatric manifestations (personality changes, psychosis, dementia, and confusion)
- Sleep disorders, uncontrolled sweating, orthostatic hypotension, gastric and urinary retention, and constipation

Diagnostic Evaluation
- Patient's history and presence of two of the three cardinal manifestations: tremor, muscle rigidity, and bradykinesia
- Positron emission tomography (PET) scanning
- Neurologic examination and response to pharmacologic management

Medical Management
The goal of treatment is to control symptoms and maintain functional independence (no approach prevents disease progression).

Pharmacotherapy

- Levodopa therapy (converts to dopamine), most effective agent to relieve symptoms, usually given in combination with carbidopa (Sinemet), which prevents levodopa breakdown
- Antihistamine drugs for allaying tremors
- Dopamine agonists (eg, pergolide [Permax], bromocriptine mesylate [Parlodel]), used to postpone the initiation of carbidopa and levodopa therapy
- Anticholinergic therapy for controlling the tremor and rigidity
- Amantadine hydrochloride, an antiviral agent, to reduce rigidity, tremor, and bradykinesia
- Monamine oxidase (MAO) inhibitors to inhibit dopamine breakdown
- Antidepressant drugs
- Trials of catechol-O-methyl-transferase (COMT) inhibitors

Surgical Intervention

- Surgery to destroy a part of the thalamus (stereotaxic thalamotomy and pallidotomy) to interrupt nerve pathways and alleviate tremor or rigidity
- Transplantation of neural cells from fetal tissue of human or animal source to reestablish normal dopamine release
- Deep brain stimulation with pacemaker-like brain implants (showing promise though not approved yet by the Food and Drug Administration)

Nursing Management

Assessment

- Note how disease affects the patient's activities of daily living and functional abilities.
- Observe changes in function throughout the day and responses to medication.
- Observe how patient moves about, walks, thinks, speaks, and drinks.

Major Nursing Diagnoses
- Impaired physical mobility related to muscle rigidity and motor weakness
- Self-care deficits (eating, drinking, dressing, hygiene) related to tremor and motor disturbance
- Constipation related to medication and reduced activity
- Altered nutrition: less than body requirements related to tremor, slowness in eating, difficulty in chewing and swallowing
- Impaired verbal communication related to decreased speech volume, slowness of speech, inability to move facial muscles
- Ineffective coping related to depression and dysfunction due to disease progression
- Sleep pattern disturbances, knowledge deficit, pneumonia, ineffective family coping, alteration in thought processes, and risk for injury

Planning and Goals
Patient goals may include improvement of mobility, maintenance of independence in activities of daily living, achievement of adequate bowel elimination, attainment and maintenance of acceptable nutritional status, achievement of effective communication, and development of positive coping mechanisms.

Nursing Interventions
IMPROVING MOBILITY
- Help patient plan progressive program of daily exercise to increase muscle strength, improve coordination and dexterity, reduce muscular rigidity, and prevent contractures.
- Encourage exercises for joint mobility (eg, stationary bike, walking).
- Instruct in stretching and range-of-motion exercises to increase joint flexibility.
- Postural exercises counter the tendency of the head and neck to be drawn forward and down. Teach patient to walk erect, watch horizon, use a wide-based gait, swing

arms with walking, walk heel-toe, and practice marching to music.
- Advise patient that warm baths and massage to help relax muscles.

ENHANCING SELF-CARE ACTIVITIES AND ENCOURAGING USE OF ASSISTIVE DEVICES
- Encourage, teach, and support patient during activities of daily living.
- Modify environment to compensate for functional disabilities.
- Enlist assistance of an occupational therapist as indicated.
- Obtain special equipment as needed to assist patient (plate stabilization, nonspill cup, eating utensils with built-up handles).

IMPROVING BOWEL FUNCTION
- Establish a regular bowel routine.
- Increase fluid intake; eat foods with moderate fiber content.
- Provide raised toilet seat to facilitate toilet activities.

IMPROVING SWALLOWING AND NUTRITION
- Facilitate swallowing and prevent aspiration by having patient sit in upright position during meal time.
- Provide semisolid diet with thick liquids that are easier to swallow.
- Remind patient to hold head upright, and make conscious effort to swallow to control buildup of saliva.
- Provide supplementary feeding and, as disease progresses, nasogastric tube feedings.
- Consult a dietitian regarding patient's nutritional needs.
- Monitor patient's weight on a weekly basis.

IMPROVING COMMUNICATION
- Remind patient to face the listener, speak slowly and deliberately, and exaggerate pronunciation of words.
- Instruct patient to speak in short sentences and take a few breaths before speaking.
- Enlist a speech therapist to assist the patient.

SUPPORTING COPING ABILITIES
- Encourage patient to maintain faithful adherence to exercise and walking program; point out activities being maintained through active participation.
- Provide continuous encouragement and reassurance.
- Assist and encourage patient to set achievable goals.
- Encourage patient to carry out daily tasks to retain independence.

Promoting Home and Community-Based Care

Teaching Patients Self-Care
Explain the nature and management of the disease and the importance of assisting the patient to remain as functionally independent as long as possible.

Continuing Care
- Acknowledge the stress the family is under living with a disabled member.
- Include caregiver in planning and counsel to learn stress-reduction techniques.
- Provide family with information about treatment and care to prevent complications.
- Encourage caregiver to obtain periodic relief from responsibilities and to have a yearly health assessment.
- Give family members permission to express feelings of frustration, anger, and guilt.

Evaluation

EXPECTED OUTCOMES
- Strives toward improved mobility
- Progresses toward self-care
- Maintains bowel function
- Attains improved nutritional status
- Achieves a method of communication

For more information, see Chapter 59 in Smeltzer and Bare: *Brunner and Suddarth's Textbook of Medical-Surgical Nursing,* 9th edition. Philadelphia: Lippincott Williams & Wilkins, 2000.

PELVIC INFECTION (PELVIC INFLAMMATORY DISEASE)

Pelvic infection is an inflammatory condition of the pelvic cavity that may involve the fallopian tubes, ovaries, pelvic peritoneum, or pelvic vascular system. Infection may be acute, subacute, recurrent, or chronic and may be localized or widespread. It is usually bacterial but may be caused by a virus, fungus, or parasite. Pathogenic organisms usually enter the body through the vagina and pass through the cervical canal into the uterus and may proceed to one or both fallopian tubes, ovaries, and into the pelvis. It is most commonly caused by sexual transmission but also may be caused by invasive procedures, such as endometrial biopsy, surgical abortion, hysteroscopy, or intrauterine device (IUD) insertion. The most common organisms involved are gonorrhea, chlamydia, and mycoplasma. The infection is usually bilateral. Risk factors include early age at first intercourse, multiple sex partners, frequent intercourse, risky sexual behaviors (intercourse without condoms, history of sexually transmitted diseases).

P

Clinical Manifestations
- Vaginal discharge, lower abdominal pelvic pain, and tenderness after menses; pain increases during voiding or defecating.
- Systemic symptoms include fever, general malaise, anorexia, nausea, headache, and possibly vomiting.
- Intense tenderness is noted on palpation of the uterus or movement of cervix (cervical motion tenderness) during pelvic examination.

Medical Management
- Broad-spectrum antibiotic therapy is instituted.
- Mild to moderate infections are usually treated on an outpatient basis.
- If acutely ill, the patient may require hospitalization.

- Once hospitalized, bed rest, intravenous fluids, and intravenous antibiotic therapy are prescribed; nasogastric intubation and suction are used if ileus is present; vital signs are modified.
- Treatment of sexual partners is necessary to prevent reinfection.

Complications
- Pelvic or generalized peritonitis, abscess formation, strictures, and obstruction of fallopian tubes
- Adhesions that eventually require removal of the uterus, tubes, and ovaries
- Bacteremia with septic shock and thrombophlebitis with possible embolization

Nursing Management
- Support patient nutritionally, and administer antibiotic therapy as prescribed.
- Note vital signs, characteristics, and amount of vaginal discharge.
- Prevent transmission of infection to others by impeccable use of hand washing, barrier precautions, and hospital guidelines for disposing of biohazardous articles (ie, pad).

Hospitalized Patient
- Maintain on bed rest.
- Place in semi-Fowler's position to facilitate dependent drainage.

🏠 Promoting Home and Community-Based Care
Teaching Patients Self-Care
- Inform patient that IUDs may increase risk for infection and that antibiotics may be prescribed.
- Instruct patient to use proper perineal care, wiping from front to back.
- Instruct patient to avoid douching, which can reduce natural flora.

- Teach patient to consult with health care provider if unusual vaginal discharge or odor is noted.
- Educate patient to maintain optimal health with proper nutrition, exercise, weight control, and safer sex practices (ie, using condoms, avoiding multiple sexual partners).
- Advise patient to have a gynecologic examination at least once a year.
- Evaluate any pelvic pain or abnormal discharge, particularly after sexual exposure, childbirth, or pelvic surgery.
- Instruct patient that before and during intercourse, a partner should wear a condom if there is any chance of transmitting infection.
- Provide information about signs and symptoms of ectopic pregnancy (pain, abnormal bleeding, faintness, dizziness, and shoulder pain).

For more information, see Chapter 43 in Smeltzer and Bare: *Brunner and Suddarth's Textbook of Medical-Surgical Nursing,* 9th edition. Philadelphia: Lippincott Williams & Wilkins, 2000.

P

PEMPHIGUS

Pemphigus is a group of serious diseases of the skin characterized by appearance of bullae (blisters) on apparently normal skin and mucous membranes (mouth, vagina). Evidence indicates that pemphigus is an autoimmune disease involving immunoglobulin G (IgG). The condition may be associated with ingestion of penicillin and captopril and with myasthenia gravis. Genetic factors may also play a role, with the highest incidence in those of Jewish or Mediterranean descent. It occurs with equal frequency in men and women in middle and late adulthood.

Clinical Manifestations
- Most cases present with oral lesions appearing as irregularly shaped erosions that are painful, bleed easily, and heal slowly.

- Skin bullae enlarge, rupture, and leave large, painful eroded areas with crusting and oozing.
- A characteristic offensive odor emanates from the bullae.
- Blistering or sloughing of uninvolved skin occurs when minimal pressure is applied (Nikolsky's sign).
- Eroded skin heals slowly, and eventually huge areas of the body are involved. Fluid and electrolyte imbalance and hypoalbuminemia may result from loss of fluid and protein.
- Bacterial superinfection is common.

Diagnostic Evaluation

Diagnosis is confirmed by histologic examination of a biopsy specimen and immunofluorescent examination of the patient's serum, which show circulating pemphigus antibodies.

Medical Management

Goals of therapy are to bring the disease under control as rapidly as possible, prevent loss of serum and development of secondary infection, and promote reepithelialization of the skin.

- Primary treatment: systemic, oral corticosteroids
- Adjunct therapy: immunosuppressive agents (eg, azathioprine [Imuran], cyclophosphamide [Cytoxan]), gold
- Plasmapheresis, generally reserved for life-threatening cases

Nursing Management

Assessment

- Monitor disease activity by examining skin for appearance of new blisters.
- Assess for signs and symptoms of infection.

Major Nursing Diagnoses

- Pain of oral cavity and skin related to blistering and erosions
- Impaired skin integrity related to ruptured bullae and denuded areas of the skin

- Anxiety and ineffective coping related to appearance of the skin and no hope of a cure
- Knowledge deficit about medications and side effects

Collaborative Problems/Potential Complications
- Infection and sepsis related to loss of protective barrier of skin and mucous membranes
- Fluid volume deficit and electrolyte imbalance related to loss of tissue fluids

Planning and Goals
The major goals may include relief of discomfort from lesions, skin healing, reduced anxiety, improved coping capacity, and absence of complications.

Nursing Interventions
RELIEVING ORAL DISCOMFORT
- Provide meticulous oral hygiene for cleanliness and regeneration of epithelium.
- Provide frequent prescribed mouthwashes to rinse mouth of debris.
- Avoid commercial mouthwashes.
- Keep lips moist with lanolin, petrolatum, or lip balm.
- Humidify environmental air.

ENHANCING SKIN INTEGRITY
- Provide cool, wet dressings or baths (protective and soothing).
- Premedicate with analgesics before skin care is initiated.
- Dry patient's skin carefully, and dust with nonirritating powder.
- Avoid use of tape, which may produce more blisters.
- Keep patient warm to avoid hypothermia.
See Nursing Management under Burn Injury for additional information.

REDUCING ANXIETY
- Demonstrate a warm and caring attitude; allow patient to express anxieties, discomfort, and feelings of hopelessness.

- Educate patient and family regarding the disease.
- Refer to psychological counseling as needed.

MONITORING AND MANAGING POTENTIAL COMPLICATIONS: INFECTION AND SEPSIS

- Keep skin clean to eliminate debris and dead skin and to prevent infection.
- Inspect oral cavity for secondary infections and *Candida albicans* infection from high-dose steroid therapy; report if noted.
- Investigate all "trivial" complaints or minimal changes because corticosteroids mask typical symptoms of infection.
- Monitor for temperature fluctuations and chills; secretions and excretions are monitored for changes suggestive of infection.
- Administer antimicrobials as prescribed, and note response to treatment.
- Employ effective hand-washing techniques for health care personnel; use protective isolation measures and standard precautions.
- Avoid environmental contamination (have housekeeping department dust with a damp cloth and wash floor with a wet mop).

ACHIEVING FLUID AND ELECTROLYTE BALANCE

- Administer saline infusion for sodium chloride depletion.
- Administer blood component therapy to maintain blood volume and hemoglobin and plasma protein concentrations if necessary.
- Encourage adequate oral intake.
- Monitor serum albumin, hemoglobin, hematocrit, and protein levels.
- Provide cool, nonirritating fluids (grape or apple juice) for hydration; provide small, frequent feedings of high-protein, high-calorie foods and snacks.
- Provide total parenteral nutrition if unable to eat.

Promoting Home and Community-Based Care

- Encourage continuing therapy because disease is characterized by recurrent relapses.
- Monitor for side effects of cortisone regularly.
- Encourage patient to report for health-care follow-up regularly.

Evaluation

EXPECTED OUTCOMES

- Achieves relief from pain of oral lesions
- Achieves skin healing
- Experiences decreased anxiety and increased ability to cope
- Experiences no infection
- Experiences no complications

For more information, see Chapter 52 in Smeltzer and Bare: *Brunner and Suddarth's Textbook of Medical-Surgical Nursing,* 9th edition. Philadelphia: Lippincott Williams & Wilkins, 2000.

P

PEPTIC ULCER

A peptic ulcer is an excavation formed in the mucosal wall of the stomach, pylorus, duodenum, or esophagus. It is frequently referred to as a *gastric, duodenal,* or *esophageal ulcer,* depending on its location. It is caused by the erosion of a circumscribed area of mucous membrane. Peptic ulcers are more likely to be in the duodenum than in the stomach. They tend to occur singly, but there may be several present at one time. Chronic gastric ulcers usually occur in the lesser curvature of the stomach, near the pylorus. Peptic ulcer has been associated with bacterial infection, such as *Helicobacter pylori* (present in 70% of patients with gastric and 95% of patients with duodenal ulcers, not associated with esophageal ulcers). The greatest frequency is noted in people between the ages of 40 and 60 years. After menopause, the incidence among women is almost equal to that in men. Predisposing factors include family history of peptic ulcer, blood type O, chronic use of nonsteroidal anti-inflammatory drugs (NSAIDs), alcohol ingestion, excessive smoking, and possibly high stress. Esophageal ulcers result from backward flow of hydrochloric acid from the stomach into the esophagus.

Zollinger-Ellison syndrome (gastrinoma) is suspected when a patient presents with severe peptic ulcer or ulcer that is resistant to standard medical therapy. This syndrome involves extreme gastric hyperacidity (hypersecretion of gastric juice), duodenal ulcer, and gastrinomas (islet cell tumors, which are gastrin-secreting, benign, or malignant tumors of the pancreas). Ninety percent of tumors are found in the gastric triangle. About one third of gastrinomas are malignant. Diarrhea and steatorrhea (unabsorbed fat in the stool) may be evident. These patients may have coexistent parathyroid adenomas or hyperplasia and exhibit signs of hypercalcemia. The patient's most frequent complaint is epigastric pain. The presence of *H. pylori* is not a risk factor.

Stress ulcer is a term given to acute mucosal ulceration of the duodenal or gastric area that occurs after physiologically stressful events, such as burns, shock, severe sepsis (particularly in ventilator-dependent posttraumatic or postsurgical patients), and multiple organ trauma. Fiberoptic endoscopy within 24 hours of injury shows shallow erosions of the stomach wall; by 72 hours, multiple gastric erosions are observed, and as the stressful condition continues, the ulcers spread. When the patient recovers, the lesions are reversed; this pattern is typical of stress ulceration.

Clinical Manifestations

- Symptoms of duodenal ulcer (most common peptic ulcer) may last days, weeks, or months and may even disappear only to reappear without cause. Many patients have asymptomatic ulcers.

- Dull, gnawing pain and a burning sensation in the mid-epigastrium or in the back are characteristic.
- Pain is relieved by eating or taking alkali; once the stomach has emptied or the alkali wears off, the pain returns.
- Sharply localized tenderness is elicited by gentle pressure on the epigastrium or slightly right of the midline; some relief is obtained with local pressure to the epigastrium.
- Also seen are pyrosis (heartburn) and a burning sensation in the esophagus and stomach, which moves up to the mouth, occasionally with sour eructation (burping).
- Vomiting is rare in uncomplicated duodenal ulcer; it may or may not be preceded by nausea and usually follows a bout of severe pain and bloating; it is relieved by ejection of the acid gastric contents.
- Constipation or diarrhea may result from diet and medications.
- Bleeding (25% of patients with gastric ulcers) and tarry stools may occur; a small portion of patients who bleed from an acute ulcer have no previous digestive complaints but develop symptoms later.

Diagnostic Evaluation
Diagnostic tests include endoscopy, stool specimens for occult blood, gastric secretory studies, and biopsy and histology with culture to determine presence of *H. pylori* (there is also a breath test for *H. pylori*).

Medical Management
The goals are to eradicate *H. pylori* and manage gastric acidity.

Stress Reduction and Rest
- The patient may identify situations that are stressful or exhausting (eg, rushed lifestyle and irregular schedules).
- The patient may benefit from suggestions regarding regular rest periods during the day, during acute phase of the disease.
- Biofeedback, hypnosis, or behavioral modification may be used.

Smoking Cessation
- Acidity of the duodenum is higher with smoking.
- Cigarette smoking significantly inhibits ulcer repair.
- The patient is strongly encouraged to stop smoking; support groups are helpful.

Dietary Modification
- Patients should eat whatever agrees with them; small, frequent meals are not necessary if antacid or histamine blocker is taken.
- Oversecretion and hypermotility of the gastrointestinal tract can be minimized by avoiding extremes of temperature and overstimulation by meat extracts. Alcohol, caffeinated beverages, coffee (including decaffeinated coffee, which stimulates acid secretion) should be avoided.
- The patient should eat three regular meals a day.
- Diets rich in milk and cream should be avoided because they are potent acid stimulators.

Pharmacologic Therapy
- Antibiotics combined with bismuth salts to suppress *H. pylori* bacteria
- H_2-receptor antagonists to decrease acid secretion in stomach; proton pump inhibitors (in high doses in patients with Zollinger-Ellison syndrome)
- Cytoprotective agents (protect mucosal cells from acid or NSAIDs)
- Antacids in combination with cimetidine (Tagamet) or ranitidine (Zantac) for treatment of stress ulcer and for prophylactic use
- Anticholinergics (inhibit acid secretion)

Duration of Treatment
- Patient should adhere to the drug program to ensure complete healing of the ulcer.
- Maintenance doses of H_2-receptor antagonists are usually recommended for 1 year.

Surgical Intervention

- With the advent of H_2-receptor antagonists, surgical intervention is less common.
- Surgery is recommended for intractable ulcers (particularly with Zollinger-Ellison syndrome), life-threatening hemorrhage, perforation, or obstruction.
- Surgical procedures include vagotomy, vagotomy with pyloroplasty, or Billroth I or II.

Nursing Management

Assessment

- Assess patient's pain and methods used to relieve it; take a thorough history, including 72-hour food intake history.
- Question whether patient has vomited. Is emesis bright red or coffee ground in appearance?
- Assess presence of blood in the stools. Test for occult blood.
- Ask patient about usual food habits, smoking, and level of tension or nervousness.
- Ask how the patient expresses anger (especially at work and with family).
- Determine whether the patient is experiencing occupational stress or problems in the family.
- Obtain a family history of ulcer disease.
- Assess patient's vital signs for indicators of anemia (tachycardia, hypotension).
- Palpate the abdomen for localized tenderness.
- Assess for malnutrition and weight loss.

Major Nursing Diagnoses

- Pain related to the effect of gastric acid secretion on damaged tissue.
- Anxiety related to coping with an acute disease.
- Knowledge deficit about prevention of symptoms and management of the condition.

P

Collaborative Problems/Potential Complications
- Hemorrhage: upper gastrointestinal
- Perforation
- Pyloric obstruction (gastric outlet obstruction)

Planning and Goals
The major goals of the patient may include relief of pain, reduction of anxiety, maintenance of nutritional requirements, acquisition of knowledge about management and prevention of ulcer recurrence, and absence of potential complications.

Nursing Interventions
RELIEVING PAIN
- Administer prescribed medications.
- Avoid aspirin and foods and beverages that contain caffeine (colas, tea, coffee, chocolate).
- Encourage regularly spaced meals in a relaxed atmosphere.
- Encourage relaxation techniques, and assist patient to cope with stress and pain and to stop smoking.

REDUCING ANXIETY
- Assess what the patient wants to know about the disease, and evaluate level of anxiety; encourage patient to express fears openly and without criticism.
- Explain diagnostic tests; administer medications on schedule.
- Assure patient that nurses are always available to help with problems.
- Interact in a relaxing manner, help in identifying stressors, and explain effective coping techniques and relaxation methods.
- Encourage participation of the patient's family in care, and give emotional support.

MONITORING AND MANAGING COMPLICATIONS: HEMORRHAGE
- Assess for faintness or dizziness and nausea, before or with bleeding.

- Test stool for occult or gross blood.
- Monitor vital signs frequently (tachycardia, hypotension, and tachypnea).
- Monitor intake and output.
- Insert and maintain an intravenous line for infusion of fluid and blood.
- Monitor laboratory values (hemoglobin and hematocrit).
- Insert and maintain a nasogastric tube and monitor drainage; provide lavage as ordered.
- Treat hypovolemic shock as indicated (see Nursing Management under Shock for additional information).

MONITORING FOR PERFORATION
AND PENETRATION
- Note and report symptoms of penetration (back and epigastric pain not relieved by medications that were effective in the past).
- Note and report symptoms of perforation (sudden abdominal pain, referred pain to shoulders, vomiting and collapse, extremely tender and rigid abdomen, hypotension and tachycardia, or other signs of shock).

P

See Preoperative and Postoperative Nursing Management for additional information.

Promoting Home and Community-Based Care

Teaching Patients Self-Care
- Assist the patient in understanding the condition and factors that help or aggravate it.

MEDICATION
- Teach patient what medications are taken at home, including name, dosage, frequency, and possible side effects.
- Teach patient what medications to avoid.

DIET
- Teach patient to be aware of particular foods that are upsetting.

- Instruct patient to avoid coffee, tea, colas, and alcohol, which have acid-producing potential.
- Encourage regular meals in a relaxed setting and avoidance of overeating.

SMOKING
- Teach patient that smoking may interfere with ulcer healing.
- Make patient aware of programs to assist with smoking cessation.

REST AND STRESS REDUCTION
- Help patient to be aware of sources of stress in family and work environments.
- Help patient to identify rest periods during the day.
- Evaluate need for extended psychological counseling.

AWARENESS OF COMPLICATIONS
- Alert patient to signs and symptoms of complications that should be reported.
  ○ Hemorrhage: cool skin, confusion, increased heart rate, labored breathing, blood in stool
  ○ Perforation: severe abdominal pain, rigid and tender abdomen, vomiting, elevated temperature, increased heart rate
  ○ Pyloric obstruction: nausea, vomiting, distended abdomen, abdominal pain

CONTINUING WITH CARE AFTER TREATMENT
- Teach patient that follow-up supervision is necessary for about 1 year.
- Tell patient that the ulcer could recur and to seek medical assistance if symptoms recur.
- Inform patient and family that surgery is no guarantee of cure.
- Discuss possible postoperative sequelae, such as intolerance to dairy products and sweet foods.

Evaluation

EXPECTED OUTCOMES
- Remains free of pain between meals
- Experiences less anxiety by avoiding stress
- Complies with therapeutic regimen
- Experiences no complications

For more information, see Chapter 34 in Smeltzer and Bare: *Brunner and Suddarth's Textbook of Medical-Surgical Nursing,* 9th edition. Philadelphia: Lippincott Williams & Wilkins, 2000.

PERICARDITIS (CARDIAC TAMPONADE)

Pericarditis refers to an inflammation of the pericardium, the membranous sac enveloping the heart. It may be primary, or develop in the course of a variety of medical and surgical disorders. Some causes include idiopathic, infection (bacterial, viral, or fungal), connective tissue disorders, hypersensitivity states, diseases of adjacent structures, neoplastic disease, radiation therapy, trauma, renal disorder association, and tuberculosis.

Clinical Manifestations
- Characteristic symptom is pain and friction rub.
- Pain is felt over the precordium or beneath the clavicle and in the neck and left scapular region.
- Pericardial pain is aggravated by breathing, turning in bed, and twisting body; it is relieved by sitting up (or forward leaning).
- Dyspnea may occur as a result of pericardial compression of the heart's movements.
- The patient may have no signs other than fever, high white blood cell count, and friction rub, or may appear extremely ill.

Cardiac Tamponade

Cardiac tamponade is a life-threatening compression of the heart as a result of fluid within the pericardial sac. It is usually caused by blunt or penetrating trauma to the chest; it may also follow invasive diagnostic cardiac procedures, certain disease processes, and high-dose radiation to the chest.

Clinical Manifestations

- Falling blood pressure, rising venous pressure (distended neck veins), and distant (muffled) heart sounds with pulsus paradoxus
- Anxious, confused, and restless state
- Dyspnea, tachypnea, and precordial pain
- Elevated central venous pressure (CVP)

Diagnostic Evaluation

Diagnosis is based on signs and symptoms, echocardiogram, and electrocardiogram (ECG).

Medical Management

The objectives of management are to determine the cause, to administer therapy for the specific cause (when known), and to watch for cardiac tamponade (compression of the heart from fluid in the pericardial sac).

- Bed rest when cardiac output is impaired, until fever, chest pain, and friction rub have disappeared
- Narcotic analgesics for pain relief during the acute phase
- Analgesics and nonsteroidal antiinflammatory drugs (NSAIDs) to relieve pain and hasten reabsorption of fluid in rheumatic pericarditis
- Corticosteroids to control symptoms, hasten resolution of the inflammatory process, and prevent recurring pericardial effusion
- Penicillin for pericarditis of rheumatic fever
- Isoniazid ethambutol, rifampin, and streptomycin for pericarditis of tuberculosis
- Amphotericin B for fungal pericarditis
- Gradual increase in activity as condition improves

Treatment of Cardiac Tamponade
- Thoracotomy for penetrating cardiac injuries
- Pericardiocentesis

Nursing Management

NURSING ALERT

Nursing assessment skills are key to anticipating and identifying the triad of symptoms of cardiac tamponade: falling arterial pressure, rising venous pressure, and distant heart sounds. Search diligently for a pericardial friction rub.

Assessment
- Assess pain by observation and evaluation while having patient vary positions to determine precipitating or intensifying factors.
- Monitor temperature frequently; pericarditis causes an abrupt onset of fever in a previously afebrile patient.
- Assess pericardial friction rub.
  - Audible on auscultation
  - Synchronous with the heartbeat
  - Best heard at the left sternal edge in the fourth intercostal space where the pericardium comes into contact with the left chest wall
  - Scratchy or leathery sound
  - Louder at the end of expiration and may be best heard with the patient in sitting position
- Note that a pericardial friction rub is continuous, distinguishing it from a pleural friction rub. Ask patient to hold breath to help in differentiation.

Major Nursing Diagnosis
- Pain related to inflammation of the pericardium

Collaborative Problems/Potential Complications
- Pericardial effusion
- Cardiac tamponade

Planning and Goals
The major goals of the patient may include relief of pain and absence of potential complications.

Nursing Interventions

RELIEVING PAIN
- Advise bed rest or chair rest in a sitting-upright and leaning-forward position.
- Instruct the patient to resume activities of daily living as the chest pain and friction rub abate.
- Administer medications; monitor and record responses.
- Instruct the patient to resume bed rest if chest pain and friction rub recur.

MONITORING AND MANAGING
POTENTIAL COMPLICATIONS
- Observe for cardiac tamponade: arterial pressure falls; systolic pressure falls while diastolic pressure remains stable; pulse pressure narrows; heart sounds progress from being distant to imperceptible.
- Observe for neck vein distention and other signs of rising central venous pressure.
- Notify physician immediately upon observing any of the above symptoms, and prepare for pericardiocentesis. Assure patient, and continue to assess and record signs and symptoms until physician arrives.

Evaluation

EXPECTED OUTCOMES
- Is free of pain
- Experiences no complications

For more information, see Chapters 26 and 27 in Smeltzer and Bare: *Brunner and Suddarth's Textbook of Medical-Surgical Nursing,* 9th edition. Philadelphia: Lippincott Williams & Wilkins, 2000.

PERIPHERAL ARTERIAL OCCLUSIVE DISEASE

Arterial insufficiency of the extremities is usually found in patients older than 50 years of age, most often in men, and predominantly in the legs. The age of onset and severity is influenced by the type and number of atherosclerotic risk factors present. Obstructive lesions are predominantly confined to segments of the arterial system extending from the aorta, below the renal arteries, to the popliteal artery.

Clinical Manifestations
Intermittent Claudication
- Claudication, the hallmark of peripheral arterial occlusive disease, is insidious and described as aching, cramping, fatigue, or weakness.
- Rest pain is persistent, aching, or boring and is usually present in distal extremities with severe disease.
- Elevation or horizontal placement of the extremity aggravates the pain; dependency of the extremity reduces pain.

Other Manifestations
- Coldness or numbness in the extremities accompanies intermittent claudication.
- Extremities may be cool and exhibit pallor on elevation or a ruddy, cyanotic color when in a dependent position.
- Skin and nail changes, ulcerations, gangrene, and muscle atrophy are present.
- Bruits may be auscultated.
- Peripheral pulses may be diminished or absent.
- Inequality of pulses between extremities or absence of a normally palpable pulse is a reliable sign of occlusion.
- Nails may be thickened and opaque, and the skin shiny, atrophic, and dry with sparse hair growth.
- Upper extremity occlusions are less symptomatic or asymptomatic.

P

- Patient may report vertigo, ataxia, syncope, and bilateral visual changes.
- Arm fatigue and pain with exercise may be experienced.

Diagnostic Evaluation

- History of symptoms and physical examination (peripheral pulses)
- Imaging studies (eg, continuous wave Doppler device ultrasonic flow studies, angiography, digital subtraction angiography [DSA])
- Treadmill testing for claudication, duplex ultrasound

Medical Management

- Maintain meticulous cleanliness of the feet; wash feet daily, dry carefully, and do not rub with a towel.
- Keep feet warm; protect feet from injury.
- Wear shoes that provide adequate comfort.
- Prevent constriction of blood vessels: do not cross legs; avoid any activity that cuts off blood supply to legs and feet.
- Promote exercise to stimulate circulation and tissue repair.
- Report redness, blistering, swelling, pain, any peeling or itching.
- Avoid tobacco in any form because it aggravates peripheral vascular circulation.
- Exercise programs combined with weight reduction and cessation of smoking often improve patient activity limitations.
- Sympathectomy to improve collateral circulation.
- Vascular grafting or endarterectomy when the limb is at risk for amputation.
- Percutaneous transluminal angioplasty (PTA) for stenosis or occlusion of the vessel (short focal lesion in upper extremity artery).

Nursing Management
Postoperative
The primary objective in postoperative management of patients who have had vascular procedures is to maintain adequate circulation through the arterial repair.

- Check pulses of affected extremity and compare with other every hour for the first 24 hours.
- Disappearance of a pulse may indicate thrombotic occlusion of the graft; notify surgeon immediately.
- Monitor color and temperature of extremity, capillary refill, sensory and motor functions for 24 hours with Doppler pulse elevation of vessels distal to bypass graft and ankle/arm indices every 2 hours, and report changes.

Nursing Interventions
MONITORING AND MANAGING
POTENTIAL COMPLICATIONS
- Monitor urine output (more than 30 mL/h), central venous pressure, mental status, and pulse rate and volume to permit early recognition and treatment of fluid imbalances.
- Instruct patient to avoid leg crossing and prolonged extremity dependence.
- Teach patient to perform leg elevation and to exercise limbs while in bed to reduce edema.
- Monitor for compartment syndrome (severe limb edema, pain, and decreased sensation).

🏠 Promoting Home and Community-Based Care
Teaching Patients Self-Care
- Assess patient's ability to manage independently or availability of family and friends to assist.
- Determine patient's motivation to make lifestyle changes needed with chronic disease.

- Assess patient's knowledge and ability to assess for postoperative complications, such as infection, occlusion of graft, and decreased blood flow.
- Determine if patient has stopped smoking.

For more information, see Chapter 28 in Smeltzer and Bare: *Brunner and Suddarth's Textbook of Medical-Surgical Nursing,* 9th edition. Philadelphia: Lippincott Williams & Wilkins, 2000.

PERITONITIS

Peritonitis is inflammation of the peritoneum, which is usually the result of bacterial infection, with the organisms coming from disease of the gastrointestinal tract, or, in women, the internal reproductive organs. It can also result from external sources, such as injury or trauma or an inflammation from an extraperitoneal organ, such as the kidney. The most common bacteria implicated are *Escherichia coli,* and *Klebsiella, Proteus,* and *Pseudomonas* species. Other common causes are appendicitis, perforated ulcer, diverticulitis, and bowel perforation. Peritonitis may also be associated with abdominal surgical procedures and peritoneal dialysis. Sepsis is the major cause of death from peritonitis (shock, from sepsis or hypovolemia). Intestinal obstruction from bowel adhesions may develop.

Clinical Manifestations

Clinical features depend on the location and extent of inflammation.

- Diffuse type of pain that becomes constant, localized, and more intense near site of the process.
- Pain is aggravated by movement.
- Affected area of the abdomen becomes extremely tender and distended, and muscles become rigid.
- Rebound tenderness and ileus may be present.
- Temperature and pulse increase; leukocyte count is elevated.

Diagnostic Evaluation
- Leukocytes, complete blood count, hemoglobin, hematocrit, and serum electrolytes
- Abdominal radiographs, computed tomography (CT) scan, and peritoneal aspiration with culture and sensitivity studies

Medical Management
- Fluid, colloid, and electrolyte replacement is the major focus of medical management.
- Analgesics are administered for pain; antiemetics are administered for nausea and vomiting.
- Intestinal intubation and suction are used to relieve abdominal distention.
- Oxygen therapy by nasal cannula or mask is instituted to improve ventilatory function.
- Occasionally, airway intubation and ventilatory assistance may be required.
- Massive antibiotic therapy may be instituted (sepsis is the major cause of death).
- Surgical objectives include removal of infected material and are directed toward excision (appendix), resection (intestine), repair (perforation), and drainage (abscess).
- Postoperative complications include wound evisceration and abscess.

Nursing Management
Pain Assessment
- Assess nature of pain, location in the abdomen, and shifts of pain and location.
- Assess vital signs, gastrointestinal function, fluid and electrolyte balance.
- Administer analgesic medication and position for comfort (ie, on side with knees flexed).
- Record intake and output and central venous pressure.
- Administer and monitor intravenous fluids closely.
- Observe and record character of any surgical drainage.
- Observe for decrease in temperature and pulse rate, softening of the abdomen, return of peristaltic sounds,

and passing of flatus and bowel movements, which indicate peritonitis is subsiding.

- Increase food and oral fluids gradually, and decrease parenteral fluid intake when peritonitis subsides.
- Observe and record character of drainage from postoperative wound drains if inserted; take care to avoid dislodging drains.
- Postoperatively, prepare patient and family for discharge; teach care of incision and drains if still in place at discharge.

For more information, see Chapter 35 in Smeltzer and Bare: *Brunner and Suddarth's Textbook of Medical-Surgical Nursing,* 9th edition. Philadelphia: Lippincott Williams & Wilkins, 2000.

PHARYNGITIS, ACUTE

Acute pharyngitis is a febrile inflammation caused by a viral organism 70% of the time. Uncomplicated viral infections usually subside promptly within 3 to 10 days after onset. When caused by bacteria, the most common organism is group A streptococcus ("strep throat"). Pharyngitis caused by streptococcus is a more severe illness because of dangerous complications, including sinusitis, otitis media, mastoiditis, cervical adenitis, rheumatic fever, and nephritis.

Clinical Manifestations
- Fiery, red pharyngeal membrane
- Tonsils and lymphoid follicles swollen and freckled with exudate
- Cervical lymph nodes enlarged and tender
- Fever, malaise, and sore throat
- Hoarseness, cough, and rhinitis

Diagnostic Evaluation
- Rapid screening test for streptococcal antigens, streptolysin titers, and throat cultures
- Nasal swabbings and blood cultures

Medical Management

- Viral pharyngitis is treated with supportive measures.
- Antimicrobial agents are used to treat the bacterial cause: penicillin for group A streptococci and cephalosporins for penicillin allergies or erythromycin resistance.
- Antibiotics are administered for at least 10 days.
- Liquid or soft diet is recommended during the acute stage.
- Intravenous fluids are administered if the patient is unable to swallow owing to sore throat.
- The patient is encouraged to drink if able to swallow (2000 to 3000 mL/day).
- Analgesic medications are given at 3- to 6-hour intervals
- Antitussive medications (codeine, dextromethorphan [Robitussin DM] or hydrocodone [Hycodan]) are given to control persistent and painful cough.

Nursing Management

- Encourage bed rest during febrile stage of illness.
- Implement secretion precautions to prevent spread of infection.
- Examine skin once or twice daily for possible rash because acute pharyngitis may precede some other communicable disease.
- Secure nasal swabbings and throat and blood cultures as needed.
- Administer warm saline gargles or irrigations to ease pain.
- Apply an ice collar for symptomatic relief.
- Administer analgesic drugs or antitussive medications.
- Perform mouth care to prevent fissures of lips and inflammation in the mouth.

P

🏠 Promoting Home and Community-Based Care

- Permit resumption of activity gradually.

- Advise patient of importance of taking the full course of antibiotic therapy.
- Inform patient and family of symptoms to watch for that may indicate development of complications, including nephritis and rheumatic fever.
- Instruct patient regarding purpose and technique for warm gargles (as warm as patient can tolerate) to promote maximum effectiveness.

For more information, see Chapter 20 in Smeltzer and Bare: *Brunner and Suddarth's Textbook of Medical-Surgical Nursing,* 9th edition. Philadelphia: Lippincott Williams & Wilkins, 2000.

PHARYNGITIS, CHRONIC

Chronic pharyngitis is common in adults who work or live in dusty surroundings, use the voice to excess, suffer from chronic cough, and habitually use alcohol and tobacco. Three types are recognized: hypertrophic, a general thickening and congestion of the pharyngeal mucous membranes; atrophic, a late stage of type 1; and chronic granular ("clergyman's sore throat"), with numerous swollen lymph follicles of the pharyngeal wall.

Clinical Manifestations
- Constant sense of irritation or fullness in the throat
- Mucus, which collects in the throat and is expelled by coughing
- Difficulty in swallowing

Medical Management
Treatment is based on symptom relief, avoidance of exposure to irritants, and correction of any upper respiratory, pulmonary, or cardiac condition that might be responsible for chronic cough.

- Nasal installations or sprays to relieve nasal congestion
- Aspirin or acetaminophen to control malaise

Nursing Management

 Promoting Home and Community-Based Care

Teaching Patients Self-Care
- Avoid contact with others until fever has subsided completely to prevent infection from spreading.
- Instruct to avoid the use of alcohol, tobacco, secondhand smoke, and exposure to cold.
- Avoid environmental and occupational pollutants or minimize through use of disposable masks.
- Encourage patient to drink plenty of fluids.
- Encourage gargling with warm saline to relieve throat discomfort and use of lozenges to keep the throat moist.

For more information, see Chapter 20 in Smeltzer and Bare: *Brunner and Suddarth's Textbook of Medical-Surgical Nursing,* 9th edition. Philadelphia: Lippincott Williams & Wilkins, 2000.

PHEOCHROMOCYTOMA

P

A pheochromocytoma is a tumor that usually is benign and originates from the chromaffin cells of the adrenal medulla. In 90% of patients, the tumor arises in the medulla; in the remaining patients, it occurs in the extraadrenal chromaffin tissue located in or near the aorta, ovaries, spleen, or other organs. It occurs at any age, but peak incidence is between 20 and 50 years of age; it affects men and women equally and has familial tendencies. Although uncommon, it is one form of hypertension that is usually cured by surgery; without detection and treatment, it is usually fatal.

Clinical Manifestations
Classic Symptoms
- Headache, diaphoresis, and palpitations (triad of symptoms)
- Blood pressures as high as 350/200 mm Hg

- Hypertension and other cardiovascular disturbances
- Intermittent or persistent hypertension (half of cases difficult to distinguish)
- May precipitate life-threatening complications: cardiac dysrhythmias, dissecting aneurysm, stroke, and acute renal failure
- Postural hypotension in most untreated cases

Other Symptoms
- Tremor
- Flushing
- Anxiety
- Hyperglycemia from epinephrine secretion; may require insulin

Symptoms of the Paroxysmal Form of Pheochromocytoma
- Acute, unpredictable attacks, lasting seconds or several hours, during which patient is extremely anxious, tremulous, and weak
- Headache, vertigo, blurring of vision, tinnitus, air hunger, and dyspnea
- Polyuria, nausea, vomiting, diarrhea, abdominal pain, and feeling of impending doom
- Palpitations and tachycardia

Diagnostic Evaluation
- Catecholamines in 24-hour urine (metanephrine [MN] and vanillylmandelic acid [VMA]) and plasma (norepinephrine and epinephrine) offer the most direct and conclusive test.
- Imaging studies (eg, computed tomography [CT] and magnetic resonance imaging [MRI] scans, ultrasound, ^{131}I-metaiodobenzylguanidine (MIBG) scintigraph to determine location of tumor).

Medical Management
- Preliminary preparation includes effective control of blood pressure and blood volume, carried out over 10

days to 2 weeks (eg, cautious use of alpha-adrenergic blocking agents or beta-adrenergic blockers and smooth muscle relaxants).

- Bed rest is recommended.
- Treatment is surgical removal of the tumor, usually with adrenalectomy (hypertension usually subsides with treatment).
- The patient is hydrated before, during, and after surgery.
- Postoperative corticosteroid replacement is required after bilateral adrenalectomy.
- Patient is monitored for several days in the intensive care unit with attention given to electrocardiogram (ECG) changes, arterial pressures, fluid and electrolyte balance, and blood glucose levels.
- Blood pressure is monitored; hypertension can persist or recur if blood vessels have been damaged or if all pheochromocytoma tissue has not been removed.
- Postoperative urine and plasma levels of catecholamines are measured; when levels return to normal, patient may be discharged.

P

Nursing Management
- Advise bed rest, with head of bed elevated to promote orthostatic decrease in blood pressure.
- Monitor ECG changes.
- Administer alpha-adrenergic blocking agents (phentolamine [Regitine]) or smooth muscle relaxants (sodium nitroprusside [Nipride]) to lower blood pressure.

🏠 Promoting Home and Community-Based Care

Teaching Patients Self-Care
- Encourage patient to schedule follow-up appointments to observe for return of normal blood pressure and serum and urine levels of catecholamines.
- Give verbal and written instructions on collecting 24-hour urine specimen.

- Give instructions regarding long-term steroid therapy, including the risk of skipping doses or stopping their medication abruptly.
- Assess compliance to the medication schedule.
- Teach patient and family how to measure the patient's blood pressure and when to notify the physician about changes in blood pressure.

Continuing Care
- Refer for home care nurse if indicated.
- Reinforce prior teaching about management and monitoring.
- Assist in dealing with problems that may result from long-term steroid use.
- Give encouragement and support because patient may remain fearful of repeated attacks.

For more information, see Chapter 38 in Smeltzer and Bare: *Brunner and Suddarth's Textbook of Medical-Surgical Nursing,* 9th edition. Philadelphia: Lippincott Williams & Wilkins, 2000.

PITUITARY TUMORS

Pituitary tumors are of three principal types, representing an overgrowth of eosinophilic cells, basophilic cells (hyperadrenalism), or chromophobic cells (cells with no affinity for either eosinophilic or basophilic stains).

Clinical Manifestations
Eosinophilic Tumors Developing Early in Life
- Gigantism: patient may be more than 7 feet tall and large in all proportions.
- Patient is weak and lethargic, hardly able to stand.

Eosinophilic Tumors Developing in Adulthood
- Acromegaly (excessive skeletal growth occurs of the feet, hands, superciliary ridges, molar eminences, nose, and chin)

- Enlargement of every tissue and organ of the body
- Severe headaches and visual disturbances because the tumors exert pressure on the optic nerves
- Loss of color discrimination, diplopia (double vision), or blindness of a portion of the field of vision
- Decalcification of the skeleton, muscular weakness, and endocrine disturbances, similar to those occurring in hyperthyroidism

Basophilic Tumors

CUSHING'S SYNDROME
- Masculinization and amenorrhea in females
- Truncal obesity, hypertension, osteoporosis, and polycythemia in males and females

Chromophobic Tumors (90% of Pituitary Tumors)

HYPOPITUITARISM
- Inclined to be obese and somnolent
- Fine, scanty hair; dry, soft skin; pasty complexion; small bones
- Headaches, loss of libido, and visual defects progressing to blindness
- Polyuria, polyphagia, lowering of the basal metabolic rate, and subnormal body temperature

Diagnostic Evaluation

- History and physical examination (visual field assessment)
- Computed tomography (CT) and magnetic resonance imaging (MRI)
- Serum levels of pituitary hormone

Medical Management of Acromegaly or Pituitary Tumors

- Surgical removal through a transphenoidal approach is the treatment of choice.
- Stereotactic radiotherapy is used to deliver an external-beam radiation therapy to the tumor with minimal effect on normal tissue.

- Traditional radiation therapy and use of bromocriptine (dopamine agonist) and octreotide (somatostatin analogue) inhibit production or release of growth hormone.
- Hypophysectomy is used for treatment of primary tumors.

For more information, see Chapter 38 in Smeltzer and Bare: *Brunner and Suddarth's Textbook of Medical-Surgical Nursing,* 9th edition. Philadelphia: Lippincott Williams & Wilkins, 2000.

PLEURAL EFFUSION

Pleural effusion, a collection of fluid in the pleural space, is rarely a primary disease process; it is usually secondary to other diseases (eg, pneumonia, pulmonary infections, nephrotic syndrome, neoplastic tumors, congestive heart failure). The effusion can be relatively clear fluid, which may be a transudate due to altered formation or reabsorption of pleural fluid or an exudate resulting from inflammation by bacterial products on tumors, or it can be blood or pus.

Clinical Manifestations

Some symptoms are caused by the underlying disease. Pneumonia causes fever, chills, and pleuritic chest pain. Malignant effusion may result in dyspnea and coughing. The size of effusion determines the severity of symptoms.

- Dullness or flatness to percussion over areas of fluid, minimal or absence of breath sounds, and tracheal deviation away from the affected side
- Large effusion: shortness of breath to acute respiratory distress
- Small to moderate effusion: dyspnea may not be present

Diagnostic Evaluation

- Chest radiographs

- Ultrasound
- Thoracentesis
- Pleural fluid cultures

Medical Management

The objectives of treatment are to discover the underlying cause, to prevent reaccumulation of fluid, and to relieve discomfort and dyspnea. Specific treatment is directed at the underlying cause.

- Thoracentesis is performed to remove fluid, collect specimen for analysis, and relieve dyspnea.
- Chest tube and water-seal drainage may be necessary for pneumothorax.
- Drugs are instilled into the pleural space to obliterate the space and prevent further accumulation of fluid.
- Other treatment modalities include surgical pleurectomy and diuretic therapy.

Nursing Management

- Implement the medical regimen: prepare and position patient for thoracentesis and offer support throughout the procedure.
- Assist patient in pain relief. Assist patient to assume positions that are least painful. Administer pain medication as prescribed and needed.
- Monitor chest tube drainage and water-seal system; record amount of drainage at prescribed intervals.
- Administer nursing care related to the underlying cause of the pleural effusion.

See Nursing Management under the disorder describing the underlying condition.

P

For more information, see Chapter 21 in Smeltzer and Bare: *Brunner and Suddarth's Textbook of Medical-Surgical Nursing,* 9th edition. Philadelphia: Lippincott Williams & Wilkins, 2000.

PLEURISY

Pleurisy refers to inflammation of both the visceral and parietal pleurae. The result is severe, sharp, knifelike pain with breathing that is intensified on inspiration. Pleurisy may develop with pneumonia or upper respiratory tract infection, tuberculosis, or a collagen disease; after chest trauma, pulmonary infarction, or embolism; in primary and metastatic cancer; and after thoracotomy.

Clinical Manifestations
- Pain usually occurs on one side and worsens with deep breaths, coughing, or sneezing.
- Pain is decreased when the breath is held. Pain is localized, or radiates to the shoulder or abdomen.
- As pleural fluid develops, pain lessens. A friction rub can be auscultated but disappears as fluid accumulates.

Diagnostic Evaluation
- Chest radiographs
- Sputum culture
- Thoracentesis, pleural fluid examination, pleural biopsy (less common)

Medical Management
The objectives of management are to discover the underlying condition causing the pleurisy and to relieve the pain.

- The patient is monitored for signs and symptoms of pleural effusion: shortness of breath, pain, and decreased excursion of the chest.
- Prescribed analgesics and applications of heat or cold are provided for symptomatic relief.
- Nonsteroidal antiinflammatory drugs (NSAIDs) are given for pain relief and effective coughing.
- Procaine intercostal block is done for severe pain.

Nursing Management
Nursing Interventions
- Enhance comfort by turning frequently on affected side to splint chest wall.
- Teach patient to use hands to splint rib cage while coughing.

See Nursing Management under Pneumonia for additional information.

For more information, see Chapter 21 in Smeltzer and Bare: *Brunner and Suddarth's Textbook of Medical-Surgical Nursing,* 9th edition. Philadelphia: Lippincott Williams & Wilkins, 2000.

PNEUMONIA

Pneumonia is an inflammation of the lung parenchyma commonly caused by microbial agents. An inflammatory reaction may occur in the alveoli and produces an exudate that interferes with gas exchange. *Bronchopneumonia,* the most common form, is distributed in a patchy fashion extending from the bronchi to surrounding lung parenchyma. *Lobar pneumonia* is the term used if a substantial part of one or more lobes is involved. Classically, pneumonia has been categorized as either being bacterial or typical, atypical, anaerobic/cavitary, or opportunistic. Another classification scheme categorizes pneumonias as community-acquired, hospital-acquired, pneumonia in the compromised host, and aspiration pneumonia. Those at risk for pneumonia often have chronic underlying disorders, severe acute illness, a suppressed immune system from disease or medications, immobility, and other factors that interfere with normal lung protective mechanisms. The elderly are also at high risk. Pneumonias are caused by a variety of microbial agents in the various settings. Common organisms include *Staphylococcus aureus, Haemophilus influenzae, Staphylococcus pneumoniae,* and enteric gram-negative bacilli, fungi, and viruses (most common in children).

Clinical Manifestations

Clinical features vary depending on the causative organism and patient's disease.

- Sudden chills, rapidly rising fever, and profuse perspiration
- Pleuritic chest pain aggravated by respiration and coughing
- Severely ill with marked tachypnea (25 to 45 minutes) and dyspnea; orthopnea when not propped up
- Pulse rapid and bounding; may increase 10 beats/min per degree of temperature elevation (Celsius)
- A relative bradycardia for the amount of fever suggests viral infection or *Mycoplasma* or *Legionella* species infection
- Sputum purulent, rusty, blood-tinged, viscous, or green relative to etiologic agent
- Other signs: fever, crackles, and signs of lobar consolidation; initial upper respiratory tract symptoms (nasal congestion, sore throat)
- Severe pneumonia: flushed cheeks; lips and nail beds demonstrating central cyanosis

Diagnostic Evaluation
- Primarily history, physical examination
- Chest radiographs, blood and sputum cultures

Medical Management
- Penicillin G is the antibiotic of choice for treatment of *S. pneumoniae.*
- Amantadine and rimantadine also reduce the duration of fever and other systemic complications.
- Supportive treatment includes with hydration, antipyretics, antihistamines, or nasal decongestants.
- Bed rest is recommended until infection shows sign of clearing.

- Oxygen therapy is given for hypoxemia, arterial blood gases (ABGs).
- Respiratory support includes endotracheal intubation, high inspiratory oxygen concentrations, and mechanical ventilation.
- Treatment of atelectasis, pleural effusion, shock, respiration failure, or superinfection is instituted, if needed.

Nursing Management
Assessment
- Assess for fever, chills, night sweats, pain, fatigue, tachypnea, use of accessory muscles, bradycardia or relative bradycardia, coughing, and purulent sputum, and auscultate breath sounds for consolidation.
- Note changes in temperature, pulse, and color of secretions.
- Assess for restlessness and excited delirium in alcoholism.
- Assess for complications, including continuing or recurring fever, failure to resolve, atelectasis, pleural effusion, cardiac complications, and superinfection.
- Assess the elderly patient for altered mental status, dehydration prostration, and congestive heart failure.

Major Nursing Diagnoses
- Ineffective airway clearance related to copious tracheobronchial secretions
- Activity intolerance related to altered respiratory function
- Risk for fluid volume deficit related to fever and dyspnea
- Altered nutrition: potential for less than body requirements
- Knowledge deficit about the treatment regimen and preventive health measures

Collaborative Problems/Potential Complications
- Hypotension and shock
- Respiratory failure

- Atelectasis
- Pleural effusion
- Delirium
- Superinfection

Planning and Goals

The major goals of the patient may include improvement in airway patency, adequate rest to conserve energy, maintenance of proper fluid volume, maintenance of adequate nutrition, an understanding of the treatment protocol and preventive measures, and absence of complications.

Nursing Interventions

IMPROVING AIRWAY PATENCY

- Encourage high fluid intake (2 to 3 L/day) to loosen secretions.
- Provide humidified air using high-humidity face mask.
- Encourage patient to cough, and provide chest physiotherapy and incentive spirometry.
- Provide nasotracheal suctioning if necessary.
- Provide appropriate method of oxygen therapy.
- Monitor effectiveness of oxygen therapy.

PROMOTING FLUID INTAKE

- Encourage fluids with electrolytes and calories.
- Administer intravenous fluids and nutrients, if necessary.

PROMOTING ACTIVITY TOLERANCE

- Counsel patient to rest and to avoid overexertion and possible exacerbation of symptoms, in initial phases, with moderate activity only.
- Assist patient into a comfortable position that maximizes breathing (eg, semi-Fowler's).
- Change position frequently (particularly in elderly patients).

MONITORING AND PREVENTING COMPLICATIONS

- Assess for signs and symptoms of shock and respiratory failure (eg, evaluate vital signs, pulse oximetry, and hemodynamic monitoring parameters).

- Administer intravenous fluids and medications and respiratory support as ordered.
- Initiate preventive measures for atelectasis.
- Assess for atelectasis and pleural effusion.
- Assist with thoracentesis, and monitor patient for pneumothorax after procedure.
- Monitor for superinfection (rise in temperature, increased cough), and assist in treatment therapy.

 ## Promoting Home and Community-Based Care

Teaching Patients Self-Care
- Advise patient to increase activities gradually after fever subsides.
- Advise patient that fatigue and weakness may linger after pneumonia.
- Encourage breathing exercises to promote expansion and clearing.
- Encourage follow-up chest radiographs.
- Encourage patient to stop smoking.
- Instruct patient to avoid fatigue, sudden changes in temperature, and excessive alcohol intake, which lower resistance to pneumonia.
- Review principles of adequate nutrition and rest.
- Recommend influenza vaccine and Pneumovax to all patients at risk (elderly and cardiac and pulmonary disease patients).
- Refer patient for home care to facilitate adherence to the therapeutic regimen, as indicated.

 ## Gerontologic Considerations

In older patients and in those with chronic obstructive pulmonary disease (COPD), symptoms may develop insidiously. Classic symptoms of cough, chest pain, sputum production, and fever are often absent. Pneumonia may also occur spontaneously or as a complication of a chronic disease. Onset of pneumonia may be signaled by general dete-

P

rioration, confusion, tachycardia, and increased respiratory rate.

Pulmonary infections are difficult to treat and are associated with a higher mortality in elderly patients than in younger patients. The presence of some signs may be misleading; chest radiography may be performed to assist in differentiating diagnosis.

Supportive treatment includes increased fluid intake (with caution regarding fluid overload); oxygen therapy; assistance with deep breathing, coughing, sputum production, and position changes; and early ambulation. Assess the elderly patient for alterations in mental status, prostration, and congestive heart failure. Vaccination against pneumococcal and influenza viral infections is recommended for people older than 50 years, nursing home residents, debilitated patients, and those with cardiovascular disease.

For more information, see Chapter 21 in Smeltzer and Bare: *Brunner and Suddarth's Textbook of Medical-Surgical Nursing,* 9th edition. Philadelphia: Lippincott Williams & Wilkins, 2000.

PNEUMOTHORAX AND HEMOTHORAX

Pneumothorax occurs when the parietal or visceral pleura is breached and the pleural space is exposed to positive atmospheric pressure. Air enters the pleural space, and a lung or a portion of it collapses. Types of pneumothorax include simple, traumatic, and tension pneumothorax. A simple pneumothorax may occur in an apparently healthy person or be associated with interstitial lung disease or emphysema. A traumatic pneumothorax can occur with blunt chest trauma, penetrating trauma to the chest, abdominal or diaphragmatic tears, or invasive thoracic procedures. An open traumatic pneumothorax includes a mediastinal swing that produces serious circulatory problems. Hemothorax is the collection of blood in the chest cavity because of torn intercostal vessels or laceration of the lungs injured through trauma. Often, both blood and air are found in the chest cavity (hemopneumothorax).

Clinical Manifestations

The signs and symptoms associated with pneumothorax depend on its size and cause:

- Pleuritic pain of sudden onset
- Minimal respiratory distress with small pneumothorax; acute respiratory distress if large
- Anxiety, dyspnea, air hunger, use of accessory muscles, and central cyanosis (with severe hypoxemia), if severe, accompanied by tachypnea, tympanic sound on percussion of the chest wall, decreased or absent breath sounds, and tactile fremitus of affected side

Medical Management

The goal is evacuation of air or blood from the pleural space while maintaining fluid balance.

- A large-diameter chest tube is inserted, usually in the fourth or fifth intercostal space, for hemothorax.
- A small chest tube is inserted near the second intercostal space for a pneumothorax.
- Autotransfusion is begun if excessive bleeding from chest tube occurs.
- Traumatic open pneumothorax is plugged (petroleum gauze); the patient is asked to inhale and strain against a closed glottis to eject air from the thorax until the chest tube is inserted, with water-seal drainage.

TENSION PNEUMOTHORAX

A tension pneumothorax occurs when air is drawn into the pleural space and is trapped with each breath. Tension is built up, causing lung collapse, and mediastinal shift (shift of the heart and great vessels and trachea toward the unaffected side of the chest) is a life-threatening medical emergency. Both respiratory and circulatory functions are compromised.

Clinical Manifestations
- Air hunger and agitation
- Increasing hypoxemia, cyanosis
- Hypotension, tachycardia, and profuse diuresis.

Medical Management
- Pulse oximetry is monitored, with high concentration of oxygen to treat hypoxia.
- Conversion to simple pneumothorax is accomplished by insertion of a large-bore needle into the pleural space to relieve pressure.
- Chest tube inserted with suction to remove remaining air and fluid.
- Surgery may be necessary to close the leak.

NURSING ALERT
Relief of tension pneumothorax is considered an emergency measure.

OPEN PNEUMOTHORAX

Open pneumothorax is an opening in the chest wall large enough to allow air to pass freely in and out of the thoracic cavity with respiration (sucking wounds). The lung is collapsed; the heart and great vessels are shifted toward the uninjured side with each inspiration and in the opposite direction with expiration (mediastinal flutter).

NURSING ALERT: EMERGENCY INTERVENTIONS TO STOP THE FLOW OF AIR THROUGH THE OPENING IN THE CHEST WALL

Use anything large enough to fill the hole (towel, handkerchief, heel of hand). Have patient inhale and strain against a closed glottis if conscious. When possible, plug the opening by sealing with petroleum-impregnated gauze. Apply pressure dressing by circumferential strapping.

Medical Management
- Chest tube to water-seal drainage for exit of air and fluid
- Antibiotics to combat infection from contamination

Nursing Management: The Patient With Pneumothorax or Hemothorax
Nursing Interventions
- Promote early detection through assessment and identification of high-risk population; report of symptoms.
- Assist in chest tube insertion; maintain chest drainage or water-seal.
- Monitor respiratory status and reexpansion of lung, with interventions (pulmonary support) performed in collaboration with other health care professionals (eg, physician, respiratory therapist, physical therapist).
- Provide information and emotional support to patient and family.

For more information, see Chapter 21 in Smeltzer and Bare: *Brunner and Suddarth's Textbook of Medical-Surgical Nursing,* 9th edition. Philadelphia: Lippincott Williams & Wilkins, 2000.

P

POLYCYTHEMIA

Polycythemia refers to an increased volume of red blood cells. The hematocrit is elevated by more than 55% in men or more than 50% in women.

Secondary Polycythemia
Secondary polycythemia is caused by excessive production of erythropoietin. This may occur in response to a hypoxic stimulus, as in chronic obstructive pulmonary disease or cyanotic heart disease, or in certain hemoglobinopathies in which the hemoglobin has an abnormally high affinity for oxygen, or it can occur from a neoplasm, such as renal cell carcinoma. Management of secondary polycythemia

involves treatment of the primary problem. If the cause cannot be corrected, phlebotomy may be necessary to reduce hypervolemia and hyperviscosity.

Polycythemia Vera

Polycythemia vera, or primary polycythemia, is a proliferative disorder in which the myeloid stem cells do not respond to normal control mechanisms. The bone marrow is hypercellular, and in the peripheral blood, the red cell count, white cell count, and platelets are often elevated. Patients typically have a ruddy complexion and splenomegaly. The symptoms are due to the increased blood volume (headache, tinnitus, paresthesias, dizziness, fatigue, and blurred vision) or to increased blood viscosity (angina, claudication, dyspnea and thrombophlebitis). Bleeding is a complication, and pruritus is another common and unexplained problem. Erythromyalgia may be reported.

Medical Management

The objective of management is to reduce the high blood viscosity.

- Phlebotomy is performed repeatedly to keep the hemoglobin within normal range; iron supplements are avoided.
- Radioactive phosphorus or chemotherapeutic agents are used to suppress marrow function (may increase risk for leukemia).
- Allopurinol is used to prevent gouty attacks, when the uric acid level is elevated.
- Antihistamines may be administered to control pruritus (not very effective).
- Dipyridamole may be used for ischemic symptoms.

Nursing Management

- Advise patient to avoid aspirin and medications containing aspirin.
- Inform patient that alcohol intake must be minimized.

- Suggest a cool or tepid bath for pruritus, along with cocoa butter-based lotions and bath products.

For more information, see Chapter 30 in Smeltzer and Bare: *Brunner and Suddarth's Textbook of Medical-Surgical Nursing,* 9th edition. Philadelphia: Lippincott Williams & Wilkins, 2000.

POSTOPERATIVE NURSING MANAGEMENT

The postoperative period extends from the time the patient leaves the operating room until the last follow-up visit with the surgeon (as short as 1 week or as long as several months). During the postoperative period, nursing care is directed at reestablishing the patient's physiologic equilibrium, alleviating pain, preventing complications, and teaching the patient self-care. Careful assessment and immediate intervention assist the patient in returning to optimal function quickly, safely, and as comfortably as possible. Ongoing care in the community through home care, clinic, or office visits facilitates an uncomplicated recovery.

Nursing Management in the Postanesthesia Care Unit

Patients still under anesthesia or recovering from it are placed in the *postanesthesia care unit* (PACU), also called the *postanesthesia recovery room* (PARR), which is located adjacent to the operating rooms. Patients may be in a PACU for as long as 4 to 6 hours or for as little as 1 to 2 hours, and in some cases, the patient may be discharged home directly from this unit.

The nursing management objectives for the patient in the PACU are to provide care until the patient has recovered from the effects of anesthesia (ie, until return of motor and sensory functions), is oriented, has stable vital signs, and shows no evidence of hemorrhage.

Obtain frequent assessments of the patient's oxygen saturation, pulse volume and regularity, depth and nature of respirations, skin color, level of consciousness, and ability to respond to commands.

Perform a baseline assessment followed by checking the surgical site for drainage or hemorrhage and connecting all drainage tubes and monitoring lines.

After the initial assessment, monitor vital signs and assess the patient's general physical status at least every 15 minutes, including assessment of cardiovascular function with the above assessments.

Note any pertinent information from the patient's history that may be significant (eg, patient is hard of hearing, has a history of seizures, has diabetes, is allergic to certain medications).

Nursing interventions in the PACU promote patient recovery and address any complications that arise.

Usually, the following measures are used to determine the patient's readiness for discharge from the PACU: uncompromised pulmonary function; pulse oximetry readings of adequate O_2 saturation; stable vital signs; orientation to place, events, and time; urine output not less than 30 mL/h; nausea and vomiting under control; and minimal pain.

Provide patients being discharged directly to home with teaching, written instructions, and information about follow-up care.

🏠 Promoting Home and Community-Based Care in the Patient Undergoing Same-Day or Ambulatory Surgery

Teaching Patients Self-Care

- Inform the patient and caregiver (ie, family member or friend) about expected outcomes and immediate postoperative changes anticipated in the patient's capacity for self-care.
- Provide written instructions about wound care, activity and dietary recommendations, medication, and follow-

up visits to the same-day surgery unit or the surgeon. Provide the patient's caregiver at home with verbal and written instructions about what to observe the patient for and about the actions to take if complications occur.

- Give prescriptions to the patient, provide the nurse's or surgeon's telephone number, and encourage the patient and caregiver to call if questions arise.
- Instruct the patient to limit activity for 24 to 48 hours (avoid driving a vehicle, drinking alcoholic beverages, or performing tasks that require energy or skill); to consume fluids as desired; and to consume smaller than normal amounts of food at mealtime.
- Caution the patient not to make important decisions at this time because the medications, anesthesia, and surgery may affect thinking ability.

Continuing Care

- Refer patients for home care as indicated (elderly or frail patients, those who live alone, and patients with other health care problems that may interfere with self-care or resumption of usual activities).
- The home care nurse assesses the patient's physical status (ie, respiratory and cardiovascular status, adequacy of pain management, the surgical incision) and the patient's and family's ability to adhere to the recommendations given at the time of discharge. Previous teaching is reinforced as needed.
- The home care nurse may change surgical dressings, monitor patency of a drainage system, administer medications, and assess for surgical complications as well as remind the patient and family about the importance of keeping follow-up appointments with the surgeon.
- Follow-up telephone calls from the nurse or surgeon may also be used to assess the patient's progress and to answer any questions.

Nursing Management in the Clinical Unit

- Prepare the patient's unit by assembling the necessary equipment and supplies: intravenous pole, drainage receptacle holder, emesis basin, tissues, disposable pads (Chux), blankets, and postoperative charting forms.

- Receive report from the PACU nurse on the baseline data of the patient's condition, including demographic data, medical diagnosis, procedure performed, comorbid conditions, unexpected intraoperative events, estimated blood loss, the type and amount of fluids received, medications administered for pain, whether patient has voided, and information patient and family have received about the patient's condition.

- Review the postoperative orders, admit the patient to the unit, perform an initial assessment, and attend to the patient's immediate needs.

Nursing Management During The First Hours After Surgery

- Interventions focus on continuing to help the patient recover from the effects of anesthesia, performing frequent assessments, monitoring for complications, managing pain, and implementing measures to promote self-care, successful management of the therapeutic regimen, discharge to home, and full recovery.

- In the initial hours after admission to the clinical unit, adequate ventilation, hemodynamic stability, incisional pain, surgical site integrity, nausea and vomiting, neurologic status, and spontaneous voiding are all primary concerns.

- Unless indicated more frequently, record the pulse, blood pressure, and respirations every 15 minutes for the first hour and every 30 minutes for the next 2 hours. Thereafter, they are measured less frequently if they remain stable. Monitor the patient's temperature every 4 hours for the first 24 hours.

Nursing Interventions

MAINTAINING A PATENT AIRWAY

- Check the orders for and apply supplemental oxygen; assess respiratory rate and depth, ease of respirations, oxygen saturation, and breath sounds.

- Monitor the patient for airway obstruction: the tongue falls backward, and the patient has choking, noisy, and irregular respirations, and, within minutes, a blue, dusky color (cyanosis) of the skin.
- Encourage the patient to turn frequently and take deep breaths and cough at least every 2 hours.
- Carefully splint an abdominal or thoracic incision site to help the patient overcome the fear that the exertion of coughing might open the incision.
- Administer pain medications to permit more effective coughing,
- Assist and encourage patient to use incentive spirometer hourly while awake (10 breaths per hour).

NURSING ALERT

Coughing is contraindicated in patients who have head injuries or who have undergone intracranial surgery, eye surgery, or plastic surgery.

MAINTAINING CARDIOVASCULAR STABILITY
- Monitor cardiovascular stability by assessing the patient's mental status; vital signs; cardiac rhythm; skin temperature, color, and moisture; and urine output.
- Assess the patency of all intravenous lines.
- On the patient's arrival in the clinical unit, observe the surgical site for bleeding, type and integrity of dressing, and drains (eg, Penrose, Hemovac, and Jackson-Pratt).
- Assess output from wound drainage systems and the amount of bloody drainage on the surgical dressing frequently; mark and time spots of drainage on the dressings; report excess drainage or fresh blood to surgeon immediately.
- Reinforce the dressing with sterile gauze bandages and record the time. *Do not change initial dressing, surgeon will usually wish to be present.*

ASSESSING AND MANAGING PAIN
- Assess pain level using a verbal or visual analog scale, and assess the characteristics of the pain.

- Discuss the options in pain relief measures with the patient to determine the best medication. Assess the effectiveness of the medication periodically beginning 30 minutes after administration or sooner if given intravenously.
- Administer medication at prescribed intervals, or if ordered as needed, before the patient's pain becomes severe or unbearable (risk of addiction is negligible with use of opioids for short-term pain control).
- Provide other pain relief measures (changing the patient's position, using distraction, applying cool washcloths to the face, and rubbing the back with a soothing lotion) to relieve general discomfort temporarily.

MAINTAINING NORMAL BODY TEMPERATURE
- Monitor body system function and vital signs with temperature every 4 hours for the first 24 hours and every shift thereafter.
- Report signs of hypothermia to the physician (a particular risk in elderly patients and with long surgeries).
- Maintain the room at a comfortable temperature, and provide blankets to prevent chilling.
- Monitor the patient for cardiac dysrhythmias.
- Take efforts to identify malignant hyperthermia and to treat it early.

ASSESSING MENTAL STATUS
- Assess the patient's mental status (level of consciousness, speech, and orientation) and compare to the preoperative baseline; change may be related to anxiety, pain, medications, oxygen deficit, or hemorrhage.
- Assess for possible causes of discomfort, such as tight, drainage-soaked bandages or distended bladder.
- Address sources of discomfort, and report signs of complications to surgeon for immediate treatment.
- Assess neurovascular status (have patient move the hand or foot distal to the surgical site through a full range of motion, ensuring that all surfaces have intact sensation and assessing peripheral pulses).

ASSESSING AND MANAGING GASTROINTESTINAL FUNCTION AND PROMOTING NUTRITION

- If in place, maintain nasogastric tube and monitor patency and drainage.
- Provide symptomatic therapy including antiemetic medications for nausea and vomiting.

☒ NURSING ALERT

At the slightest indication of nausea, the patient is turned completely on one side to promote mouth drainage to prevent aspiration of vomitus, which can cause asphyxiation and death.

- Administer phenothiazine medications as prescribed for severe, persistent hiccups.
- Assist the patient to return to normal dietary intake gradually at the pace set by the patient (liquids first, then soft foods, such as gelatin, junket, custard, milk, and creamed soups, are added gradually, then solid food).
- Note that paralytic ileus and intestinal obstruction are potential postoperative complications that occur more frequently in patients undergoing intestinal or abdominal surgery. (See specific gastrointestinal disorders for discussion of treatment.)
- Arrange for the patient to consult with the dietitian to plan appealing, high-protein meals that provide sufficient fiber, calories, and vitamins. Nutritional supplements, such as Ensure or Sustacal, may be recommended.
- Instruct the patient to take multivitamins, iron, and vitamin C supplements if prescribed postoperatively.

ASSESSING AND MANAGING VOLUNTARY VOIDING

- Assess for bladder distention and urge to void on the patient's arrival in the unit and frequently thereafter (patient should void within 8 hours of surgery).
- Obtain order for catheterization if the patient has an urge to void and cannot, or if the bladder is distended

P

and no urge is felt or the patient cannot void, without delaying until 8 hours have passed.

- Initiate methods to encourage the patient to void (eg, letting water run, applying heat to the perineum).
- Warm the bedpan to reduce discomfort and automatic tightening of muscles and urethral sphincter.
- Assist patient who complains of not being able to use the bedpan to use a commode or stand or sit to void (males), unless contraindicated.
- Take safeguards to prevent the patient from falling or fainting due to loss of coordination from medications or orthostatic hypotension.
- Note the amount of urine voided, and palpate the suprapubic area for distention or tenderness, or use a portable ultrasound device to assess residual volume.
- Continue intermittent catheterization every 4 to 6 hours until patient can void spontaneously and postvoid residual is less than 100 mL.

ENCOURAGING ACTIVITY

- Encourage surgical patients (most) to ambulate as soon as possible.
- Remind patient of the importance of early mobility in preventing complications (helps overcome fears).
- Anticipate and avoid orthostatic hypotension (postural hypotension: 20 mm Hg fall in systolic blood pressure or 10 mm Hg fall in diastolic blood pressure, weakness, dizziness, and fainting).
- Assess the patient's feelings of dizziness and his or her blood pressure first in the supine position, after the patient sits up, again after the patient stands, and 2 to 3 minutes later.
- Assist patient to change position gradually; if patient becomes dizzy, return to the supine position and delay getting out of bed for several hours.
- Once out of bed, remain at the patient's side to give physical support and encouragement.
- Take care not to tire the patient.
- Initiate and encourage patient to perform bed exercises

to improve circulation (range of motion to arms, hands and fingers, feet, and legs; leg flexion and leg lifting; abdominal and gluteal contraction).

• Encourage frequent position changes early in the postoperative period to stimulate circulation. Avoid positions that compromise venous return (raising the knee gatch or placing a pillow under the knees, sitting for long periods, and dangling the legs with pressure at the back of the knees).

• Apply antiembolism stockings, and assist patient in early ambulation. Check postoperative activity orders before getting the patient out of bed; sit on the edge of bed for a few minutes initially, advance as tolerated.

PROMOTING FLUID BALANCE

• Monitor closely to detect and correct conditions such as fluid volume deficit, altered tissue perfusion, and decreased cardiac output.

• Assess the patency of the intravenous lines, ensuring that the appropriate fluids are administered at the prescribed rate (up to 24 hours or until patient is tolerating oral fluids).

• Record intake and output, including emesis and output from wound drainage systems, separately and add them to determine fluid balance (with indwelling urinary catheter, monitor outputs hourly and report rates of less than 30 mL/h; if the patient is voiding, report an output of less than 240 mL per shift).

• Monitor electrolyte levels and hemoglobin and hematocrit levels.

PROMOTING SELF-CARE

• Have the patient perform as much routine hygiene care as possible on the first postoperative day (setting up the patient to bathe with a bedside wash basin, or, if possible, assisting the patient to the bathroom to sit at a chair at the sink).

• Assist the patient to build ability to ambulate a functional distance (length of the house or apartment), get in and out of bed unassisted, and be independent with toileting, to prepare for discharge to home.

- Ask the patient to perform as much as possible and then to call for assistance. Collaborate with the patient for progressive activity, and assess the patient's vital signs before, during, and after a scheduled activity.
- Provide physical support to maintain the patient's safety, and provide a positive attitude about the patient's ability to perform the activity, promoting the patient's confidence.
- While changing the dressing, teach the patient how to care for the incision and change the dressings at home. Observe for indicators of the patient's readiness to learn, such as looking at the incision, expressing interest, or assisting in the dressing change.

MAINTAINING A SAFE ENVIRONMENT
- Keep side rails up and the bed in the low position.
- Assess the patient's level of consciousness and orientation.
- Determine whether the patient needs his or her eyeglasses or hearing aid and provide them as soon as possible.
- Place all objects the patient may need within reach, including, of course, the call bell.
- Implement any immediate postoperative orders concerning special positioning, equipment, or intervention.
- Ask the patient to seek assistance with any activity.
- Only use restraints if absolutely needed (disoriented patient), and assess neurovascular status frequently.

PROVIDING EMOTIONAL SUPPORT TO THE
PATIENT AND FAMILY
- Help the patient and family work through their anxieties by providing reassurance and information and by spending time listening to and addressing their concerns.
- Describe hospital routines and what to expect in the ensuing hours and days until discharge.
- Explain the purpose of nursing assessments and interventions.

- Inform patients when they can take fluids or eat, when they will be getting out of bed, when tubes and drains will be removed, and so forth, to help them gain a sense of control and participation in recovery.
- Acknowledge family's concerns, and accept and encourage their participation in the patient's care.
- Manipulate the environment to enhance rest and relaxation: provide privacy, reduce noise, adjust lighting, provide enough seating for family members, and perform any other supportive measures.

MONITORING AND PREVENTING POSTOPERATIVE COMPLICATIONS

Preventing Deep Vein Thrombosis

- Monitor for symptoms of deep vein thrombosis (DVT), which may include a pain or a cramp in the calf elicited on ankle dorsiflexion (Homans' sign); pain and tenderness may be followed by a painful swelling of the entire leg and may be accompanied by a slight fever and sometimes chills and perspiration.
- Administer prophylactic treatment for postoperative patients at risk (low-dose subcutaneous heparin, and then warfarin, external pneumatic compression, and thigh-high elastic pressure stockings).
- Avoid the use of blanket rolls, pillow rolls, or any form of elevation that can constrict vessels under the knees. Even prolonged "dangling" (having the patient sit on the edge of the bed with legs hanging over the side) can be dangerous and is not recommended in susceptible patients.
- Encourage adequate hydration (offer juices and water throughout the day).

Monitoring and Treating Hypotension and Shock

- Monitor closely for signs of shock (a fall in venous pressure, a rise in peripheral resistance, and tachycardia, or a fall in blood pressure). If the amount of blood loss exceeds 500 mL (especially if the loss is rapid), replacement is usually indicated.

- Monitor for the classic signs of shock: pallor; cool, moist skin; rapid breathing; cyanosis of the lips, gums, and tongue; a rapid, weak, thready pulse; decreasing pulse pressure; low blood pressure; and concentrated urine.
- Prevent hypovolemic shock by timely administration of intravenous fluids, blood, and medications that elevate blood pressure.
- Control pain by making the patient as comfortable as possible and by using opioids judiciously. Avoid exposure, and maintain normothermia to prevent vasodilation.
- Administer volume replacement as ordered (lactated Ringer's solution or blood component therapy).
- Administer oxygen by nasal cannula, face mask, or mechanical ventilation.
- Administer cardiotonics, vasodilators, or steroids to improve cardiac function and reduce peripheral vascular resistance. Keep the patient warm; however, avoid overheating to prevent vessels dilation.
- Place the patient flat in bed with legs elevated.
- Monitor respiratory and pulse rate, blood pressure, O_2 concentration, urinary output, level of consciousness, central venous pressure, pulmonary artery pressure, pulmonary capillary wedge pressure, and cardiac output to provide information about the patient's respiratory and cardiovascular status.
- Monitor vital signs continuously until the patient's condition has stabilized.

Detecting and Minimizing Hemorrhage
- Note signs of extreme blood loss (apprehensiveness, restless, and thirst; cold, moist, pale skin; increased pulse rate; decreasing temperature; and rapid and deep respirations, often of the gasping type spoken of as "air hunger").
- If the hemorrhage progresses untreated, cardiac output decreases, arterial and venous blood pressure and hemoglobin level fall rapidly, the lips and the conjunctivae become pallid, spots appear before the

eyes, a ringing is heard in the ears, and the patient grows weaker but remains conscious until near death.

- Administer blood or blood product transfusion of blood, and determine the cause of hemorrhage.
- Inspect the surgical site and incision for bleeding. If bleeding is evident, apply a sterile gauze pad and a pressure dressing, and elevate the site of the bleeding to the level of the heart, if possible; place the patient in the shock position (lying flat on back with legs elevated at a 20-degree angle while knees are kept straight). If indicated, prepare the patient for return to surgery.
- Give special considerations to patients who decline blood transfusions, such as Jehovah's Witnesses, and to those who identify specific requests on their advanced directives or living will.

NURSING ALERT
Giving too large a quantity or administering the intravenous fluid too rapidly may raise the blood pressure enough to start the bleeding again.

NURSING ALERT
A systolic blood pressure of less than 90 mm Hg is usually considered reportable at once. However, the patient's preoperative or baseline blood pressure is used to make informed postoperative comparisons. A previously stable blood pressure that shows a downward trend of 5 mm Hg at each 15-minute reading should also be reported.

Managing Wound Complications
HEMATOMA

- Monitor for bleeding beneath the skin at the surgical site, which may result in clot formation (hematoma) within the wound. (If clot is large, the wound may bulge, and healing is delayed unless the clot is removed).
- Prepare patient for removal of several sutures by the

physician, evacuation of the clot, and light wound packing with gauze. Healing occurs usually by granulation, or a secondary closure may be performed.

INFECTION (WOUND SEPSIS)

- Monitor for (or instruct patient and family to monitor for) wound infection, which may not present until at least postoperative day 5 (pulse rate and temperature elevation; white blood cell elevation; wound swelling, warmth, tenderness, or discharge; and incisional pain). Local signs may be absent if the infection is deep.

- Note risk factors for wound sepsis, which include wound contamination, foreign body, faulty suturing technique, devitalized tissue, hematoma, debilitation, dehydration, malnutrition, anemia, advanced age, extreme obesity, shock, length of preoperative hospitalization, duration of surgical procedure, and associated disorders (eg, diabetes mellitus, immunosuppression).

- Take extreme care if wound infection due to beta-hemolytic *Streptococcus* or *Clostridium* species infection occurs, to prevent spread of infection to others; provide intensive nursing care.

- Provide care for open incision and drain if present.

- Prepare patient as needed; if the infection is deep, incision and drainage may be necessary.

- Administer antimicrobial therapy, and initiate wound care regimen.

Monitoring for Wound Dehiscence and Evisceration

- Monitor for wound *dehiscence* (disruption of surgical incision or wound) and *evisceration* (protrusion of wound contents), which are serious complications (especially when they involve abdominal incisions or wounds). The earliest sign may be a gush of bloody (serosanguineous) peritoneal fluid from the wound; coils of intestine may push out of the abdomen, pain and vomiting may be noted, and frequently, the patient may say that "something gave way."

- Monitor patients with risk factors closely (patients with infection, marked distention, strenuous cough, increasing age, poor nutritional status, and the presence of pulmonary or cardiovascular disease in patients who undergo abdominal surgery).

- When wound disruption occurs, place patient in low Fowler's position, and instruct to lie quietly to minimize protrusion of body tissues.
- Cover the protruding tissue or coils of intestine with sterile dressings moistened with sterile saline, and notify the surgeon at once.
- Apply an abdominal binder as a prophylactic measure against an abdominal incision evisceration.

Promoting Home and Community-Based Care

- Although certain needs are germane to individual patients and the specific procedures they have undergone, the scope of patient education needs for postoperative care have been identified.

Teaching Patients Self-Care

- Provide detailed discharge instructions to assist the patient to become proficient in special self-care needs after surgery.

Continuing Care

- Arrange for care by community-based services, such as a home care nurse, if necessary (older patients, patients who live alone, or patients without family support).
- Arrange for necessary services early in the acute care hospitalization.
- Wound care, drain management, catheter care, infusion therapy, and physical or occupational therapy are some of the needs addressed by community health care providers.
- Instruct the patient to continue to perform bed exercises, wear antiembolic hose when in bed, and rests as needed. Spray silicone over the adhesive used to hold dressings in place; the silicone waterproofs the

P

dressing so that the patient can bathe or swim, and it isolates the area from contamination.

- The home care nurse coordinates activities and services and assesses for postoperative complications, evaluates the adequacy of pain management, and assesses the patient's progress in returning to preoperative status.
- The home care nurse assesses the patient's and family's ability to manage dressing changes, drainage systems, and other devices and to administer prescribed medications and may change dressings or catheters if needed.
- The home care nurse determines if any additional services are needed and assists the patient and family to arrange for them (how to obtain needed supplies, and resources or support groups the patient may want to contact).
- The home care nurse reinforces previous teaching and reminds the patient to keep follow-up appointments. The patient and family are instructed about signs and symptoms to be reported to the surgeon.

☘ Gerontologic Considerations

Elderly patients continue to be at increased risk for postoperative complications. Age-related physiologic changes in respiratory, cardiovascular, and renal function and the increased incidence of comorbid conditions demand skilled assessment to detect early signs of deterioration. Anesthetics and opioids can cause confusion in the older adult, and altered pharmacokinetics results in delayed excretion and prolonged respiratory depressive effects. Careful monitoring of electrolyte, hemoglobin, and hematocrit levels and urine output is essential because the older adult is less able to correct and compensate for fluid and electrolyte imbalances. Elderly patients may need frequent reminders and demonstrations to participate in care effectively.

- Maintain physical activity while the patient is confused (physical deterioration can worsen delirium and place the patient at increased risk for other complications).

- Avoid restraints because they can also worsen confusion. If possible, family or staff member is asked to sit with the patient instead.
- Administer haloperidol (Haldol) or lorazepam (Ativan) as ordered during episodes of acute confusion; however, these medications should be discontinued as soon as possible to avoid side effects.
- Assist the patient in early and progressive ambulation to prevent the development of other problems confronting the older postoperative patient, such as pneumonia, altered bowel function, DVT, weakness, and functional decline; avoid sitting positions that promote venous stasis in the lower extremities.
- Provide adequate assistance to keep the patient from bumping into objects and falling. A physical therapy referral may be indicated to promote safe, regular exercise for the older adult.
- Provide easy access to call bell and the commode, and prompt voiding to prevent urinary incontinence.
- Provide extensive discharge planning to coordinate both professional and family care providers; the nurse, social worker, or nurse case manager may institute the plan for continuing care.

Evaluation

EXPECTED OUTCOMES
- Indicates that pain is decreased in intensity
- Maintains optimal respiratory function
- Does not develop DVT
- Exercises and ambulates as prescribed
- Wound heals without complication
- Resumes oral intake and normal bowel function
- Acquires knowledge and skills necessary to manage therapeutic regimen
- Experiences no complications and has normal vital signs

For more information, see Chapter 18 in Smeltzer and Bare: *Brunner and Suddarth's Textbook of Medical-Surgical Nursing,* 9th edition. Philadelphia: Lippincott Williams & Wilkins, 2000.

PREOPERATIVE NURSING MANAGEMENT

Surgery, whether elective or emergency, is a stressful, complex event. Surgery may be performed for a variety of reasons. It may be diagnostic, such as when a biopsy is obtained or an exploratory laparotomy is performed; it may be curative, such as when a tumor mass is excised; it may be reparative, such as when multiple wounds must be repaired; it may be reconstructive or cosmetic, such as when a face lift is performed; or it may be palliative, such as when pain must be relieved. Surgery may also be classified according to the degree of urgency involved, with use of the terms *emergency, urgent, required, elective,* and *optional.*

Nursing Management
Promoting Informed Consent
- After the surgeon explains the surgery, the nurse reinforces information.
- Notify the physician if the patient needs additional information to make his or her decision.
- Ascertain that the consent form has been signed before administering psychoactive premedication.
- Arrange for a responsible family member or legal guardian to be available to give consent, when the patient is a minor or is unconscious or incompetent (an emancipated minor—married or independently earning own living—may sign his or her own permit).
- Place the signed consent form in a prominent place on the patient's chart.

Assessment
- Obtain a health history, and perform a physical examination to establish vital signs and a database for future comparisons.
- Determine the existence of allergies, previous allergic reactions, any sensitivities to medications, and past

adverse reactions to these agents; report a history of bronchial asthma to the anesthesiologist.

- During the physical examination, note significant physical findings, such as pressure ulcers, edema, or abnormal breath sounds, that further describe the patient's overall condition.

- Obtain and document a medication history; include dosage and frequency of prescribed and over-the-counter (OTC) preparations, particularly the following: adrenal corticosteroids, diuretics, phenothiazines, antidepressants, tranquilizers, insulin, and antibiotics.

- Assess the usual level of functioning and typical daily activities to assist in the patient's care and rehabilitation plans.

- Determine nutritional needs by the patient's height and weight, body mass index (BMI), triceps skin fold, upper arm circumference, serum protein levels, or nitrogen balance.

- Assess the mouth for dental caries, dentures, and partial plates; decayed teeth or dental prostheses may become dislodged during intubation and occlude the airway.

- Determine the value and reliability of all available support systems; determine the role of the patient's family or friends.

- Elicit patient concerns that can have a bearing on the course of the surgical experience.

- Monitor the older person undergoing surgery for subtle clues that indicate underlying problems, considering the principle that the elderly patient has less physiologic reserve (cardiac, renal, and hepatic function and gastrointestinal activity) than the younger patient.

- Identify the ethnic group to which the patient relates and the customs and beliefs the patient holds about illness and health care providers.

- Monitor obese patients for abdominal distention; phlebitis; and cardiovascular, endocrine, hepatic, and biliary diseases, which occur more readily in obese patients.

P

- Monitor elderly patients for dehydration, hypovolemia, and electrolyte imbalances, which can be a significant problem in the elderly population.
- Be alert for a history of drug or alcohol abuse, taking care and attention when obtaining the patient's history; maintain patience, ask frank questions, and maintain a nonjudgmental attitude.
- Investigate the mildest symptoms or slightest temperature elevation in patients with disorders affecting the immune system (eg, acquired immunodeficiency syndrome [AIDS], leukemia); use strict asepsis.

ASSESSING THE AMBULATORY SURGICAL PATIENT
- Obtain the health history of the ambulatory or same-day surgical patient by telephone interview or at the time of preadmission testing. Include questions relating to recent and past health history, allergies, medications, preoperative preparation, and psychosocial and demographic factors.
- Complete the physical assessment the day of surgery.

Major Nursing Diagnoses
- Anxiety related to the surgical experience (anesthesia, pain) and the outcome of surgery
- Risk for ineffective management of therapeutic regimen related to knowledge deficit regarding preoperative procedures and protocols and postoperative expectations

Planning and Goals
The surgical patient's major goals may include relief of preoperative anxiety and increased knowledge of preoperative preparations and postoperative expectations.

Nursing Interventions
REDUCING PREOPERATIVE ANXIETY: PROVIDING PSYCHOSOCIAL SUPPORT AND ALLEVIATING FEAR
- Be a good listener, be empathetic, and provide information that helps alleviate concerns.
- During preliminary contacts with the health care team, provide the patient with opportunities to ask questions

and to become acquainted with those who might be providing care during and after surgery.

- Acknowledge patient concerns or worries about impending surgery by listening and communicating therapeutically.
- Explore any fears with the patient, and arrange for the assistance of other health professionals if required.
- Teach the patient cognitive strategies that may be useful for relieving tension, overcoming anxiety, and achieving relaxation, including imagery, distraction, or optimistic self-recitation.

MANAGING NUTRITION AND FLUIDS

- Provide nutrition support as ordered to correct any nutrient deficiency before surgery to provide enough protein for tissue repair.
- Instruct patient that oral intake of food or water should be withheld 8 to 10 hours before the operation (most common), unless physician allows clear fluids up to 3 to 4 hours before surgery.
- Inform the patient that a light meal may be permitted on the preceding evening when surgery is scheduled in the morning, or provide a soft breakfast, if prescribed, when the surgery is scheduled to take place after noon and does not involve any part of the gastrointestinal tract.
- In dehydrated patients, and especially in older patients, encourage fluids by mouth, as ordered, before surgery, and administer fluids intravenously, as ordered.
- Monitor the patient with a history of chronic alcoholism for malnutrition and other systemic problems that increase the surgical risk as well as for alcohol withdrawal delirium (delirium tremens up to 72 hours after alcohol withdrawal).

PROMOTING OPTIMAL RESPIRATORY AND CARDIOVASCULAR STATUS

- Urge patient to stop smoking 4 to 6 weeks before surgery.
- Teach the patient breathing exercises and how to use an incentive spirometer if indicated.

P

- Assess patient with underlying respiratory disease (eg, asthma, chronic obstructive pulmonary disease [COPD]) carefully for current threats to the pulmonary status; assess patient's use of medications that may affect postoperative recovery.
- In the patient with cardiovascular disease, avoid sudden changes of position, prolonged immobilization, hypotension or hypoxia, and overloading of the circulatory system with fluids or blood.

SUPPORTING HEPATIC AND RENAL FUNCTION

- If patient has a disorder of the liver, carefully assess various liver function tests and acid–base status.
- Frequently monitor the blood glucose levels of the patient with diabetes before, during, and after surgery.
- Report the use of steroid medications for any purpose by the patient during the preceding year to the anesthesiologist and surgeon.
- Monitor the patient for signs of adrenal insufficiency.
- Assess patients with uncontrolled thyroid disorders for a history of thyrotoxicosis (with hyperthyroid disorders) or respiratory failure (with hypothyroid disorders).

ENCOURAGING MOBILITY AND ACTIVE BODY MOVEMENT

- Explain the rationale for frequent position changes after surgery (to improve circulation, prevent venous stasis, and promote optimal respiratory function) and show the patient how to best turn from side to side and how to assume the lateral position without causing pain or disrupting intravenous lines, drainage tubes, or other apparatus.
- Discuss any special position the patient will need to maintain after surgery (eg, adduction or elevation of an extremity) and the importance of maintaining as much mobility as possible despite restrictions.
- Instruct the patient in exercises of the extremities, including extension and flexion of the knee and hip joints (similar to bicycle riding while lying on the side);

foot rotation (tracing the largest possible circle with the great toe), and range of motion of the elbow and shoulder.
- Use proper body mechanics, and instruct the patient to do the same. Maintain the patient's body in proper alignment when the patient is placed in any position.

RESPECTING SPIRITUAL AND CULTURAL BELIEFS
- Help the patient obtain the spiritual help that he or she requests; respect and support the beliefs of each individual patient.
- Ask if the patient's spiritual adviser knows about the impending surgery.
- When assessing pain, consider the pattern of self-control that some cultural groups exhibit (some are unaccustomed to expressing feelings openly).
- Understand that as a sign of respect, individuals from other cultural groups may not make direct eye contact with others; this lack of eye contact is not avoidance or a lack of interest.
- Listen carefully to the patient, especially when obtaining the patient's history, using communication and interviewing skills to acquire invaluable information and insight; remain unhurried, understanding, and caring.

Gerontologic Considerations

- Assess the older patient for and report dehydration, constipation, and malnutrition.
- Maintain a safe environment for the older client with sensory limitations such as impaired vision or hearing and reduced tactile sensitivity.
- Initiate protective measures for the older patient who may have arthritis, which may affect mobility and comfort. Include adequate padding for tender areas, move the patient slowly and protect bony prominences from prolonged pressure, and provide gentle massage to promote adequate circulation.

- Take added precautions when moving an elderly person because decreased perspiration leads to dry, itchy, fragile skin that is easily abraded.
- Apply a lightweight cotton blanket as cover when an elderly patient is moved to and from the operating room because decreased subcutaneous fat makes older people more susceptible to temperature changes.
- Provide the elderly patient with an opportunity to express fears to enable the patient to gain some peace of mind and a sense of being understood.

PROVIDING PREOPERATIVE PATIENT EDUCATION

- Teach each patient as an individual, with consideration for any unique concerns or learning needs.
- Begin teaching as soon as possible, starting in the physician's office and continuing during the preadmission visit, when diagnostic tests are being performed, through arrival in the operating room.
- Space instruction over a period of time to allow the patient to assimilate information and ask questions.
- Combine teaching sessions with various preparation procedures to allow for an easy flow of information; include descriptions of the procedures and explanations of the sensations the patient will experience.
- During the preadmission visit, arrange for the patient to meet and ask questions of the perianesthesia nurse, view audiovisuals, receive written materials, and provide a telephone number for patient to call as questions arise closer to the date of surgery.
- Reinforce information about the possible need for a ventilator and the presence of drainage tubes or other types of equipment to help the patient adjust during the postoperative period.
- Inform the patient when family and friends will be able to visit after surgery and that a spiritual advisor will be available if desired.

TEACHING THE AMBULATORY SURGICAL PATIENT

- Present preoperative education for the same-day or ambulatory surgical patient, including discharge and follow-up home care, using a videotape or by telephone or during a group meeting, night classes, preadmission testing, or the preoperative interview.

- Answer questions and describe what to expect, and tell the patient when and where to report, what to bring (insurance card, list of medications and allergies), what to leave at home (jewelry, watch, medications, contact lenses), and what to wear (loose-fitting, comfortable clothes; flat shoes).
- During the last preoperative phone call, remind the patient not to eat or drink as directed; brushing teeth is permitted, but no fluids should be swallowed.

TEACHING DEEP BREATHING AND COUGHING EXERCISES

- Teach the patient how to promote optimal lung expansion and consequent blood oxygenation after anesthesia by assuming a sitting position, taking deep and slow breaths (maximal sustained inspiration), exhaling slowly.
- Demonstrate how the incision line can be splinted so that pressure is minimized and pain is controlled if there will be a thoracic or abdominal incision.
- Inform the patient that medications are available to relieve pain and that they should be taken regularly for pain relief to enable effective deep breathing and coughing exercises.

EXPLAINING PAIN MANAGEMENT

- Instruct the patient to take medication as frequently as prescribed during the initial postoperative period for pain relief.
- Discuss oral analgesic agents with the patient before surgery, and assess the patient's interest and willingness to participate in use of those pain-relief methods.
- Instruct the patient in the use of a pain ratio scale to promote effective postoperative pain management.

PREPARING THE BOWEL FOR SURGERY

- If ordered preoperatively, administer or instruct the patient to take the antibiotic and to take a cleansing

enema or laxative the evening before surgery and repeat it the morning of surgery.
- Use the toilet or bedside commode rather than the bed-pan for evacuation of the enema, unless the condition of the patient presents some contraindication.

PREPARING THE PATIENT FOR SURGERY
- Instruct patient in use of detergent-germicide for several days at home, if the surgery is not an emergency.
- If hair is to be removed, remove it immediately before the operation using electric clippers.
- Dress the patient in a hospital gown that is left untied and open in the back.
- Cover the patient's hair completely with a disposable paper cap, if the patient has long hair, it may be braided; hairpins are removed.
- Inspect the patient's mouth, and remove dentures or plates.
- Remove jewelry, including wedding rings, but if the patient objects, securely fasten the ring with tape.
- Give all articles of value, including dentures and prosthetic devices, to family members, or if needed, label articles clearly with the patient's name and store in a safe place according to agency policy.
- Assist patients (except those with urologic disorders) to void immediately before going to the operating room.
- Administer preanesthetic medication as ordered, and keep the patient in bed with the side rails raised; observe the patient for any untoward reaction to the medications, and keep the immediate surroundings quiet to promote relaxation.

TRANSPORTING THE PATIENT TO OPERATIVE AREA
- Send the completed chart with the patient to the operating room; attach the surgical consent form and all laboratory reports and nurses' records, noting any unusual last-minute observations that may have a bearing on the anesthesia or surgery at the front of the chart in a prominent place.

- Take the patient to the preoperative holding area, and keep the area quiet, avoiding unpleasant sounds or conversation.

NURSING ALERT

It is important that someone be with the preoperative patient at all times. The person who is present should ensure safety and provide reassurance (verbally as well as nonverbally by facial expression, manner, or the warm grasp of a hand).

ATTENDING TO THE FAMILY'S NEEDS
- Assist the family to the surgical waiting room where the surgeon may meet the family after surgery.
- Assure the family they should not judge the seriousness of an operation by the length of time the patient is in the operating room.
- Inform those waiting to see the patient after surgery that the patient may have certain equipment or devices in place when returned to the room (ie, intravenous lines, indwelling urinary catheter, nasogastric tube, suction bottles, oxygen lines, monitoring equipment, and blood transfusion lines).
- When the patient returns to the room, provide explanations regarding the frequent postoperative observations.

Evaluation

EXPECTED OUTCOMES
- Is relieved of anxiety
- Prepares for surgical intervention

For more information, see Chapter 16 in Smeltzer and Bare: *Brunner and Suddarth's Textbook of Medical-Surgical Nursing,* 9th edition. Philadelphia: Lippincott Williams & Wilkins, 2000.

PROSTATITIS

Prostatitis is an inflammation of the prostate gland caused by infectious agents (bacteria, fungi, mycoplasma) or by various other problems (eg, urethral stricture, prostatic hyperplasia). Micro-organisms are usually carried to the prostate from the urethra. Prostatitis may be classified as bacterial or abacterial, depending on the presence or absence of micro-organisms in the prostatic fluid. *Escherichia coli* is the most commonly isolated organism.

Clinical Manifestations
- Perineal discomfort, burning, urgency, frequency, and pain with or after ejaculation
- Prostatodynia (pain in the prostate) manifested by painful voiding or by perineal pain without evidence of inflammation or bacterial growth in prostatic fluid

Symptoms of Acute Bacterial Prostatitis
Note that some patients do not develop symptoms.
- Sudden fever and chills
- Perineal, rectal, or low back pain
- Urinary symptoms of frequency, urgency, nocturia, and dysuria

Symptoms of Chronic Prostatitis
In addition to the above symptoms, occasional urethral discharge may be noted.

Diagnostic Evaluation
- History, culture of prostatic fluid or tissue
- Histologic examination of tissue (occasionally), segmental urine culture

Medical Management
The goal of management is to avoid the complications of abscess formation and septicemia.

- Broad-spectrum antimicrobial agents are given for 10 to 14 days.
- The patient is encouraged to remain on bed rest to alleviate symptoms rapidly.
- Comfort is promoted with analgesics, antispasmodics, bladder sedatives, sitz baths, and stool softeners.

Management of Chronic Bacterial Prostatitis

Chronic bacterial prostatitis is a major source of relapsing urinary tract infection.

- Pharmacologic therapy includes antimicrobials (trimethoprim-sulfamethoxazole, tetracycline, minocycline, doxycycline).
- Continuous suppressive treatment with low-dose antimicrobial drugs may be indicated.
- Comfort measures are the same as for acute bacterial prostatitis.

Management of Nonbacterial Prostatitis

- Symptomatic relief includes sitz baths and analgesics.

Nursing Management

COLLABORATIVE PROBLEMS/POTENTIAL
COMPLICATIONS

- Urinary retention from prostate swelling
- Epididymitis
- Bacteremia
- Pyelonephritis

Nursing Interventions

- Administer antibiotics as prescribed.
- Provide comfort measures: analgesics, sitz bath.

Promoting Home and Community-Based Care

- Instruct patient to complete prescribed course of antibiotics.

- Advise patient to take hot sitz baths for 10 to 20 minutes several times daily.
- Encourage fluids to satisfy thirst but not "forced" because effective drug level must be maintained in urine.
- Instruct patient to avoid foods and drinks that have diuretic action or increase prostatic secretions, including alcohol, coffee, tea, chocolate, cola, and spices.
- Instruct patient to avoid sexual arousal and intercourse during periods of acute inflammation.
- Teach patient that ejaculation by sexual intercourse or masturbation may be beneficial for chronic prostatitis by reducing retention of prostatic fluids.
- Advise patient to avoid sitting for long periods to minimize discomfort.
- Emphasize that medical follow-up is necessary for at least 6 months to 1 year.

For more information, see Chapter 45 in Smeltzer and Bare: *Brunner and Suddarth's Textbook of Medical-Surgical Nursing,* 9th edition. Philadelphia: Lippincott Williams & Wilkins, 2000.

PRURITUS

Pruritus (itching) is one of the most common complaints in dermatologic disorders. Although pruritus usually is due to primary skin disease, it may also reflect systemic disease, such as diabetes mellitus; renal, hepatic, thyroid, or blood disorders; or cancer. Pruritus may be caused by certain oral medications, contact with irritating agents (soaps, chemicals), or prickly heat (miliaria). It may also be a side effect of radiation therapy, a reaction to chemotherapy, or a symptom of infection. It may occur in elderly patients as a result of dry skin. It may also be caused by psychological factors (emotional stress).

Clinical Manifestations
- Itching and scratching, often more severe at night (itch-scratch-itch cycle)
- Excoriations, redness, raised areas on the skin (wheals), as a result of scratching
- Infections or changes in pigmentation
- Debilitating itching, if severe

Medical Management
- The cause of pruritus should be identified and treated (removed).
- The patient should avoid washing with soap and hot water.
- Cold compresses, ice cubes, or cool agents that contain soothing menthol and camphor may be applied.
- Bath oils (Lubriderm or Alpha Keri) are prescribed, except for elderly patients or those with impaired balance, who should not add oil to the bath because of slipping danger.
- Topical steroids are prescribed to decrease itching.
- Oral antihistamines (diphenhydramine [Benadryl]) are sometimes used.
- Tricyclic antidepressants (doxepin [Sinequan]) may be prescribed when pruritus is of neuropsychogenic origin.

Nursing Management
- Reinforce reasons for the prescribed therapeutic regimen.
- Remind the patient to use tepid (not hot) water and to shake off excess water and blot between intertriginous areas with a towel.
- Advise patient to avoid rubbing vigorously with towel, which overstimulates skin, causing more itching.
- Instruct patient to avoid scratching and to trim nails short to prevent skin damage and infection.
- Advise patient to avoid situations that cause vasodilation (warm environment, ingestion of alcohol).
- Lubricate skin with an emollient that traps moisture.

P

- Keep room cool and humidified.
- Advise patient to wear soft cotton clothing next to skin.

For more information, see Chapter 52 in Smeltzer and Bare: *Brunner and Suddarth's Textbook of Medical-Surgical Nursing,* 9th edition. Philadelphia: Lippincott Williams & Wilkins, 2000.

PSORIASIS

Psoriasis is a chronic, noninfectious, inflammatory disease of the skin in which the production of epidermal cells occurs at a rate that is about six to nine times faster than normal. The basal skin cells divide too quickly, and the newly formed cells become evident as profuse scales or plaques of epidermal tissue. There appears to be a hereditary defect that causes overproduction of keratin. The primary defect is unknown. Periods of emotional stress and anxiety aggravate the condition, and trauma, infections, and seasonal and hormonal changes are trigger factors. Onset may occur at any age but is most common between the ages of 15 and 50 years. Main sites of the body affected are the scalp, area over the elbows and knees, lower part of the back, and genitalia. Bilateral symmetry often exists. Psoriasis may be associated with asymmetric rheumatoid factor–negative arthritis of multiple joints. An exfoliative psoriatic state may develop in which the disease progresses to involve the total body surface (erythrodermic psoriatic state).

Clinical Manifestations

Symptoms range from a cosmetic annoyance to a physically disabling and disfiguring affliction.

- Lesions appear as red, raised patches of skin covered with silvery scales.
- If scales are scraped away, the dark red base of lesion is exposed, with multiple bleeding points.

- Patches are dry and may or may not itch.
- The condition may involve nail pitting, discoloration, crumbling beneath the free edges, and separation of the nail plate.
- If psoriasis occurs on the palms and soles, pustular lesions may develop.

Psychological Considerations

- Psoriasis may cause despair and frustration; observers may stare, comment, ask embarrassing questions, or even avoid the person.
- The condition can eventually exhaust resources, interfere with job, and make life miserable in general.
- Teenagers are especially vulnerable to its psychological effects.
- It can cause family disruption because of time-consuming treatments, messy salves, and constant shedding of scales.

Diagnostic Evaluation

- Classic plaque-type lesions
- Signs of nail and scalp involvement and positive family history

Medical Management

The goals of management are to slow the rapid turnover of epidermis and to promote resolution of the psoriatic lesions. There is no known cure. The therapeutic approach should be understandable, cosmetically acceptable, and not too disruptive of lifestyle.

Topical Therapy

- Topical treatment is used to slow the overactive epidermis without affecting other tissues.
- Medications include tar preparations and anthralin (irritating), salicylic acid, and corticosteroids; calcipotriene (Dovonex) and tazarotene (Tazorac) may require occlusive dressings. Medications may be in lotions, ointments, pastes, creams, and shampoos.

NURSING ALERT

Assess the flammability of any plastic substances used; caution patient not to smoke or go near open flame.

Intralesional Therapy
- Intralesional injections of triamcinolone acetonide (Aristocort, Kenalog-10, Trymex)

Systemic Therapy
- Systemic cytotoxic preparations (methotrexate) may be used.
- Laboratory studies are monitored to ensure that hepatic, hematopoietic, and renal systems are functioning adequately.
- Patient should avoid drinking alcohol while taking methotrexate, (increases possibility of liver damage).
- Oral retinoids (synthetic derivatives of vitamin A and vitamin A acid) may be prescribed.

Photochemotherapy
- Psoralen and ultraviolet A (PUVA) therapy may be used for severely debilitating psoriasis.
- Photochemotherapy is associated with long-term risks of skin cancer, cataracts, and premature aging of the skin.
- Ultraviolet B (UVB) light therapy may be used to treat generalized plaque and may be combined with topical coal tar (Goeckerman's therapy).

Nursing Management
Assessment
Assessment focuses on how the patient is coping with the skin condition, the appearance of "normal" skin, and the appearance of skin lesions.
- Note major skin manifestations.
- Examine areas especially affected: elbows, knees, scalp, gluteal cleft, fingers, and toenails (for small pits).

Major Nursing Diagnoses
- Knowledge deficit of the disease process and treatment
- Impaired skin integrity related to lesions and inflammatory response
- Body image disturbance related to embarrassment over appearance and self-perception of uncleanliness

Collaborative Problems/Potential Complications
- Psoriatic arthritis
- Infection

Planning and Goals
The major goals of the patient may include increased understanding of psoriasis and the treatment regimen, achievement of smoother skin with control of lesions, development of self-acceptance, and absence of complications.

Nursing Interventions
PROMOTING UNDERSTANDING
- Explain with sensitivity that there is no cure and that lifetime management is necessary; the disease process can usually be controlled.
- Review pathophysiology of psoriasis and factors that provoke it: any irritation or injury to the skin (cut, abrasion, sunburn), any current illness, emotional stress, unfavorable environment (cold), and drug (caution patient about nonprescription medication).
- Review and explain treatment regimen to ensure compliance; provide patient education materials in addition to face-to-face discussions.

INCREASING SKIN INTEGRITY
- Advise patient not to pick or scratch areas.
- Encourage patient to prevent the skin from drying out; dry skin causes psoriasis to worsen.
- Inform patient that water should not be too hot and skin should be dried by patting with a towel.

P

- Teach patient to use bath oil or emollient cleansing agent for sore and scaling skin.

IMPROVING SELF-CONCEPT AND BODY IMAGE
- Introduce coping strategies and suggestions for reducing or coping with stressful situations to facilitate a more positive outlook and acceptance of the disease.

MONITORING AND MANAGING COMPLICATIONS
- Psoriatic arthritis: note joint discomfort and evaluate further.
- Assist patient to rest joint, apply heat, and take salicylates.
- Educate patient about the care and treatment and need for compliance.

🏠 Promoting Home and Community-Based Care

Teaching Patients Self-Care
- Advise patient that the topical agent anthralin leaves a brownish purple stain; will subside when treatment stops; cover lesions to avoid staining clothing.
- Advise patient that topical corticosteroid preparations on face and around eyes predispose to cataract development; use strict guidelines to avoid overuse.
- Provide helpful tips on application of tar preparations.
- Teach patient to avoid exposure to sun when undergoing PUVA treatments.
- Remind patient to schedule ophthalmic examinations on regular basis.
- Instruct patient to prevent nausea by taking food with methoxsalen.
- Instruct patient to use lubricants and bath oils to remove scales and dryness.
- Advise female patient to use contraceptives to prevent the teratogenic effect of PUVA (fetal defects).
- Encourage patient to belong to a support group and to contact the National Psoriasis Foundation for information.

Evaluation

EXPECTED OUTCOMES

- Acquires knowledge and understanding of disease process and its treatment
- Achieves smoother skin and control of lesion
- Experiences relief of itching and discomfort
- Experiences no complications

For more information, see Chapter 52 in Smeltzer and Bare: *Brunner and Suddarth's Textbook of Medical-Surgical Nursing,* 9th edition. Philadelphia: Lippincott Williams & Wilkins, 2000.

PULMONARY EDEMA, ACUTE

Pulmonary edema is the abnormal accumulation of fluid in the lung tissue or alveoli. Fluid leaks through the capillary walls, permeating the airways and giving rise to severe dyspnea. This is a severe, life-threatening condition, usually resulting from increased pulmonary vascular pressure due to abnormal cardiac function. Noncardiac pulmonary edema has a wide variety of causes, including sudden increase in intravascular pressure in the lung, such as after pneumonectomy, and rapid inflation of the lungs after aspiration of a pneumothorax or evacuation of a pleural effusion, toxic inhalants, drug overdose, and neurogenic pulmonary edema. The most common cause of pulmonary edema is cardiac disease: atherosclerotic, hypertensive, valvular, myopathic. If appropriate measures are taken promptly, attacks can be aborted, and patients can survive this complication.

Clinical Manifestations

- A typical attack occurs at night after lying down for a few hours and is usually preceded by increasing restlessness, anxiety, and inability to sleep.
- The patient experiences sudden onset of breathlessness and a sense of suffocation; the hands become cold and

moist, nailbeds become cyanotic, and skin color turns gray.
- Pulse is weak and rapid; neck veins are distended.
- Incessant coughing produces increasing quantities of mucoid sputum.
- As pulmonary edema progresses, anxiety develops into near panic; the patient becomes confused, then stuporous.
- Breathing is noisy and moist; the patient can suffocate with blood-tinged, frothy fluid (can drown in own fluid).

Diagnostic Evaluation
- Clinical manifestations
- Hemodynamic testing: pulmonary artery capillary pressure and wedge pressure, and cardiac output by pulmonary artery catheter

Medical Management
The goals of medical management are to reduce total circulating volume and to improve respiratory exchange.

Oxygenation
- Oxygen in concentrations adequate to relieve hypoxia and dyspnea
- Oxygen by intermittent or continuous positive pressure, if signs of hypoxemia persist
- Endotracheal intubation and mechanical ventilation, if respiratory failure occurs
- Positive end-expiratory pressure (PEEP)
- Monitoring of pulse oximetry and arterial blood gases (ABGs)

Pharmacotherapy
- Morphine given intravenously in small doses to reduce anxiety and dyspnea; contraindicated in cerebral vascular accident, chronic pulmonary disease, or cardiogenic shock; naloxone hydrochloride (Narcan) available for excessive respiratory depression

- Diuretics: furosemide (Lasix) or hydrochlorothiazide (HydroDIURIL) to produce a rapid diuretic effect
- Digitalis: to improve cardiac contractility; administered with extreme caution to patients with acute myocardial infarction
- Amrinone to dilate the arteries, or dobutamine to increase cardiac contractility

Nursing Management
Nursing Interventions
POSITIONING THE PATIENT TO
PROMOTE CIRCULATION
- Position the patient upright (in bed if necessary) or with legs and feet down.
- Preferably position the patient with legs dangling over the side of bed.

PROVIDING PSYCHOLOGICAL SUPPORT
- Reassure patient, touching to offer a sense of concrete reality.
- Maximize time at the bedside.
- Give frequent, simple, concise information about what is being done to treat the condition and what the responses to treatment mean.

MONITORING MEDICATION
- Observe patient for excessive respiratory depression, hypotension, and vomiting.
- Keep a morphine antagonist available (eg, naloxone hydrochloride [Narcan]).
- Insert and maintain an indwelling catheter if ordered.

PREVENTING COMPLICATIONS
- Recognize early stages when presenting signs and symptoms are those of pulmonary congestion; auscultate lung fields of patients with cardiac disease.
- Place patient in an upright position with feet and legs dependent.
- Eliminate overexertion and emotional stress to reduce left ventricular load.

- Administer morphine to reduce anxiety, dyspnea, and preload.
- Direct long-range approach at its precursor, pulmonary congestion.
- Use patient teaching and measures to prevent congestive heart failure.
- Advise patient to sleep with head of bed elevated on 25-cm (10-inch) blocks.
- Teach patient that surgical treatment is used to eliminate or minimize valvular defects that limit flow of blood into or out of left ventricle.

☰ NURSING ALERT

Use extreme caution when administering infusions and transfusions to cardiac patients and elderly people. To prevent circulatory overload, administer intravenous fluids at a slower rate; position patient upright in bed, and place under close nursing surveillance. Use intravenous control devices to restrict volume of fluid that can be delivered.

For more information, see Chapter 27 in Smeltzer and Bare: *Brunner and Suddarth's Textbook of Medical-Surgical Nursing,* 9th edition. Philadelphia: Lippincott Williams & Wilkins, 2000.

PULMONARY EMBOLISM

Pulmonary embolism refers to the obstruction of the base or one or more branches of the pulmonary arteries by a thrombus (or thrombi) that originates somewhere in the venous system or in the right side of the heart. Massive pulmonary embolism is life-threatening and can cause death within the first 1 to 2 hours after the embolic event. It is a common disorder associated with trauma, surgery (orthopedic, major abdominal, pelvic, gynecologic), pregnancy, oral contraceptive use, congestive heart failure, advanced age (older than 50 years), hypercoagulable states, and prolonged immobility. Most thrombi originate in the deep veins of the legs.

Clinical Manifestations

Symptoms depend on the size of the thrombus and the area of the pulmonary artery occlusion.

- Dyspnea is the most common symptom.
- Tachypnea is the most frequent sign.
- Chest pain is common, usually sudden in onset and pleuritic in nature; it can be substernal and may mimic angina pectoris.
- Fever, tachycardia, apprehension, cough, diaphoresis, hemoptysis, syncope, shock, and sudden death may occur.
- Multiple small emboli in the terminal pulmonary arterioles simulate symptoms of bronchopneumonia or heart failure.
- Sudden pain or swelling of the proximal or distal extremity is relieved with elevation.

Diagnostic Evaluation

- Ventilation-perfusion scan, pulmonary angiography, chest radiograph
- Electrocardiogram (ECG), peripheral vascular studies, impedance plethysmography, and arterial blood gases (ABGs)

Medical Management

The immediate objective is to stabilize the cardiorespiratory system.

- Nasal oxygen is administered immediately to relieve hypoxemia, respiratory distress, and cyanosis.
- An infusion is started to establish intravenous route for drugs or fluids.
- In some circumstances pulmonary angiography, perfusion lung scans, hemodynamic measurements, and ABGs are performed.

- An indwelling urethral catheter is inserted to monitor urinary output, if embolism is massive and patient is hypotensive.
- Hypotension is treated by infusion of dobutamine or dopamine.
- The ECG is monitored continuously for dysrhythmias and right ventricular failure.
- Digitalis glycosides, intravenous diuretics, and antidysrhythmic agents are administered when appropriate.
- Blood is drawn for serum electrolytes, complete blood count, and hematocrit.
- Patient is placed on a volume-controlled ventilator if clinical assessment and ABGs indicate.
- Small doses of intravenous morphine are given to relieve anxiety, alleviate chest discomfort, help the patient tolerate the endotracheal tube, and ease adaptation to mechanical ventilator.

Anticoagulation Therapy
- The partial thromboplastin time (PTT) is maintained at 1.5 to 2.5 times normal, prothrombin time (PT) 1.5 to 2.5 hours normal, or an INR of 2.0 to 3.0.
- Heparin is administered for 5 to 7 days.
- Warfarin (Coumadin) is begun within 24 hours following the start of heparin therapy and continued for 3 to 6 months.

Thrombolytic Therapy
- Thrombolytic therapy may include urokinase and streptokinase (tissue plasminogen activator).
- It is reserved for pulmonary embolism affecting a significant area and causing hemodynamic instability.
- Bleeding is a significant side effect; nonessential invasive procedures are avoided.

Surgical Intervention
- Embolectomy by means of thoracotomy with cardiopulmonary bypass technique
- Interruption of inferior vena cava

- Transvenous catheter embolectomy with or without insertion of an inferior vena caval filter

Prevention
- Anticoagulant therapy before abdominothoracic surgery and every 8 to 12 hours until discharge from hospital
- Intermittent pneumatic leg compression devices

Nursing Management
Assessment
- Examine for a positive Homans' sign, which may indicate impending thrombosis of the leg veins.
- Identify those who are at high risk to minimize risk of pulmonary embolism.
- Suspect pulmonary embolism in conditions predisposing to slowing of venous return.
- Assess frequently for signs of hypoxia; monitor pulse oximetry values.
- Be alert for potential complication of cardiogenic shock or right ventricular failure.

Major Nursing Diagnoses
- Impaired gas exchange related to pulmonary vessel obstruction
- Risk for altered tissue perfusion related to thrombus formation
- Pain related to vascular obstruction and decreased tissue perfusion
- Anxiety related to uncertain outcome and lack of knowledge about condition and treatment
- Risk for infection related to surgical wound
- Risk for injury: hemorrhage related to decreased clotting

Nursing Interventions
PROVIDING GENERAL CARE
- Ensure understanding of need for continuous oxygen therapy.

- Provide nebulizers, incentive spirometry, or percussion and postural drainage,
- Encourage deep-breathing exercises.

PREVENTING THROMBUS FORMATION
- Encourage early ambulation and active and passive leg exercises.
- Instruct patient to move legs in a "pumping" exercise.
- Advise patient to avoid prolonged sitting, immobility, and constrictive clothing.
- Do not permit dangling of legs and feet in a dependent position.
- Instruct patient to place feet on floor or chair and to avoid crossing legs.
- Do not leave intravenous catheters in veins for prolonged periods.

MONITORING THROMBOLYTIC AND ANTICOAGULANT THERAPY
- Advise bed rest, monitor vital signs every 2 hours, limit invasive procedures.
- Measure PT or activated PTT every 3 to 4 hours after thrombolytic infusion is started to confirm activation of fibrinolytic systems.
- Perform only essential ABG studies on upper extremities, with manual compression of puncture site for at least 30 minutes.

MINIMIZING CHEST PAIN, PLEURITIC
- Place patient in semi-Fowler's position; turn and reposition patient frequently.
- Administer analgesics as prescribed for severe pain.

HELPING PATIENT TO COPE WITH ANXIETY
- Encourage patient to express feelings and concerns.
- Answer questions concisely and accurately.
- Explain therapy, and describe how to recognize unfound effects early.

PROVIDING POSTOPERATIVE NURSING CARE
- Measure pulmonary arterial pressure and urinary output.
- Assess insertion site of arterial catheter for hematoma formation and infection.
- Maintain blood pressure to ensure profusion of vital organs.
- Encourage isometric exercises, elastic stockings, and walking when permitted out of bed; elevate the foot of the bed, when resting.
- Discourage sitting; hip flexion causes compression of large veins in the legs.

🏠 Promoting Home and Community-Based Care

Teaching Patients Self-Care
- Before discharge and at follow-up clinic or home visits, instruct patient in how to prevent recurrence and what signs and symptoms should alert patient to seek medical attention.
- Teach patient to look for bruising and bleeding when taking anticoagulants; protect from bumping into objects that can cause bruising.
- Teach patient to use a toothbrush with soft bristles.
- Instruct patient not to take aspirin or antihistamine drugs while taking warfarin sodium (Coumadin) and always to check with physician before taking any medication, including over-the-counter drugs.
- Advise patient to continue wearing antiembolism stockings as long as directed.
- Instruct patient to avoid laxatives, which affect vitamin K absorption.
- Teach patient to avoid sitting with legs crossed or for prolonged periods.
- Recommend that patient change position regularly when traveling, walk occasionally, and do active exercises of legs and ankles.
- Advise patient to drink plenty of liquids.

- Teach patient to report dark, tarry stools immediately.
- Recommend that patient wear identification stating that anticoagulants are being taken.

For more information, see Chapter 21 in Smeltzer and Bare: *Brunner and Suddarth's Textbook of Medical-Surgical Nursing,* 9th edition. Philadelphia: Lippincott Williams & Wilkins, 2000.

PULMONARY HEART DISEASE (COR PULMONALE)

Cor pulmonale is a condition in which the right ventricle enlarges (with or without failure) as a result of diseases that affect the structure or function of the lung or its vasculature. The most frequent cause is chronic obstructive pulmonary disease (COPD). Other causes are conditions that restrict or compromise ventilatory function (massive obesity) and deformities of the thoracic cage, or that reduce the pulmonary vascular bed (pulmonary embolus), causing primary pulmonary hypertension. Certain disorders of the nervous system, respiratory muscles, chest wall, and pulmonary arterial tree may also be responsible for cor pulmonale. Prognosis depends on reversing the hypertensive process.

Clinical Manifestations
Symptoms are usually those of the underlying lung disease.

- Clinical features include COPD, shortness of breath, and cough.
- Right ventricular failure develops (edema of the feet and legs, distended neck veins, enlarged palpable liver, pleural effusion, ascites, and a heart murmur).
- Headache, confusion, and somnolence from carbon dioxide narcosis may occur.

Medical Management

The objectives of treatment are to improve the patient's ventilation and to treat both the underlying lung disease and the manifestations of heart disease.

- Oxygen is given to reduce pulmonary arterial pressure and pulmonary vascular resistance.
- Continuous (24-h/day) oxygen therapy is provided for severe hypoxia.
- Pulse oximetry and arterial blood gases (ABGs) are assessed.
- Bronchial hygiene, bronchodilators, and chest physical therapy may be instituted.
- If respiratory failure occurs, intubation and mechanical ventilation may be necessary.
- If heart failure occurs, hypoxemia and hypercapnia are improved.
- Peripheral edema and circulatory load on the right side of the heart are reduced with bed rest, sodium restriction, and diuretics.
- If indicated (eg, left ventricular failure), digitalis may be given.
- The electrocardiogram (ECG) is monitored.
- Pulmonary infection (precipitates cor pulmonale) is treated.

Nursing Management

See Nursing Management of Cardiac Failure for additional information.

Nursing Interventions

- If intubation and mechanical ventilation are required, assist. Support patient physically and emotionally.
- Assess the patient's respiratory and cardiac status.
- Instruct patient about the importance of close monitoring and adherence to the therapeutic regimen, especially oxygen.

- Explain and address factors that affect the patient's adherence to the treatment regime.

 Promoting Home and Community-Based Care

Teaching Patients Self-Care
- Advise patient and family that management is long-term and that most care and monitoring are performed at home for this chronic disorder.
- Advise patient to avoid activities that irritate airway if COPD exists.
- Administer continuous oxygen and instruct how to use.
- Urge patient to stop smoking; refer patient to smoking cessation or community support group.
- Counsel patient about nutrition if on a sodium-restricted diet or taking diuretics.
- If the patient's physical condition warrants close assessment or the patient cannot manage self-care, refer the patient for home care.

NURSING ALERT

If the patient has coincident left ventricular failure, supraventricular dysrhythmia, or right ventricular failure and is nonresponsive to other therapy, give digitalis with extreme caution because pulmonary heart disease appears to enhance susceptibility to digitalis toxicity.

For more information, see Chapter 21 in Smeltzer and Bare: *Brunner and Suddarth's Textbook of Medical-Surgical Nursing,* 9th edition. Philadelphia: Lippincott Williams & Wilkins, 2000.

PULMONARY HYPERTENSION

Pulmonary hypertension is a condition that is not clinically evident until late in the disease progression. The systolic pulmonary arterial pressure exceeds 30 mm Hg, and the mean pulmonary artery pressure is higher than 25 mm Hg. There are two forms: primary (idiopathic) and secondary. Primary pulmonary hypertension is uncommon; diagnosis is made by exclusion. The exact cause is unknown. The clinical presentation exists with no evidence of pulmonary and cardiac disease or pulmonary embolism. It occurs most often in women between 20 and 40 years of age and is usually fatal within 5 years of diagnosis. Secondary pulmonary hypertension is more common and results from existing cardiac or pulmonary disease. The prognosis depends on the severity of the underlying disorder and the changes in the pulmonary vascular bed. A common cause is pulmonary artery constriction due to hypoxia from chronic obstructive pulmonary disease (COPD).

Clinical Manifestations
- Dyspnea, the main symptom, is noticed first with exertion and then rest.
- Substernal chest pain is common.
- Weakness, fatigability, and syncope may occur.
- Signs of right-sided heart failure (peripheral edema, ascites, distended neck veins, liver engorgement, crackles, heart murmur) are noted.
- Electrocardiogram (ECG) changes (right ventricular hypertrophy) are seen, with right axis deviation and tall, peaked ranges in inferior leads and tall anterior ranges and ST-segment depression or T-wave inversion anteriorly.
- PaO_2 is decreased (hypoxemia).

Diagnostic Evaluation
- Chest radiograph
- ECG

- Cardiac catheterization
- Ventilation-perfusion scan
- Pulmonary function studies
- Lung biopsy
- Echocardiogram, open-lung biopsy (in some cases)

Medical Management
The objective of treatment is to manage the underlying cardiac or pulmonary condition. In all cases, management includes continuous oxygen therapy.

When Caused by Cor Pulmonale
- Fluid restriction
- Cardiac glycosides (digitalis)
- Rest
- Diuretics to decrease fluid accumulation

When Caused by Primary Pulmonary Hypertension
- Vasodilators
- Anticoagulants (warfarin [Coumadin])
- Heart-lung transplantation when not responsive to other therapies

Nursing Management
Nursing Interventions
- Identify patients who are at high risk for developing pulmonary hypertension (ie, those with COPD, pulmonary emboli, congenital heart disease, and mitral valve disease).
- Be alert for signs and symptoms.
- Administer oxygen therapy appropriately.

For more information, see Chapter 21 in Smeltzer and Bare: *Brunner and Suddarth's Textbook of Medical-Surgical Nursing,* 9th edition. Philadelphia: Lippincott Williams & Wilkins, 2000.

PYELONEPHRITIS, ACUTE

Pyelonephritis is a bacterial infection of the renal pelvis, tubules, and interstitial tissue of one or both kidneys. Bacteria reach the bladder through the urethra and ascend to the kidney. It is frequently secondary to urine backup (reflux) into the ureters, usually at the time of voiding. Urinary tract obstruction and renal diseases are other causes. Pyelonephritis may be acute or chronic.

Clinical Manifestations
- Chills and fever, flank pain, costovertebral angle tenderness
- Leukocytosis, bacteria and white blood cells in the urine, frequent symptoms of lower urinary tract involvement (dysuria and frequency)
- Enlarged kidneys

Diagnostic Evaluation
- Ultrasound or computed tomography (CT) scan
- Urine culture and sensitivity
- Radionuclide imaging with gallium if other studies not conclusive

Medical Management
- Intensive antimicrobial therapy: 2 to 3 days of parenteral therapy if patient is dehydrated, has nausea or vomiting, shows signs of sepsis, or is pregnant; followed with oral agents once patient is afebrile and showing clinical improvement; 2-week course of antibiotics for outpatients
- Continuous antimicrobial treatment after initial regimen until there is no evidence of infection, all causative factors have been treated or controlled, and kidney function has stabilized

P

Nursing Management

The plan of care is the same as that for upper urinary tract infections; see Nursing Management under Cystitis for additional information.

For more information, see Chapter 41 in Smeltzer and Bare: *Brunner and Suddarth's Textbook of Medical-Surgical Nursing,* 9th edition. Philadelphia: Lippincott Williams & Wilkins, 2000.

PYELONEPHRITIS, CHRONIC

Repeated bouts of acute pyelonephritis may lead to chronic pyelonephritis (chronic interstitial nephritis). Complications of chronic pyelonephritis include end-stage renal disease (from progressive loss of nephrons secondary to chronic inflammation and scarring), hypertension, and formation of kidney stones (from chronic infection with urea-splitting organisms, resulting in stone formation).

Clinical Manifestations
- Patient usually has no symptoms of infection unless an acute exacerbation occurs.
- Fatigue, headache, and poor appetite may occur.
- Polyuria, excessive thirst, and weight loss may result.
- Persistent and recurring infection, which may produce progressive scarring resulting in renal failure; however, evidence suggests chronic pyelonephritis is less frequently a cause of chronic renal failure.

Diagnostic Evaluation
- Intravenous urogram
- Measurement of blood urea nitrogen (BUN), creatinine levels, creatinine clearance

Medical Management

The goal of treatment is to eradicate bacteria from the urine.

- Antimicrobial medication based on pathogen identification by culture
- Nitrofurantoin or a combination of sulfamethoxazole and trimethoprim to suppress bacterial growth

Nursing Management

The plan of care is the same as that for upper urinary tract infections; see Nursing Management under Cystitis for additional information.

Nursing Interventions

- Recognize patients at risk for infection.
- Teach preventive measures and early recognition of symptoms.
- Instruct patient to complete full prescription of antibiotics and have a follow-up urine culture 2 weeks after completion of antibiotic therapy (additional weeks of antibiotics will be needed if relapse is seen).
- Monitor with serum creatinine determinations and blood counts for duration of long-term therapy.
- Monitoring for and teach patient signs of compromised renal function in excretion of antimicrobial agents, particularly with nephrotoxic antimicrobial agents.

P

For more information, see Chapter 41 in Smeltzer and Bare: *Brunner and Suddarth's Textbook of Medical-Surgical Nursing*, 9th edition. Philadelphia: Lippincott Williams & Wilkins, 2000.

R

RAYNAUD'S DISEASE

Raynaud's disease is a form of intermittent arteriolar vaso-constriction. The cause is unknown, but episodes may be triggered by emotional factors or by unusual sensitivity to cold. Raynaud's disease is most common in women between the ages of 16 and 40 years and is seen much more frequently in cold climates and during the winter months. The term *Raynaud's phenomenon* is currently used to refer to localized, intermittent episodes of vasoconstriction of small arteries of the feet and hands, causing color and temperature changes. It is generally unilateral and affects only one or two digits. It is always associated with an underlying systemic disease. The prognosis for Raynaud's disease varies: some patients slowly improve, some grow slowly worse, and others show no change.

Clinical Manifestations
- Coldness, pain, and pallor brought on by sudden vasoconstriction followed by cyanosis followed by vasodilation; the progression follows the characteristic color change: white, blue, and red.
- Numbness, tingling, and burning pain occur as color changes.
- Involvement tends to be bilateral and symmetric.

Medical Management
- The prime objective in controlling Raynaud's disease is avoiding the particular stimuli that provoke vasoconstriction.
- Calcium-channel blockers may be effective.

- Sympathectomy (interruption of sympathetic nerves by removal of sympathetic ganglia or division of their branches).

Nursing Management

 Promoting Home and Community-Based Care

Teaching Patients Self-Care

- Instruct patient to avoid situations that may be upsetting, stressful, or unsafe.
- Reassure patient that serious complications (gangrene and amputation) are not usual.
- Emphasize the importance of smoking cessation; assist in finding support group.
- Advise patient to minimize exposure to cold, remain indoors as much as possible, and wear protective clothing when outdoors during cold winter and fall weather.
- Advise patient to handle sharp objects carefully to avoid injuring the fingers.
- Caution about postural hypotension (results from drugs and is increased by alcohol, exercise, and hot weather).

R

For more information, see Chapter 28 in Smeltzer and Bare: *Brunner and Suddarth's Textbook of Medical-Surgical Nursing*, 9th edition. Philadelphia: Lippincott Williams & Wilkins, 2000.

REGIONAL ENTERITIS (CROHN'S DISEASE)

Regional enteritis is a subacute and chronic inflammation that extends through all layers of the bowel wall. It commonly occurs in adolescents or young adults and is seen frequently in the older population (50 to 80 years) but can appear at any time of life. Although the most common areas in which it is found are the distal ileum and colon, it can occur anywhere along the gastrointestinal tract. Formation of fistulas, fissures, and abscesses occurs as the inflammation extends into the peritoneum. In advanced cases, the intestinal mucosa has a cobblestone-like appearance. As the disease advances, the bowel wall thickens and becomes fibrotic, and the intestinal lumen narrows. The clinical course and symptoms vary. In some patients, periods of remission and exacerbation occur; in others, the disease follows a fulminating course.

Clinical Manifestations

- Onset of symptoms is usually insidious, with prominent abdominal pain and diarrhea unrelieved by defecation.
- Diarrhea is present in 90% of patients.
- Crampy pains occur after meals; the patient tends to limit intake, causing weight loss, malnutrition, and secondary anemia.
- Chronic diarrhea may occur, resulting in an uncomfortable person who is thin and emaciated from inadequate food intake and constant fluid loss. The inflamed intestine may perforate and form intraabdominal and anal abscesses.
- Fever and leukocytosis occur.
- Abscesses, fistulas, and fissures are common.
- Symptoms extend beyond the gastrointestinal tract to include joint problems (arthritis), skin lesions (erythema nodosum), ocular disorders (conjunctivitis), and oral ulcers.

Diagnostic Evaluation

- Barium study of the upper gastrointestinal tract (most conclusive diagnostic aid shows the classic "string sign" of the terminal ileum—constriction of segment of intestine—as well as cobblestone appearance, fistulas, and fissures)
- Proctosigmoidoscopic examination, computed tomography (CT) scan
- Stool examination for occult blood and steatorrhea

- Complete blood count, sedimentation rate, albumin, and protein levels

Medical Management
See Medical Management under Ulcerative Colitis for additional information.

Nursing Management
See Nursing Management: The Patient With Inflammatory Bowel Disease under Ulcerative Colitis for additional information.

For more information, see Chapter 35 in Smeltzer and Bare: *Brunner and Suddarth's Textbook of Medical-Surgical Nursing,* 9th edition. Philadelphia: Lippincott Williams & Wilkins, 2000.

RENAL FAILURE, ACUTE

Renal failure results when the kidneys are unable to remove the body's metabolic waste and perform their regulatory functions. Acute renal failure (ARF) is a sudden and almost complete loss of kidney function (decreased glomerular filtration rate). Three major categories of ARF are (1) prerenal (hypoperfusion of the kidney commonly due to volume depletion states, extreme vasodilation, and impaired cardiac performance), (2) intrarenal (actual parenchymal damage to the glomeruli or kidney tubules from conditions such as burns, crush injuries, and infections as well as transfusion reactions on nephrotoxic agents, which may lead to acute tubular necrosis [ATN]), and (3) postrenal (urinary tract obstruction such as that due to calculi [stones], tumor, strictures, prostatic hyperplasia, or blood clots).

Clinical Manifestations
Four Clinical Phases of Acute Renal Failure
- The *initiation period* begins with the initial insult and ends when oliguria develops.

- The *period of oliguria* (urine volume less than 400 mL/24 h): uremic symptoms first appear, and hyperkalemia may develop.
- The *period of diuresis:* gradual increase in urinary output, which signals glomerular filtration has started to recover. Laboratory values stabilize and start to decrease.
- The *period of recovery:* improvement of renal function may take 3 to 12 months.

Signs and Symptoms
- Patient appears critically ill and lethargic with persistent nausea, vomiting, and diarrhea.
- Skin and mucous membranes are dry; breath may have odor of urine (uremic fetor).
- Central nervous system manifestations include drowsiness, headache, muscle twitching, and seizures.
- Urinary output is scanty to normal; urine may be bloody and of low specific gravity.
- A steady rise in blood urea nitrogen (BUN) may occur, depending on degree of catabolism. Serum creatinine values increase with disease progression.
- Hyperkalemia may lead to dysrhythmias and cardiac arrest.
- Progressive acidosis, increase in serum phosphate concentrations, and low serum calcium levels may be noted.
- Anemia may result from blood loss due to uremic gastrointestinal lesions, reduced red blood cell life-span, and reduced erythropoietin production.

Diagnostic Evaluation
- BUN, creatinine, electrolytes
- Urinary output

Medical Management
The objectives of treatment are to restore normal chemical balance and prevent complications until repair of renal tissue and restoration of renal function can take place. All possible causes of damage are identified, treated, and eliminated, if possible.

- Management of fluid balance based on daily body weight; serial measurements of central venous pressure; serum and urine concentrations; fluid losses; blood pressure; and clinical status
- Detection of fluid excesses and treatment using mannitol, furosemide, or ethacrynic acid to initiate a diuresis and prevent or minimize subsequent renal failure
- Restoration of adequate blood flow to the kidneys in prerenal ARF by intravenous fluids, an infusion of albumin or blood product transfusions
- Initiation of dialysis to prevent serious complications of uremia, including hyperkalemia, pericarditis, and seizures; use of hemodialysis, hemofiltration, or peritoneal dialysis
- Administration of ion exchange resins (sodium polystyrene sulfonate [Kayexalate]) orally or by retention enema
- Administration of intravenous glucose and insulin or calcium glutamate as an emergency and temporary measure to treat hyperkalemia
- Administration of sodium bicarbonate to promote an elevation of plasma pH
- Treatment of reduced levels of erythropoietin production with parenteral form of erythropoietin (Epogen) to prevent anemia
- Administration of sorbitol orally or as an enema; assessment for development of fecal impaction
- Treatment of shock and infection, if present
- Monitoring of arterial blood gases (ABGs) when severe acidosis is present
- Institution of appropriate ventilatory measures if respiratory problems develop (may require sodium bicarbonate therapy or dialysis)
- Control of elevated serum phosphate concentration with phosphate-binding agents (aluminum hydroxide)
- Limitation of dietary protein to about 1 g/kg during oliguric phase to minimize protein breakdown and to prevent accumulation of toxic end products

R

- Achievement of caloric requirements with high-carbohydrate feedings; total parenteral nutrition (TPN) may be required
- Restriction of foods and fluids containing potassium and phosphorus (bananas, citrus fruits and juices, coffee); restriction or potassium intake to 40 to 60 mEq/day
- Restriction of sodium to 2 g/day
- Evaluation of blood chemistry to determine the amounts of sodium, potassium, and water needed for replacement during oliguric phase
- After the diuretic phase, adoption of a high-protein, high-calorie diet with gradual resumption of activities

Nursing Management
Assessment
- Note information in nursing history and physical assessment indicating possible renal failure, particularly in patients at risk, and report to physician.
- Monitor intake and output for indications of failing renal function.
- Assess laboratory values and monitor regularly for patient response to therapy.
- Note clinical manifestations of renal failure and need for nursing care to address patient concerns.
- Assess patient's progress and response to treatment.
- Direct attention to patient's primary disorder; monitor for complications.

Major Nursing Diagnoses
- Fluid volume excess related to decreased urine output
- Activity intolerance related to fatigue, toxins, and fluid buildup
- Risk for impaired akin integrity related to edema, toxins, or impaired tissue perfusion
- Risk for infection related to invasive lines or uremic toxins
- Knowledge deficit regarding condition and treatment

Collaborative Problems/Potential Complications

- Pericarditis
- Anemia
- Bone disease
- Hyperkalemia, or risk for hyperkalemia

Planning and Goals

The major goals of the patient may include maintenance of ideal fluid balance, body weight, and electrolyte levels; increased knowledge about condition and treatment; participation in activities within patient tolerance; and absence of complications.

Nursing Interventions

- Direct attention to patient's primary disorder; monitor for complications.
- Participate in emergency treatment of fluid and electrolyte imbalances.
- Assess patient's progress and response to treatment.
- Provide physical and emotional support.
- Keep patient's family informed about condition, assist in understanding the treatments, and provide psychological support.
- Continue to include in the plan of care those nursing measures indicated for the patient's primary disorder (eg, burns, shock, trauma, obstruction of the urinary tract).

MONITORING FLUID AND ELECTROLYTES

- Screen parenteral fluids, all oral intake, and all medications carefully to ensure that hidden sources of potassium are not inadvertently administered or consumed.
- Monitor cardiac function and musculoskeletal status closely for changes suggestive of hyperkalemia. Monitor serum electrolyte levels and electrocardiogram (ECG) assessment (peaked T waves).
- Monitor fluid status by careful attention to parenteral and oral intake, urine output, gastric and stool output, wound drainage and perspiration, changes in body weight, presence of edema, distention of jugular veins,

alterations in heart sounds and breath sounds, and increasing difficulty in breathing.
- Use flowchart to record pertinent information to indicate degree to which condition is improving or deteriorating.
- Auscultate lungs for signs of moist crackles.
- Assess for generalized edema by examining presacral and pretibial areas several times daily.
- Report immediately to physician indicators of deterioration of fluid and electrolyte status; prepare for emergency treatment, including medications to treat hyperkalemia and initiation of hemodialysis, peritoneal dialysis, or hemofiltration to correct fluid and electrolyte disturbances.

REDUCING METABOLIC RATE
- Reduce exertion and metabolic rate during most acute stage with bed rest.
- Prevent or treat fever and infection promptly.

PROMOTING PULMONARY FUNCTION
- Assist patient to turn, cough, and take deep breaths frequently.
- Encourage and assist patient to move and turn.

AVOIDING INFECTION
- Practice asepsis with invasive lines and catheters.
- Avoid an indwelling catheter if possible.

PROVIDING SKIN CARE
- Give meticulous skin care.
- Massage bony prominences, turn frequently, bathe with cool water for comfort, and prevent skin breakdown.

PROVIDING SUPPORT DURING DIALYSIS
- Assist, explain, and support patient and family; do not ignore psychological needs and concerns.
- Explain rationale of treatment to patient and family.
- Repeat explanation and clarify questions after physician teaching.

- Encourage family members to touch and talk to patient during dialysis.
- Continually assess patient for complications (eg, pericarditis, bone disease, anemia) and their precipitating causes.

🍁 Gerontologic Considerations

- Changes in kidney function with normal aging increase susceptibility to kidney dysfunction and renal failure.
- Alterations in renal blood flow, glomerular filtration rate, and renal clearance increase the risk for drug-associated changes in renal function; take precautions with the administration of all medications.
- The kidney is less able to respond to fluid and electrolyte changes; recognize and treat problems quickly to avoid kidney damage.
- Use precautions when elderly patient must undergo extensive diagnostic tests or when new medications (eg, diuretics) are added, to prevent dehydration leading to acute renal failure.
- The mortality rate of ARF is slightly higher in elderly patients. Its etiology includes prerenal causes (eg, dehydration) and intrarenal causes (eg, nephrotoxic agents, such as nonsteroidal antiinflammatory drugs [NSAIDs], and contrast agents or media).
- Diabetes mellitus increases contrast agent–induced renal failure because of preexisting renal insufficiency and imposed fluid restriction.

R

For more information, see Chapter 41 in Smeltzer and Bare: *Brunner and Suddarth's Textbook of Medical-Surgical Nursing*, 9th edition. Philadelphia: Lippincott Williams & Wilkins, 2000.

RENAL FAILURE, CHRONIC (END-STAGE RENAL DISEASE)

Chronic renal failure, or end-stage renal disease (ESRD), is a progressive, irreversible deterioration in renal function in which the body's ability to maintain metabolic and fluid and electrolyte balance fails, resulting in uremia. It may be caused by diabetes; hypertension; chronic glomerulonephritis; pyelonephritis; hereditary lesions, such as in polycystic disease; vascular disorders; obstruction of the urinary tract; infections; or toxic agents. Environmental and occupational agents that have been implicated in chronic renal failure include lead, cadmium, mercury, and chromium. Dialysis or kidney transplantation eventually becomes necessary for patient survival. The rate of decline and progression of ESRD is related to the underlying disorder, urinary excretion of protein, and the presence of hypertension.

Clinical Manifestations

■ Signs and Symptoms of Chronic Renal Failure

Cardiovascular
Hypertension; pitting edema (feet, hands, sacrum); periorbital edema; pericardial friction rub; engorged neck veins; pericarditis; pericardial effusion; pericardial tamponade; hyperkalemia; hyperlipidemia

Integumentary
Gray-bronze skin color; dry, flaky skin; pruritus: ecchymosis; purpura; thin, brittle nails; coarse, thinning hair

Pulmonary
Crackles; thick, tenacious sputum; depressed cough reflex; pleuritic pain; shortness of breath; tachypnea; Kussmaul-type respirations; uremic pneumonitis ("uremic lung")

Gastrointestinal
Ammonia odor to breath ("fetor uremicus"); metallic taste; mouth ulcerations and bleeding; anorexia, nausea, and vomiting; hiccups; constipation or diarrhea; bleeding from GI tract

continued

■ **Signs and Symptoms of Chronic Renal Failure** (Continued)

Neurologic
Weakness and fatigue; confusion; inability to concentrate; disorientation; tremors; seizures; asterixis; restlessness of legs; burning of soles of feet; behavior changes

Musculoskeletal
Muscle cramps; loss of muscle strength; renal osteodystrophy; bone pain; bone fractures; foot drop

Reproductive
Amenorrhea; testicular atrophy; infertility; decreased libido

Hematologic
Anemia; thrombocytopenia

Medical Management

The goals of management are to retain kidney function and maintain homeostasis for as long as possible. All factors that contribute to ESRD and those that are reversible (eg, obstruction) are identified and treated.

- Complications can be prevented or delayed by administering prescribed antihypertensives, cardiovascular agents, anticonvulsants, erythropoietin (Epogen), iron supplements, phosphate-binding agents (antacids), and calcium supplements.
- Dietary intervention is needed, with careful regulation of protein intake, fluid intake to balance fluid losses, and sodium intake and with some restriction of potassium.
- Adequate calorie intake and vitamin supplementation are ensured.
- Protein is restricted; allowed protein must be of high biologic value: dairy products, eggs, meats.
- Calories are supplied with carbohydrates and fats to prevent wasting.
- Vitamin supplementation is provided.
- Hyperphosphatemia and hypocalcemia are treated with aluminum-based antacids or calcium carbonate; both must be given with food.

- Fluid allowance is 500 to 600 mL of fluid or more than the 24-hour urine output.
- Hypertension is managed by intravascular volume control and antihypertensive medication.
- Congestive heart failure and pulmonary edema are treated with fluid restriction, low-sodium diet, diuretics, inotropic agents (eg, digitalis or dobutamine), and dialysis.
- Metabolic acidosis is treated, if necessary, with sodium bicarbonate supplements or dialysis.
- Hyperkalemia is treated with dialysis; medications are monitored for potassium content; patient is placed on potassium-restricted diet; Kayexalate is administered as needed.
- Patient is observed for early evidence of neurologic abnormalities (eg, slight twitching, headache, delirium, or seizure activity).
- The onset of seizures, type, duration, and general effect on patient are recorded; physician is notified immediately.
- Patient is protected from injury with padded bed side rails.
- Intravenous diazepam (Valium) or phenytoin (Dilantin) is administered to control seizures.
- Anemia is treated with recombinant human erythropoietin (Epogen); hematocrit is monitored frequently. Heparin is adjusted as necessary to prevent clotting of the dialysis lines during treatments.
- Serum iron and transferrin levels are monitored to assess iron states (iron is necessary for adequate response to erythropoietin).
- Blood pressure and serum potassium levels are monitored.
- Patient is referred to a dialysis and transplantation center early in the course of progressive renal disease.
- Dialysis is initiated when patient cannot maintain a reasonable lifestyle with conservative treatment.

Nursing Management
- Address fluid volume excess (assess fluid status, help patient limit fluid intake to prescribed limit).
- Maintain adequate nutritional intake (assess nutritional status, address factors contributing to altered nutritional intake).
- Address the patient's knowledge deficit regarding condition and treatment (assess understanding, provide explanation of renal function, assist patient to identify ways to incorporate lifestyle changes related to illness and its treatment).
- Address the patient's activity intolerance (assess factors contributing to fatigue).
- Address self-esteem disturbance (assess patient's and family's responses and reaction to illness and treatment, encourage open discussion of concerns about changes produced by disease and treatment).
- Monitor and address collaborative problems (eg, hyperkalemia, pericarditis, pericardial effusion and pericardial tamponade, hypertension, anemia, bone disease, and metastatic calcifications).

Nursing Interventions
- Assess fluid status and identify potential sources of imbalance.
- Implement a dietary program to ensure proper nutritional intake within the limits of the treatment regimen.
- Provide explanations and information to the patient and family concerning ESRD, treatment options, and potential complications.
- Provide emotional support to patient and family.

Promoting Home and Community-Based Care

Teaching Patients Self-Care
- Provide ongoing education and reinforcement of previous teaching.

- Monitor the patient's progress and compliance with the treatment regimen.
- Provide a referral for nutritional consult.
- Teach patient and family what problems to report: worsening signs of renal failure, signs of hyperkalemia, signs and symptoms of access problems.
- Provide medication teaching.
- Teach patient how to assess vascular access for patency and precautions to take (no venipunctures or blood pressure on access arm).

Continuing Care
- Provide assistance and support to patient and family in dealing with dialysis and its long-term implications.
- Stress the importance of follow-up examinations and treatment.
- Refer patient to home care nurse for continued monitoring and support.

Evaluation
EXPECTED OUTCOMES
- Demonstrates fluid balance
- Maintains adequate nutritional intake
- Tolerates activity of daily living
- Experiences absence of complications

Gerontologic Considerations

Diabetes mellitus and hypertension are the leading causes of chronic renal failure in elderly patients. The symptoms of other disorders (congestive heart failure, dementia) can mask the symptoms of renal disease and delay or prevent diagnosis and treatment. The patient often complains of signs and symptoms of nephrotic syndrome, such as edema and proteinuria.

Hemodialysis and peritoneal dialysis have been used effectively in treating elderly patients. Concomitant disorders have made transplantation a less common treatment for the elderly.

The elderly patient may develop nonspecific signs of disturbed renal function and fluid and electrolyte imbalances.

For more information, see Chapter 41 in Smeltzer and Bare: *Brunner and Suddarth's Textbook of Medical-Surgical Nursing,* 9th edition. Philadelphia: Lippincott Williams & Wilkins, 2000.

R

S

SEBORRHEIC DERMATOSES

Seborrhea is an excessive production of sebum. Seborrheic dermatitis is a chronic inflammatory disease of the skin with a predilection for areas that are well supplied with sebaceous glands or that lie between folds of the skin, where the bacterial count is high. Seborrheic dermatitis has a genetic predisposition; hormones, nutritional status, infection, and emotional stress influence its course. There are remissions and exacerbations of this condition.

Clinical Manifestations
Two forms can occur: an oily form and a dry form; either form may start in childhood with fine scaling of scalp or other areas.
- Oily form: moist or greasy patches of sallow, greasy-appearing skin, with or without scaling, and slight erythremia; small pustules or papulopustules on trunk, resembles acne
- Dry form: flaky desquamation of the scalp (dandruff)
- Asymptomatic mild forms
- Scaling often accompanied by pruritus, leading to scratching and secondary complications (ie, infection and excoriation)

Medical Management
Because there is no known cure for seborrhea, the objectives of therapy are to control the disorder and allow the skin to repair itself.

- Administration of topical corticosteroid cream to body and face.

- Maximum aeration of skin and careful cleansing of areas where there are creases or folds are ensured to avoid candida yeast infection.
- Hair is shampooed daily or at least three times weekly with medicated shampoos. Two or three different types of shampoo are used in rotation to prevent the seborrhea from becoming resistant to a particular shampoo.

Nursing Management

- Advise patient to remove external irritants and to avoid excess heat and perspiration; rubbing and scratching prolong the disorder.
- Instruct patient to avoid secondary infections by airing the skin and keeping skin folds clean and dry.
- Instruct on use of medicated shampoo.
- Caution patient that seborrheic dermatitis is a chronic problem that tends to wax and wane. The goal is to keep it under control.
- Encourage patient to adhere to treatment program.
- Treat patients with sensitivity and an awareness of their need to express their feelings when they become discouraged by the effect on body image.

For more information, see Chapter 52 in Smeltzer and Bare: *Brunner and Suddarth's Textbook of Medical-Surgical Nursing,* 9th edition. Philadelphia: Lippincott Williams & Wilkins, 2000.

S

SHOCK, CARDIOGENIC

Cardiogenic shock occurs when the heart's ability to pump blood is impaired. The result is a marked reduction in cardiac output with inadequate perfusion to the heart, brain, and kidneys. Causes of cardiogenic shock are either coronary or noncoronary. Coronary cardiogenic shock is more common and is seen most often in patients with myocardial infarction. Noncoronary causes include cardiac tamponade, cardiomyopathy, valvular damage, and dysrhythmias.

Clinical Manifestations
• Dysrhythmias are common and result from a decrease in oxygen to the myocardium.
• Angina pain may be experienced.

Classic Signs
• Low blood pressure, rapid and weak pulse
• Cerebral hypoxia manifested by confusion and agitation
• Decreased urinary output and cold, clammy skin

Medical Management
The goals of medical treatment include limiting further myocardial damage, preserving the healthy myocardium, and improving the heart's ability to pump effectively.

• First-line treatment of cardiogenic shock includes supplying supplemental oxygen, controlling chest pain, administering vasoactive drugs, and selective fluid support.
• Oxygenation needs of heart muscle are addressed.
• Hemodynamic monitoring is performed.
• Pharmacologic therapy (eg, dopamine, nitroglycerine, dobutamine, and various antidysrhythmics) may be used.
• Mechanical support (eg, intraaortic balloon counterpulsation [IABC]) may be necessary.
• Coronary cardiogenic shock is treated with thrombolytic therapy, angioplasty, or coronary artery bypass graft surgery.
• Noncoronary cardiogenic shock is treated with cardiac valve replacement or correction of a dysrhythmia.

Nursing Management
Prevention
• Identify patients at risk early.
• Promote adequate oxygenation of the heart muscle, and decrease cardiac workload.

Hemodynamic Monitoring
- Monitor patient's hemodynamic and cardiac status: arterial lines and electrocardiogram (ECG).
- Anticipate need for medications, intravenous fluids, and other equipment.
- Document and report promptly changes in hemodynamic, cardiac, and pulmonary status.

Fluids Administration
- Provide for safe and accurate administration of intravenous fluids and medications.

Intraaortic Balloon Counterpulsation
- Provide ongoing timing adjustments of the balloon pump for maximum effectiveness.

Safety and Comfort
- Take an active role in ensuring patient's safety and physical comfort and in reducing anxiety.

For more information, see Chapter 14 in Smeltzer and Bare: *Brunner and Suddarth's Textbook of Medical-Surgical Nursing,* 9th edition. Philadelphia: Lippincott Williams & Wilkins, 2000.

S

SHOCK, HYPOVOLEMIC

Hypovolemic shock is a condition in which there is loss of effective circulating blood volume. It is the most common type of shock. Hypovolemic shock is caused by external fluid losses from hemorrhage; internal fluid shifts (eg, severe dehydration, severe edema, or ascites); and fluid losses from prolonged vomiting or diarrhea.

Clinical Manifestations
- Fall in venous pressure, rise in peripheral resistance, tachycardia

- Cold, moist skin; pallor; thirst; diaphoresis
- Altered sensorium, oliguria, metabolic acidosis, tachypnea
- Most dependable criterion: level of arterial blood pressure

Medical Management

The goals of treatment are to restore intravascular volume, redistribute fluid volume, and correct the underlying cause.

Fluid and Blood Replacement

- Ringer's lactate, colloids, and 0.9% NaCl are administered to restore intravascular volume.
- Blood products are used only if other alternatives are unavailable or blood loss is extensive and rapid; autotransfusion methods may be considered for closed cavity hemorrhage.

Redistribution of Fluids

- Patient is positioned properly to assist in fluid redistribution (modified Trendelenburg).
- Military antishock trousers (MAST) are used in extreme emergency situations when bleeding cannot be controlled.

Treatment of Underlying Cause

- If hemorrhaging, the bleeding is stopped by application of pressure or surgery.
- Diarrhea and vomiting are treated with medications.

Medications

- The same medications are used that are given in cardiogenic shock.
- The type of medication depends on the underlying cause.

Nursing Management
Primary Prevention

- Closely monitor patients who are at risk for fluid deficits (patients younger than 1 year and older than 65 years of age).

- Assist with fluid replacement before intravascular volume is depleted.

General Nursing Measures
- Assure safe administration of prescribed fluids and medications, and document effects.
- Monitor and report signs of complications and side effects of treatment.

Administering Blood Transfusions
- Monitor patient closely for adverse effects.

Fluid Replacement Complications
- Monitor for cardiovascular overload and pulmonary edema (eg, hemodynamic pressure monitoring, vital signs, arterial blood gases [ABGs], fluid intake and output).

Oxygen
- Reduce fear and anxiety about the need for oxygen mask by giving patient explanation and frequent reassurance.

For more information, see Chapter 14 in Smeltzer and Bare: *Brunner and Suddarth's Textbook of Medical-Surgical Nursing,* 9th edition. Philadelphia: Lippincott Williams & Wilkins, 2000.

S

SHOCK, SEPTIC

Septic shock is the most common type of distributive shock and is caused by widespread infection (gram-negative bacteria is the most common cause). Other infectious agents, such as gram-positive bacteria and viruses, can also cause septic shock. Conditions placing patients at risk for septic shock are immunosuppression, extremes of age (younger than 1 year and older than 65 years of age), malnourishment, extensive trauma or burns, chronic illness, and invasive procedures.

Clinical Manifestations

First Phase: Hyperdynamic or "Warm" Phase

- High cardiac output with vasodilation
- Hyperthermia with warm, flushed skin
- Heart and respiratory rates elevated
- Urinary output increased or normal
- Gastrointestinal status compromised (eg, nausea, vomiting, or diarrhea)
- Possible fever, hypotension, or subtle changes in status

Later Phase: Hypodynamic or "Cold" Phase

- Low cardiac output with vasoconstriction
- Decreased blood pressure
- Skin cool and pale
- Temperature normal or below normal
- Heart and respiratory rates rapid
- Anuria and multiple organ failure possible

Medical Management

- The cause of infection is identified and eliminated.
- Specimens are collected of urine, blood, sputum, and wound drainage.
- Broad-spectrum antibiotics are begun immediately.
- Potential routes of infection are eliminated (intravenous lines rerouted if necessary).
- Abscesses are drained and necrotic areas débrided.
- Fluid replacement is instituted.
- Aggressive nutritional supplementation (high protein) is provided. Enteral feedings are preferred.

Nursing Management

- Carry out all invasive procedures with correct aseptic technique and follow with careful hand washing.
- Monitor for signs of infection at intravenous lines, arterial and venous puncture sites, surgical incisions, trauma wounds, urinary catheters, and pressure ulcers.
- Identify patients at risk for sepsis and septic shock.
- Reduce patient's temperature when ordered for temperatures above 104°F or 40°C or if the patient is uncom-

fortable by administering salicylates, ice bags, and
hypothermia blankets; monitor closely for shivering.
- Administer prescribed intravenous fluids and
  medications.
- Monitor and report blood levels (antibiotic levels, blood
  urea nitrogen [BUN], creatinine, white blood count).
- Monitor hemodynamic status, fluid intake and output,
  and nutritional status.
- Monitor daily weights and serum albumin levels for
  daily protein requirements.

Gerontologic Considerations

Septic shock may be manifested in atypical or confusing
clinical signs. Suspect septic shock in any elderly person
who develops an unexplained acute confused state, tachypnea, or hypotension.

For more information, see Chapter 14 in Smeltzer and Bare: *Brunner and
Suddarth's Textbook of Medical-Surgical Nursing,* 9th edition. Philadelphia:
Lippincott Williams & Wilkins, 2000.

S

SPINAL CORD INJURY

Spinal cord injury is a major health problem, with an estimated 10,000 new injuries occurring each year. Half of
these injuries result from motor vehicle accidents; most of
the others occur from falls, sporting, and industrial accidents and gunshot wounds. Sixty percent of the victims are
16 to 30 years of age. Other risk factors include gender
(male) and substance abuse (alcohol and drugs). There is a
high frequency of associated injuries and medical complications. The vertebrae most frequently involved in spinal cord
injuries are the 5th, 6th, and 7th cervical, the 12th thoracic,
and the 1st lumbar. These vertebrae are the most susceptible because there is a greater range of mobility in the vertebral column in these areas. Damage to the spinal cord

ranges from transient concussion (patient recovers fully) to contusion, laceration, and compression of the cord substance (either alone or in combination), to complete transection of the cord (paralysis below the level of injury). Injury can be categorized as primary (usually permanent) or secondary (nerve fibers swell and disintegrate with ischemia, hypoxia, edema, and hemorrhagic lesions).

Clinical Manifestations

The consequences of spinal cord injury depend on the level of injury of the cord. The type of injury refers to the extent of injury to the spinal cord itself.

Neurologic Level

The neurologic level refers to the lowest level at which sensory and motor functions are normal.

- Total sensory and motor paralysis below the neurologic level
- Loss of bladder and bowel control (usually with urinary retention and bladder distention)
- Loss of sweating and vasomotor tone below the neurologic level
- Marked reduction of blood pressure from loss of peripheral vascular resistance
- If conscious, complains of acute pain in the back or neck

Respiratory Problems

- Related to compromised respiratory function; severity depends on level of injury
- Acute respiratory failure: leading cause of death in high cervical cord injury

Diagnostic Evaluation

Detailed neurologic examination, radiographic examinations (lateral cervical spine radiographs and computed tomography [CT] scanning).

Emergency Management

- Immediate management of the patient at the scene of the accident is crucial. Improper handling can cause further damage and loss of neurologic function.
- Consider any victim of a motor vehicle or driving accident, a contact sports injury, a fall, or any direct trauma to the head and neck as a spinal cord injury until ruled out.
- Initial care includes rapid assessment, immobilization, extrication, stabilization or control of life-threatening injuries, and transportation to an appropriate medical facility.
- Maintain patient in an extended position (no sitting); no body part should be twisted or turned.

Medical Management: Acute Phase

The goals of management are to prevent further spinal cord injury and to observe for symptoms of progressive neurologic deficits.

- Patient is resuscitated as necessary, and oxygenation and cardiovascular stability are maintained.

Pharmacotherapy
- High-dose steroids (methylprednisolone) are administered to counteract cord edema.

Respiratory Measures
- Oxygen is administered to maintain a high arterial PO_2.
- Extreme care is taken to avoid flexing or extending the neck if endotracheal intubation is necessary.
- Diaphragm pacing (electrical stimulation of the phrenic nerve) may be considered for patients with a high cervical lesion.

Skeletal Reduction and Traction
- Spinal cord injury requires immobilization, reduction of dislocations, and stabilization of the vertebral column.

S

○ The cervical fracture is reduced and the cervical spine aligned with a form of skeletal traction (using skeletal tongs or calipers or the halo-vest technique).
○ Weights are hung freely so as not to interfere with the traction.
- Surgical intervention: laminectomy may be performed to reduce spinal fracture or dislocation or to decompress the cord.

Complications of Spinal Injury: Spinal Shock

Spinal shock represents a sudden depression of reflex activity in the spinal cord (areflexia) below the level of injury. In this condition, the muscles innervated by the part of the cord segment situated below the level of the lesion become completely paralyzed and flaccid, and the reflexes are absent. Blood pressure and heart rate fall, and parts of the body below the level of the cord lesion are paralyzed and without sensation.

- Intestinal decompression is used to treat bowel distention and paralytic ileus caused by depression of reflexes.
- Close observation is provided to patient who does not perspire on paralyzed portion of body and for early detection of an abrupt onset of fever.
- Body defenses are maintained and supported until the spinal shock abates and the system has recovered from the traumatic insult (3 to 6 weeks).
- Special attention is paid to the respiratory system (may not be enough intrathoracic pressure to cough effectively).
- Chest physical therapy and suctioning are implemented to help clear pulmonary secretions.
- The patient is monitored for respiratory complications (respiratory failure, pneumonia).

Deep Vein Thrombosis and Its Complications

- The patient is monitored for autonomic hyperreflexia (characterized by pounding headache, profuse sweating, nasal congestion, piloerection [gooseflesh], bradycardia, and hypertension).

- Constant surveillance is maintained for signs and symptoms of pressure ulcers and infection (urinary, respiratory, local infection at the pin sites).
- The patient is observed for deep vein thrombosis (DVT), a complication of immobility (eg, pulmonary embolism). Symptoms include pleuritic chest pain, anxiety, shortness of breath, and abnormal blood-gas values.
- Thigh and calf measurements are assessed daily.
- Low-dose anticoagulation therapy is initiated to prevent DVT and pulmonary embolism.
- Thigh-high elastic stockings or pneumatic compression devices are used.

Nursing Management

Assessment

- Observe breathing pattern; assess strength of cough; auscultate lungs.
- Monitor constantly for any changes in motor or sensory function and symptoms of progressive neurologic damage.
- Determine motor and sensory function by careful neurologic examination; record these findings so that changes in or progression from the baseline can be evaluated accurately.
- Test motor ability by asking patient to spread fingers, squeeze examiner's hand, and move toes or turn the feet.
- Evaluate sensation by pinching the skin or pricking it with the broken end of a cotton swab, starting at shoulder and working down both sides. Ask patient where sensation is felt.
- Report immediately any decrease in neurologic function.
- Assess for the presence of spinal shock.
- Palpate bladder for signs of urinary retention and overdistention.
- Assess for gastric dilation and ileus due to atonic bowel.
- Monitor temperature (hypothermia may result due to autonomic disruption).

S

Major Nursing Diagnoses

- Ineffective breathing patterns related to weakness or paralysis of abdominal and intercostal muscles and inability to clear secretions
- Ineffective airway clearance related to weakness of intercostal muscles
- Impaired physical mobility related to motor and sensory impairment
- Risk for impaired skin integrity related to immobility or sensory loss
- Urinary retention related to inability to void spontaneously
- Constipation related to presence of atonic bowel as a result of autonomic disruption
- Pain and discomfort related to treatment and prolonged immobility
- Sensory-perceptual alterations related to immobility and sensory loss

Collaborative Problems/Potential Complications

- DVT
- Orthostatic hypotension
- Autonomic hyperreflexia

Planning and Goals

The major goals of the patient may include improvement of breathing pattern, improvement of mobility, maintenance of skin integrity, relief of urinary retention, improvement of bowel function, promotion of comfort, and absence of complications.

Nursing Interventions

PROMOTING ADEQUATE BREATHING

- Detect possible impending respiratory failure by observing patient, measuring vital capacity, and monitoring oxygen saturation through pulse oximetry and ABG values.
- Prevent retention of secretions and resultant atelectasis with early and vigorous attention to clearing bronchial and pharyngeal secretions.

- Employ suctioning with caution. This procedure can stimulate the vagus nerve, producing bradycardia and resulting in cardiac arrest.
- Initiate chest physical therapy and quad-assisted coughing for ineffective cough.
- Supervise breathing exercises that increase strength and endurance of inspiratory muscles, particularly the diaphragm.
- Ensure proper humidification and hydration to maintain thin secretions.
- Assess for signs of respiratory infection: cough, fever, and dyspnea.
- Discourage smoking.
- Monitor respiratory status frequently.

IMPROVING MOBILITY
- Maintain proper body alignment; place patient in dorsal or supine position.
- Turn patient every 2 hours; monitor for hypotension in patients with lesions above the mid-thoracic level.
- Do not turn patient if not on a turning frame unless physician has indicated that it is safe to do so.
- Give passive range-of-motion exercises within 48 to 72 hours after injury to avoid complications, such as contractures and atrophy.
- Provide a full range of motion at least four to five times daily to toes, metatarsals, ankles, knees, and hips.

MAINTAINING SKIN INTEGRITY
- Change patient's position every 2 hours, and inspect the skin.
- Assess for redness or breaks in skin over pressure points; check perineum for soilage; observe catheter for adequate drainage; assess general body alignment and comfort.
- Wash skin every few hours with a mild soap, rinse well, and blot dry. Keep pressure-sensitive areas well lubricated and soft with bland cream or lotion; gently perform massage with a circular motion.

S

- Teach patient danger of pressure ulcers and encourage to participate in preventive measures.

PROMOTING URINARY ELIMINATION

- Perform intermittent catheterization to avoid over-stretching the bladder and infection; if not feasible, insert indwelling catheter.
- Show family members how to catheterize, and encourage them to participate in this facet of care.
- Teach patient to record fluid intake, voiding pattern, amounts of residual urine after catheterization, quality of urine, and any unusual feelings that may be occurring.

PROMOTING ADAPTATION TO SENSORY-PERCEPTUAL ALTERATIONS

- Stimulate the area above the level of the injury through aromas, flavorful food, conversation, and music.
- Provide prism glasses to enable patient to see in supine position.
- Encourage use of hearing aids, if applicable.
- Provide emotional support; teach patient strategies to compensate for or cope with these deficits.

IMPROVING BOWEL FUNCTION

- Monitor patient's reactions to gastric intubation.
- Give a high-calorie, high-protein, and high-fiber diet, with amount of food gradually increased after bowel sounds resume.
- Administer prescribed stool softener to counteract effects of immobility and pain medications.
- Institute a bowel program as early as possible.

PROVIDING COMFORT

- Assess patient's skull for signs of infection, including drainage around the tongs.
- Check back of head periodically for signs of pressure and massage at intervals, taking care not to move the neck.
- Shave hair around tongs to facilitate inspection; avoid probing under encrusted areas.

- Reassure patient in halo traction that adapting to steel frame (ie, feeling caged in and hearing noises) will occur.
- Cleanse pin sites daily, and observe for redness, drainage, and pain; observe for loosening; keep a torque screwdriver readily available.
- Inspect skin under halo vest for excessive perspiration, redness, and skin blistering, especially on the bony prominences.
- Open vest at the sides to allow the patient's torso to be washed; do not allow vest to become wet; do not use powder inside vest.

MONITORING AND MANAGING
POTENTIAL COMPLICATIONS

Thrombophlebitis

Refer to the Medical Management heading for care.

Orthostatic Hypotension

- Reduce frequency of hypotensive episodes by providing vasopressor medications, thigh-high elastic stockings, time for slow position change, and tilt tables.

Autonomic Hyperreflexia

- Remove the triggering stimulus.
- Place patient immediately in a sitting position to lower blood pressure.
- Empty bladder immediately (ie, catheterize).
- Examine rectum for fecal mass after the symptoms subside. Apply topical anesthetic for 10 to 15 minutes before removal of fecal mass.
- Examine skin for areas of pressure, irritation, or broken skin.
- Give a ganglionic blocking agent (hydralazine [Apresoline]) if the above measures do not relieve hypertension and excruciating headache.
- Instruct patient in prevention and management measures. Inform patient with lesion above T-6 that episode can occur years after initial injury.
- Label medical record about the risk.

S

Promoting Home and Community-Based Care

Teaching Patients Self-Care

- Shift emphasis from ensuring patient is stable and free of complications to specific assessment and planning for independence and skills necessary for activities of daily living.
- Coordinate the management team, and serve as the liaison with rehabilitation centers and home care agencies.

Continuing Care

- Support patient and family, and assist them in assuming responsibility for increasing aspects of patient care and management.
- Provide assistance in dealing with the psychological impact of the spinal cord injury and its consequences.
- Refer for home care nursing support as indicated or desired.
- Refer patient to psychiatric clinical nurse specialist or other mental health care professional as indicated.

Evaluation

EXPECTED OUTCOMES

- Demonstrates improvement in gas exchange and clearance of secretions
- Moves within limits of the dysfunction, and demonstrates completion of exercises within functional limitations
- Demonstrates adaptation to sensory and perceptual alterations
- Demonstrates optimal skin integrity
- Regains urinary bladder function
- Regains bowel function
- Reports absence of pain and discomfort
- Is free of complications

For more information, see Chapter 58 in Smeltzer and Bare: *Brunner and Suddarth's Textbook of Medical-Surgical Nursing,* 9th edition. Philadelphia: Lippincott Williams & Wilkins, 2000.

SYNDROME OF INAPPROPRIATE ANTIDIURETIC HORMONE SECRETION (SIDH)

The syndrome of inappropriate antidiuretic hormone secretion (SIADH) refers to excessive antidiuretic hormone (ADH) secretion from the pituitary gland. Patients with this disorder cannot excrete or dilute urine. They retain fluids and develop a sodium deficiency (dilutional hyponatremia). SIADH is often of nonendocrine origin. The syndrome may occur in patients with bronchogenic carcinoma in which malignant lung cells synthesize and release ADH. Other causes include severe pneumonia, pneumothorax, other disorders of the lungs, and malignant tumors that affect other organs. Disorders of the central nervous system (head injury, brain surgery or tumor, or infection) are thought to produce SIADH by direct stimulation of the pituitary gland. Some medications (vincristine, diuretics, phenothiazines, tricyclic antidepressants) have been implicated in SIADH.

Medical Management
- This syndrome is generally managed by eliminating the underlying cause if possible and restricting the patient's fluid intake.
- Diuretics are used with fluid restriction for severe hyponatremia.

Nursing Management
- Monitor fluid intake and output, daily weight, urine and blood chemistries, and neurologic status.
- Provide supportive measures and explanations of procedures and treatments to assist patient to deal with this disorder.

S

For more information, see Chapter 38 in Smeltzer and Bare: *Brunner and Suddarth's Textbook of Medical-Surgical Nursing,* 9th edition. Philadelphia: Lippincott Williams & Wilkins, 2000.

SYSTEMIC LUPUS ERYTHEMATOSUS

Systemic lupus erythematosus (SLE) is a chronic, inflammatory autoimmune collagen disease that is the result of disturbed immune regulation that causes an exaggerated production of autoantibodies. This disturbance is brought about by some combination of genetic, hormonal (as evidenced by the usual onset during the childbearing years), and environmental factors (sunlight, thermal burns). Certain medications, such as hydralazine (Apresoline), procainamide (Pronestyl), isoniazid, chlorpromazine, and some anticonvulsants, have been implicated in chemical- or drug-induced SLE, as have foods such as alfalfa sprouts. In SLE, the increase in autoantibody production is thought to result from abnormal suppressor T-cell function, leading to immune complex deposition and tissue damage. Inflammation stimulates antigens, which in turn stimulate additional antibodies, and the cycle repeats (remissions and exacerbations).

Clinical Manifestations

- Onset is insidious or acute; SLE can be undiagnosed for many years.
- The clinical course is one of exacerbations and remissions. Features include nephritis, cardiopulmonary disease, skin rashes, and more indirect evidence of systemic inflammation (fever, fatigue, and weight loss).
- Musculoskeletal system: arthralgias and arthritis (synovitis) are common presenting features. Joint swelling, tenderness, and pain on movement are common, accompanied by morning stiffness.
- Several different types of skin manifestations are seen (eg, subacute cutaneous lupus erythematosus [SCLE], and discoid lupus erythematosus [DLE]).
- A butterfly rash across the bridge of the nose and cheeks occurs in less than half of patients and may be precursor to systemic involvement.

- Lesions worsen during exacerbations ("flares") and may be provoked by sunlight or artificial ultraviolet light.
- Oral ulcers may involve buccal mucosa or hard palate.
- Pericarditis is the most common clinical cardiac manifestation.
- Pleuritis or pleural effusions may occur.
- Papular, erythematosus, and purpuric lesions may occur on fingertips, elbows, toes, and extensor surfaces of forearms or lateral sides of hands and may progress to necrosis.
- Lymphadenopathy occurs in half of all SLE patients.
- Renal involvement (glomeruli) occurs in about 32% of patients.
- SLE has varied and frequent neuropsychiatric presentations, generally demonstrated by subtle changes in behavior patterns. Depression and psychosis are frequent.

Diagnostic Evaluation

Diagnosis is based on a complete history, physical examination, and analysis of blood work; no single laboratory test confirms SLE.

Medical Management

Treatment includes management of acute and chronic disease. The goals of treatment include preventing progressive loss of organ function, reducing the likelihood of acute disease, minimizing disease-related disabilities, and preventing complications from therapy.

- Nonsteroidal antiinflammatory drugs (NSAIDs) are used with corticosteroids to minimize corticosteroid requirements.
- Corticosteroids are used topically for cutaneous manifestations.
- Bolus intravenous administration is an alternative to traditional high-dose oral use.
- Cutaneous, musculoskeletal, and mild systemic features of SLE are managed with antimalarial drugs.

S

• Monitoring is performed to assess disease activity and therapeutic effectiveness. Immunosuppressive agents are generally reserved for serious forms of SLE.

Nursing Management

• Perform a thorough, systematic physical assessment, inspecting skin for erythematosus rashes and cutaneous erythematosus plaques with an adherent scale on scalp, face, or neck.
• Note areas of hyperpigmentation or depigmentation, depending on the phase and type of the disease, and question patient about skin changes, specifically about sensitivity to sunlight or artificial ultraviolet light.
• Inspect scalp for alopecia.
• Examine mouth and throat for ulcerations; provide appropriate oral care.
• Check for presence of pericardial friction rub and abnormal lung sounds (pleural effusion).
• Assess for vascular involvement: papular erythematosus and purpuric lesions.
• Observe for signs of musculoskeletal involvement: joint swelling, tenderness, warmth, pain on movement, and stiffness. Joint involvement is often symmetric.
• Observe for edema and hematuria, indicative of renal involvement.
• Facilitate interactions with patient and family to provide further evidence of systemic involvement.
• Direct neurologic assessment at identifying and describing central nervous system involvement.
• Question family members regarding behavioral changes, neuroses, or psychoses.
• Note signs of depression and reports of seizures, chorea, or other central nervous system manifestations.
• Assess knowledge of disease process and self-management.
• Assess patient's perception of and coping with fatigue, body image, and other problems caused by disease.

The nursing care of the patient with SLE is generally the same as the basic care plan for the patient with rheumatic disease (See Nursing Management under Arthritis, Rheumatoid). The primary nursing diagnoses address fatigue, impaired skin integrity, body image disturbance, and lack of knowledge for self-management decisions.

For more information, see Chapter 50 in Smeltzer and Bare: *Brunner and Suddarth's Textbook of Medical-Surgical Nursing,* 9th edition. Philadelphia: Lippincott Williams & Wilkins, 2000.

S

THROMBOCYTOPENIA

Thrombocytopenia is the most common cause of abnormal bleeding. It can result either from decreased production of platelets within the bone marrow or from increased destruction or consumption of platelets. Causes include failure of production as a result of certain anemias, septicemia, and cytotoxic medications; increased destruction as a result of idiopathic thrombocytopenia purpura, lupus erythematosus, malignant lymphoma, medications (digoxin, phenytoin, aspirin), and postviral infections; and increased utilization such as results from disseminated intravascular coagulopathy (DIC).

Diagnostic Evaluation
- Bone marrow aspiration and biopsy, if platelet deficiency is secondary to a decreased production
- Increased megakaryocytes and normal platelet production in bone marrow, when peripheral destruction is the cause

Clinical Manifestations
- Bleeding and petechiae (with platelet count below $50,000/mm^3$)
- Nosebleeds, gingival bleeding, excessive menstrual bleeding, and hemorrhage occur after surgery or dental extractions (platelet count below $20,000/mm^3$)
- Spontaneous fatal central nervous system hemorrhage or gastrointestinal hemorrhage (platelet count below $5000/mm^3$)

Medical Management

- The management of secondary thrombocytopenia is usually treatment of the underlying disease.
- Platelet transfusions are used to raise platelet count.
- If excessive destruction is the cause, patient is treated as indicated for idiopathic thrombocytopenia purpura.

Nursing Management

- Interventions focus on prevention of injury (eg, use soft toothbrush and electric razors, minimize needlestick procedures), stopping or slowing bleeding (eg, pressure, cold), and administration of medication and platelets as ordered, as well as patient teaching.

  See Nursing Management under Idiopathic Thrombocytopenia Purpura for additional information.

For more information, see Chapter 30 in Smeltzer and Bare: *Brunner and Suddarth's Textbook of Medical-Surgical Nursing,* 9th edition. Philadelphia: Lippincott Williams & Wilkins, 2000.

THYROID STORM (THYROTOXIC CRISIS)

Thyroid storm (thyrotoxic crisis) is a form of severe hyperthyroidism, usually of abrupt onset and characterized by high fever (hyperpyrexia), extreme tachycardia, and altered mental state, which frequently appears as delirium. Thyroid storm is a life-threatening condition that is usually precipitated by stress, such as injury, infection, nonthyroid surgery, thyroidectomy, tooth extraction, insulin reaction, diabetic acidosis, pregnancy, digitalis intoxication, abrupt withdrawal of antithyroid drugs, extreme emotional stress, or vigorous palpation of the thyroid. These factors precipitate thyroid storm in the partially controlled or completely untreated hyperthyroid patient. Untreated thyroid storm is almost always fatal, but with proper treatment, the mortality rate can be reduced substantially.

Clinical Manifestations
- Tachycardia (more than 130 beats/min)
- Temperature above 38.5°C (101.3°F)
- Exaggerated symptoms of hyperthyroidism
- Disturbances of a major system, such as gastrointestinal (weight loss, diarrhea, abdominal pain), neurologic (psychoses, somnolence, coma), or cardiovascular (edema, chest pain, dyspnea, palpitations)

Medical Management
The immediate objectives are to reduce body temperature and heart rate and prevent vascular collapse.

- Hypothermia mattress or blanket, ice packs, cool environment, hydrocortisone, and acetaminophen are employed.
- Humidified oxygen is administered to improve tissue oxygenation and meet high metabolic demands.
- Respiratory status is monitored with arterial blood gases (ABGs) or pulse oximetry.
- Intravenous fluids containing dextrose are administered to replace liver glycogen stores.
- Hydrocortisone is given to treat shock or adrenal insufficiency.
- Propylthiouracil (PTU) or methimazole is given to impede formation of thyroid hormone.
- Iodine is administered to decrease output of thyroxine (T_4) from thyroid gland.
- Sympatholytic agents are given for cardiac problems.

Nursing Management
- Provide astute observation and aggressive and supportive nursing care during and after acute stage of illness.
- Care of the patient with hyperthyroidism is the basis for nursing management for patients with thyroid storm or crisis.

NURSING ALERT

Salicylates are not used in the management of thyroid storm because they displace thyroid hormone from binding proteins and worsen the hypermetabolism.

For more information, see Chapter 38 in Smeltzer and Bare: *Brunner and Suddarth's Textbook of Medical-Surgical Nursing,* 9th edition. Philadelphia: Lippincott Williams & Wilkins, 2000.

THYROIDITIS

Thyroiditis is inflammation of the thyroid and can be acute, subacute, or chronic in nature. Each type of thyroiditis is characterized by inflammation, fibrosis, or lymphocytic infiltration of the thyroid gland. Acute thyroiditis is a rare disorder caused by infection of the thyroid gland. The causes are bacteria (*Staphylococcus aureus* most common), fungi, mycobacteria, or parasites. Subacute cases may be granulomatous thyroiditis (de Quervain's thyroiditis) or painless thyroiditis (silent thyroiditis or subacute lymphocytic thyroiditis). This form occurs in the postpartum period and is thought to be an autoimmune reaction.

Clinical Manifestations

Acute Thyroiditis
- Anterior neck pain and swelling, fever, dysphagia, and dysphonia
- Pharyngitis or pharyngeal pain
- Warmth, erythema, and tenderness of the thyroid gland

Subacute Thyroiditis
- Thyroid enlarges symmetrically and occasionally is painful.

- Overlying skin is often reddened and warm.
- Swallowing may be difficult and uncomfortable.
- Irritability, nervousness, insomnia, and weight loss, which are manifestations of hyperthyroidism, are common.
- Chills and fever may be experienced.

Medical Management
Acute Thyroiditis
- Antimicrobial agents and fluid replacement
- Surgical incision and drainage if abscess is present

Subacute Thyroiditis
- Control of inflammation; nonsteroidal antiinflammatory agents (NSAIDs) to relieve neck pain
- Beta-blocking agents to control symptoms of hyperthyroidism
- Oral corticosteroids to relieve pain and reduce swelling; do not usually affect the underlying cause
- Follow-up monitoring

For more information, see Chapter 38 in Smeltzer and Bare: *Brunner and Suddarth's Textbook of Medical-Surgical Nursing,* 9th edition. Philadelphia: Lippincott Williams & Wilkins, 2000.

THYROIDITIS, CHRONIC (HASHIMOTO'S THYROIDITIS)

Chronic thyroiditis occurs most frequently in women 30 to 50 years of age and is termed *Hashimoto's disease*. Diagnosis is based on the histologic appearance of the inflamed gland. The chronic forms are usually accompanied by pain, pressure symptoms, or fever, and thyroid activity is usually normal or low. Cell-mediated immunity plays a significant role in the pathogenesis of thyroiditis. A genetic predisposition also appears to be significant in its etiology. If untreated, the disease slowly progresses to hypothyroidism.

Medical Management

The objectives of treatment are to reduce the size of the thyroid gland and to prevent myxedema.

- Thyroid hormone therapy is prescribed to reduce thyroid activity and production of thyroglobulin.
- Thyroid hormone is given when hypothyroid symptoms are present.
- Surgery is performed when pressure symptoms persist.

For more information, see Chapter 38 in Smeltzer and Bare: *Brunner and Suddarth's Textbook of Medical-Surgical Nursing,* 9th edition. Philadelphia: Lippincott Williams & Wilkins, 2000.

TOXIC EPIDERMAL NECROLYSIS (TEN) AND STEVENS-JOHNSON SYNDROME (SJS)

Toxic epidermal necrolysis and Stevens-Johnson syndrome are potentially fatal skin disorders and the most severe forms of erythema multiforme. Both conditions are triggered by a reaction to medications or are secondary to a viral infection. Antibiotics, anticonvulsants, butazones, and sulfonamides are the most frequent medications implicated. The complete body surface may be involved, with widespread areas of erythema and blisters. Sepsis and keratoconjunctivitis are complications that may occur.

Clinical Manifestations

- Initial signs are conjunctival burning or itching, cutaneous tenderness, fever, headache, cough, sore throat, extreme malaise, and myalgia (aches and pains)
- Rapid onset of erythema follows, involving the skin surface and mucous membranes; large, flaccid bullae in some areas; in other areas, large sheets of epidermis are shed, exposing underlying dermis; fingernails, toenails, eyebrows, and eyelashes may all shed, along with surrounding epidermis.

- Excruciatingly tender skin and loss of skin leads to weeping surface similar to that of a total-body second-degree burn; this condition may be referred to as *scalded skin syndrome.*
- In severe cases of mucosal involvement, there may be danger of damage to the larynx, bronchi, and esophagus from ulcerations.

Diagnostic Evaluation
- Frozen histologic studies of skin cells
- Cytodiagnosis of cells of a denuded area
- Immunofluorescent studies for atypical epidermal autoantibodies

Medical Management
The goals of treatment include control of fluid and electrolyte balance, prevention of sepsis, and prevention of ophthalmic complications. The mainstay of treatment is supportive care.

- All nonessential medications are discontinued immediately.
- Patient is treated in a regional burn center.
- Surgical débridement or hydrotherapy is used initially to remove involved skin.
- Cultures are taken of nasopharynx, eyes, ears, blood, urine, skin, and unruptured blisters to identify pathogens.
- Intravenous fluids are prescribed to maintain fluid and electrolyte balance.
- Fluid replacement is accomplished by nasogastric tube and orally.
- Systemic corticosteroids are given early in the disease process.
- Skin is protected with topical agents.
- Topical antibacterial and anesthetic agents are used to prevent wound sepsis.
- Temporary biologic dressings (pig skin, amniotic membrane) or plastic semipermeable dressing (Vigilon) is applied.

Nursing Management

Assessment

- Inspect appearance and extent of involvement of skin. Monitor skin for amount, color, and odor.
- Inspect oral cavity for blistering and erosive lesions daily. Determine patient's ability to drink fluids and speak normally.
- Assess eyes daily for itching, burning, and dryness.
- Monitor vital signs, paying special attention to fever and respiratory status.
- Monitor urine volume, specific gravity, and color.
- Inspect intravenous insertion sites for local signs of infection.
- Record daily weight.
- Question patient about fatigue and pain levels.
- Assess level of anxiety and coping mechanisms; identify new effective coping skills.

Major Nursing Diagnoses

- Impaired tissue integrity (oral, eye, and skin) related to epidermal shedding
- Fluid volume deficit and electrolyte losses related to loss of fluids from denuded skin
- Risk for altered body temperature (hypothermia) related to heat loss, secondary to skin loss
- Pain related to denuded skin, oral lesions, and possible infection
- Anxiety related to the physical appearance of the skin and prognosis

Collaborative Problems/Potential Complications

- Sepsis
- Conjunctival retraction, scars, and corneal lesions

Planning and Goals

The major goals of the patient may include achievement of skin and oral tissue healing, attainment of fluid balance, prevention of heat loss, relief of pain, reduction of anxiety, and absence of complications.

Nursing Interventions

MAINTAINING SKIN AND MUCOUS
MEMBRANE INTEGRITY

- Place patient on a circular turning frame to prevent skin denudement.
- Apply prescribed topical agents that reduce wound bacteria.
- Apply warm compresses gently, if prescribed, to denuded areas.
- Use topical antibacterial agent in conjunction with hydrotherapy; monitor treatment, and encourage the patient to exercise extremities during hydrotherapy.
- Perform oral hygiene carefully. Use prescribed mouthwashes frequently to rid mouth of debris, soothe ulcerative areas, and control odor. Inspect oral cavity frequently, note changes, and report. Apply petrolatum to lips.

ATTAINING FLUID BALANCE

- Observe for signs of hypovolemia: vital signs, urine output, and sensorium.
- Evaluate laboratory tests, and report abnormal results.
- Weigh patient daily.
- Provide fluid replacement.
- Provide enteral nourishment or, if necessary, total parenteral nutrition (TPN).
- Record intake and output and daily calorie count.

PREVENTING HYPOTHERMIA

- Maintain patient's comfort and body temperature with cotton blankets, ceiling-mounted heat lamps, or heat shields.
- Work rapidly and efficiently when large wounds are exposed for wound care to minimize shivering and heat loss.
- Monitor temperature carefully.

RELIEVING PAIN

- Assess for presence and character of pain, behavioral responses, and factors that influence the pain.

- Administer prescribed analgesics, and observe for pain relief and side effects.
- Administer analgesics before painful treatments.
- Provide proper explanations and speak soothingly to the patient during treatments to allay anxiety that may intensify pain.
- Provide measures to promote rest and sleep; provide emotional support and reassurance to achieve pain control.
- Teach self-management techniques for pain relief, such as progressive muscle relaxation and imagery.

REDUCING ANXIETY
- Assess emotional state: anxiety, fear of dying, and depression; reassure patient that these reactions are normal.
- Give support, honesty, and hope that the situation can improve.
- Encourage patient to express feelings to someone he or she trusts.
- Listen to patient's concerns; be available with skillful, compassionate care.
- Provide emotional support during the long recovery period with psychiatric nurse, chaplain, psychologist, or psychiatrist.

MONITORING AND MANAGING
POTENTIAL COMPLICATIONS
- Sepsis: monitor vital signs and note adverse changes related to body systems for quick detection of infection; maintain strict asepsis, and if a large portion of the body is involved, place patient in private room with protective isolation.
- Conjunctival retraction, scars, and corneal lesions: inspect eyes for progression of disease to keratoconjunctivitis (itching, burning, and dryness); administer eye lubricant; use eye patches; avoid rubbing eyes; document and report progression of symptoms.

Evaluation

EXPECTED OUTCOMES
- Achieves increasing skin and oral tissue healing
- Attains fluid balance
- Attains thermoregulation
- Reports lessening of pain intensity
- Appears less anxious
- Experiences no complication, such as sepsis and impaired vision

---

For more information, see Chapter 52 in Smeltzer and Bare: *Brunner and Suddarth's Textbook of Medical-Surgical Nursing,* 9th edition. Philadelphia: Lippincott Williams & Wilkins, 2000.

TOXIC SHOCK SYNDROME

Toxic shock syndrome (TSS) is an infrequent condition caused by a toxin produced by strains of the bacterium *Staphylococcus aureus* and usually occurs in menstruating women. About half of cases are not related to menstruation. Other risk factors include chronic vaginal infection, pelvic infection, lung abscess, surgical wound infection, soft tissue infection, postpartum and gynecologic infection, use of intravenous (injectable) drugs, and used of superabsorbent tampons. Barrier methods of contraception (eg, diaphragm) have also been implicated, whereas oral contraceptives appear to reduce the risk. TSS may recur (usually within 2 months after initial illness, may appear during menstruation).

Clinical Manifestations
- Sudden fever (38.9°C [102°F]), chills, malaise, myalgia, dizziness, and muscle pain or vomiting, diarrhea, hypotension, headache, and signs suggesting early septic shock
- Red, macular rash similar to sunburn; may become scaly or peel in 7 to 10 days; inflammation of mucous membranes

- Decreased urine output; increased blood urea nitrogen (BUN) level, resulting in disorientation
- Leukocytosis and elevated bilirubin
- Uncontrollable hypotension; clinical picture of shock
- Disseminated intravascular coagulopathy (DIC)
- Respiratory distress as a result of pulmonary edema
- Adult respiratory distress syndrome (ARDS)—outlook becomes grave
- About 2% to 3% mortality rate

Diagnostic Evaluation
- Cultures of blood, urine, throat, vagina, and possibly cervix
- BUN, white blood cell count, bilirubin, and coagulation studies (DIC)

Medical Management
Patient is placed on bed rest, and the treatment plan is directed primarily at controlling the infection with antibiotics and restoration of circulating blood volume.

- Oxygen therapy if there is respiratory distress
- Sodium bicarbonate if signs of acidosis appear
- Calcium for hypocalcemia
- Hemodynamic monitoring, intravenous dopamine, and military antishock trousers (MAST) to manage shock
- Support of patient's emotional and psychological concerns

Nursing Management
Assessment
Direct nursing history toward determining whether patient used tampons recently, the type used, how long tampon was retained before changing it, and whether any problems were noted when inserting the tampon, which may have injured the vaginal tissue. Also include any history of diaphragm use.

T

Major Nursing Diagnoses
- Anxiety related to the severity and suddenness of the symptoms and to concerns about recovery
- Fluid volume deficit related to vomiting and diarrhea
- Fatigue related to severity of illness and of shock, prolonged immobility, excessive nutritional demands, and stress
- Knowledge deficit about risk factors and behaviors

Collaborative Problems/Potential Complications
- Septic shock
- DIC

Planning and Goals
The major goals of the patient may include reduction of anxiety and emotional stress, absence of vomiting and diarrhea, acquisition of relevant knowledge, and absence of complications.

Nursing Interventions
RELIEVING ANXIETY
- Provide emotional support and reassurance to reduce anxiety and apprehension.
- Keep patient and family informed about diagnostic procedures and treatments.
- Give opportunity for self-care and decision making when able.

IMPROVING FLUID VOLUME STATUS
- Monitor intake and output; assess for fluid deficit.
- Administer intravenous and oral fluids as prescribed; document changes in fluid status.
- Administer antiemetics and antidiarrheal agents if necessary.
- Give comfort measures (eg, frequent oral hygiene).

DECREASING FATIGUE
- Assist with self-care efforts; gradually resume activities to increase stamina.

- Counteract weight loss with nutritious diet.
- Monitor weight and caloric intake; give dietary supplements, if needed.
- Plan with patient and physical therapist an exercise and activity program to build stamina.

MONITORING AND MANAGING COMPLICATIONS
- Monitor and document vital signs and blood-gas levels.
- Culture body excretions to determine antibiotic therapy.
- Evaluate hydration and kidney function (note skin changes, fluid intake and loss).
- Be observant for DIC symptoms: hematomas; petechiae; oozing from needle puncture sites; cyanosis; and coolness of nose, fingertips, and toes. Protect patient from injury, and administer prescribed medications to treat DIC if needed.
- Be alert for changes indicative of severe shock (level of consciousness, vital signs, and laboratory values).

🏠 Promoting Home and Community-Based Care

Teaching Patients Self-Care
- Teach patient and caregiver how to detect and prevent complications associated with immobility and to increase participation in self-care activities gradually.
- Explain the possible causes of TSS and how to prevent its recurrence.
- Recommend that superabsorbent tampons not be used. If other tampons are used, change frequently (every 4 hours). Insert tampons carefully to avoid abrasions (applicators with rough edges should be avoided).
- Do not leave a diaphragm in place longer than 8 to 10 hours.
- Discourage tampon use if patient has had TSS.
- Discourage use of diaphragm or cervical cap during menses or in the first 3 months postpartum.
- Teach that risk for TSS is increased when a woman bleeds vaginally (ie, during menses and postpartum).

Continuing Care

- Refer for home care nurse, if circumstances indicate.
- Reinforce the need for keeping follow-up appointments with health care providers.

Evaluation

EXPECTED OUTCOMES
- Exhibits reduced anxiety and emotional stress
- Is free of fluid loss and imbalance
- Experiences decreased fatigue level
- Demonstrates knowledge of risk factors for TSS, and avoids using tampons
- Reports absence of complications

For more information, see Chapter 43 in Smeltzer and Bare: *Brunner and Suddarth's Textbook of Medical-Surgical Nursing,* 9th edition. Philadelphia: Lippincott Williams & Wilkins, 2000.

TRANSIENT ISCHEMIC ATTACK

Transient ischemic attack (TIA) is a temporary episode of neurologic dysfunction commonly manifested by a sudden loss of motor, sensory, or visual function. It may last a few seconds or minutes but no longer than 24 hours. Complete recovery usually occurs between attacks. A TIA may serve as a warning of impending stroke, which often occurs within the first month after the first attack. The cause is a temporary impairment of blood flow to a specific region of the brain. Reasons may include atherosclerosis of the vessels supplying the brain, obstruction of cerebral microcirculation by a small embolus, a fall in cerebral perfusion pressure, and cardiac dysrhythmias. Risk factors include hypertension, insulin-dependent diabetes mellitus, cardiac disease, history of smoking, family history of stroke, and chronic alcoholism.

Clinical Manifestations

Signs and symptoms depend on the location of the affected vessel.

- Interrupted anterior circulation can result in amaurosis fugax (fleeting blindness) occurring without warning. Sudden, painless loss of vision of one eye, aphasia, or contralateral weakness may occur.
- If ischemia occurs in the vertebral basilar system, vertigo, diplopia, numbness or paresthesia, dysphagia, or ataxia may be exhibited.

Diagnostic Evaluation

- Carotid phonoangiography provides auscultation, direct visualization, and photographic recording of carotid bruits.
- Oculoplethysmography measures pulsation in blood flow through the ophthalmic artery.
- Carotid angiography visualizes intracranial and cervical vessels.
- Digital subtraction angiography is used to define carotid artery obstruction.

Medical Management

- Anticoagulant therapy to prevent future attacks if patient is not a candidate for surgical intervention
- Platelet-inhibiting drugs (aspirin) to decrease the occurrence of cerebral infarction
- Common surgical intervention procedures: endarterectomy and angioplasty

Nursing Management

Prevention

- Assess for, report, and assist in treatment of hypertension and hyperglycemia.
- Promote cessation of smoking; assist patient to find a program or support group.

Nursing Interventions for Carotid Endarterectomy

- Keep flowchart to maintain close assessment of patient's neurologic status after procedures, and notify neurosurgeon immediately if patient develops deficits.
- Be aware of primary complications of carotid endarterectomy: stroke, cranial nerve injuries, infection or hematoma of the wound, and carotid artery disruption.
- Maintain adequate blood pressure levels in immediate postoperative period.
- Avoid hypotension to prevent cerebral ischemia and thrombosis.
- Prevent excessive hypertension, which may precipitate cerebral hemorrhage; use sodium nitroprusside.
- Assess for difficulty in swallowing, hoarseness, or other signs of cranial nerve dysfunction; have a tracheostomy set available.
- Monitor cardiac status closely because of high incidence of coronary artery disease.
- Be aware of long-term complications: recurrent stroke and myocardial infarction.

For more information, see Chapter 57 in Smeltzer and Bare: *Brunner and Suddarth's Textbook of Medical-Surgical Nursing,* 9th edition. Philadelphia: Lippincott Williams & Wilkins, 2000.

TRIGEMINAL NEURALGIA (TIC DOULOUREUX)

Trigeminal neuralgia is a condition of the fifth cranial nerve characterized by paroxysms of pain similar to an electric shock in the area innervated by one or more branches of the trigeminal nerve. Each pain episode can be described as stabbing, lasting from a few seconds to minutes, and producing contraction of some of the facial muscles (ie, sudden closing of the eye or a twitch of the mouth); hence the name tic douloureux (painful twitch). The cause is not certain. Chronic compression or irritation of the trigeminal nerve or degenerative changes in the gasserian ganglion are suggested causes. Early attacks, appearing most often in the fifth decade of life, are usually mild and brief. Pain-free intervals may be measured in terms of minutes, hours, days, or longer. With advancing years, the painful episodes tend to become more and more frequent and agonizing. The patient lives in constant fear of attacks.

Clinical Manifestations
- Pain is felt in the skin, not in the deeper structures, and is more severe at the peripheral areas of distribution of affected nerve, notably over the lip, chin, and nostrils and in the teeth.
- Paroxysms are aroused by any stimulation of terminals of the affected nerve branches (eg, washing the face, shaving, brushing the teeth, eating, and drinking).
- Draft of cold air and direct pressure against the nerve trunk may also cause pain.
- Trigger points are certain areas where the slightest touch immediately starts a paroxysm.

Diagnostic Evaluation
Diagnosis is based on characteristic behavior: avoiding stimulating trigger point areas (eg, trying not to touch or wash the face, shave, chew, or do anything else that might cause an attack).

Medical Management
Pharmacologic Treatment
- Anticonvulsive agents carbamazepine (Tegretol) and phenytoin (Dilantin) reduce transmission of impulses at certain nerve terminals and relieve pain in most patients.
- Carbamazepine is given with meals, in doses gradually increased until relief is obtained.
- Patient is observed for side effects including nausea, dizziness, drowsiness, and hepatic dysfunction.
- Patient is monitored for bone marrow depression during long-term drug therapy.

- Patient is monitored for phenytoin side effects, including nausea, dizziness, nystagmus, somnolence, ataxia, gum hyperplasia, and skin rashes or eruptions.

Alcohol or Phenol Injection
- Injection of gasserian ganglion and peripheral branches of the trigeminal nerve relieves pain for several months.
- Pain returns after the nerve regenerates.

Surgical Management
Percutaneous radiofrequency trigeminal gangliolysis (interruption of the gasserian ganglion) is the surgical procedure of choice. Small unmyelinated and thinly myelinated fibers that conduct pain are thermally destroyed (touch and proprioceptive function intact). In microvascular decompression of the trigeminal nerve, an intracranial approach (craniotomy) to decompress the trigeminal nerve is used. This procedure relieves facial pain while preserving normal sensation.

Nursing Interventions
- Recognize in preoperative management that certain factors may aggravate excruciating facial pain (eg, too hot or cold food or water, jarring the patient's bed). Lessen these discomforts by using cotton pads and room-temperature water to wash face.
- Instruct patient to rinse mouth after eating when tooth brushing causes pain.
- Perform personal hygiene during pain-free intervals.
- Advise patient to take food and fluids at room temperature, to chew on unaffected side, and to ingest soft foods.
- Recognize that anxiety, depression, and insomnia often accompany chronic painful conditions, and use appropriate interventions and referrals.

Providing Postoperative Care
- Conduct postoperative neurologic assessments to evaluate for facial motor and sensory deficits.

- Instruct patient not to rub the eye if the surgery results in sensory deficits to the affected side of the face because pain will not be felt in the event there is injury.
- Assess the eye for irritation or redness.
- Insert artificial tears, if prescribed, to prevent dryness to the affected eye.
- Caution the patient not to chew on the affected side until numbness has diminished.
- Observe the patient carefully for any difficulty in eating and swallowing foods of different consistencies.

For more information, see Chapter 59 in Smeltzer and Bare: *Brunner and Suddarth's Textbook of Medical-Surgical Nursing,* 9th edition. Philadelphia: Lippincott Williams & Wilkins, 2000.

TUBERCULOSIS

Tuberculosis (TB) is an infectious disease affecting the lung parenchyma. It is most often caused by *Mycobacterium tuberculosis.* It may spread to almost any part of the body, including the meninges, kidney, bones, and lymph nodes. The initial infection usually occurs 2 to 10 weeks after exposure. The person may then develop active disease because of a compromised or inadequate immune system response. The active process may be prolonged and characterized by long remissions when the disease is arrested, only to be followed by periods of renewed activity. TB is a worldwide public health problem. Mortality and morbidity rates continue to rise.

Transmission and Risk Factors

TB is transmitted from a person with active pulmonary disease who expels the organisms while talking, coughing, sneezing, or singing. A susceptible person inhales the droplets and becomes infected. The following people are at high risk for acquiring the infection:

- People in close contact with someone who has active TB.

- Injection drug users and alcoholics.
- People living in overcrowded, substandard housing.
- Immunocompromised patients (elderly people, patients with cancer, those on corticosteroid therapy, and those infected with the human immunodeficiency virus [HIV]).
- People with preexisting medical conditions, including diabetes, chronic renal failure, silicosis, and malnourishment.
- Immigrants from countries with a high incidence of TB (eg, Haiti, southeast Asia).
- People who are without adequate health care (eg, homeless or impoverished people, ethnic and racial minorities, children, and young adults).
- People who are institutionalized (eg, long-term care patients, psychiatric patients, prison inmates).
- Health care workers (particularly those performing high-risk activities).

Clinical Manifestations
- Insidious onset
- Low-grade fever, fatigue, anorexia, weight loss, night sweats, chest pain, and cough
- Nonproductive cough, which may progress to mucopurulent sputum with hemoptysis

Diagnostic Evaluation
- TB skin test, sputum culture, chest radiograph

Medical Management
The goals of management are to relieve pulmonary and systemic symptoms; to return the patient to health, work, and family life as quickly as possible; and to prevent transmission of the infection.

Chemotherapy
- Therapy for 6 to 12 months
- First-line medications: isoniazid (INH), rifampin (RIF), streptomycin (SM), ethambutol (EMB), and

pyrazinamide (PZA) for 4 months, with INH and RIF continuing for an additional 2 months
- Second-line medications: capreomycin, kanamycin, ethionamide, para-aminosalicylate sodium, amikacin, cyclizine
- Patient is considered noninfectious after 2 to 3 weeks of continuous therapy
- Vitamin B_6 (pyridoxine) usually administered with INH

Preventive Treatment
- Identification of people at risk: INH for preventive therapy given in a single daily dose for 6 to 12 months

Nursing Management
Assessment
- Perform complete history and physical examination.
- Perform respiratory assessment, exploring presence of fever, anorexia, weight loss, night sweats, fatigue, cough, and sputum production.
- Assess change in temperature, respiratory rate, amount and color of secretions, frequency and severity of cough, and chest pain.
- Evaluate breath sounds for consolidation (diminished, bronchial, or bronchovesicular sounds, crackles), fremitus, egophony, and percussion (dullness).
- Assess for enlarged, painful lymph nodes.
- Assess patient's living arrangements.
- Assess patient's emotional readiness to learn and perceptions and understanding of TB and its treatment.
- Review results of physical and laboratory evaluations.

Major Nursing Diagnoses
- Ineffective airway clearance related to copious tracheobronchial secretions
- Nonadherence to treatment regimens
- Knowledge deficit about preventive health measures and treatment regimen

T

Collaborative Problems/Potential Complications

- Malnutrition
- Side effects of medication therapy: hepatitis, neurologic changes (deafness or neuritis), skin rash, gastrointestinal upset
- Multidrug resistance
- Spread of TB infection (miliary TB)

Planning and Goals

The major goals of the patient include maintenance of a patent airway, knowledge about the disease and treatment regimen, adherence to the medication regimen, increased activity tolerance, and absence of complications.

Nursing Interventions

PROMOTING AIRWAY CLEARANCE

- Instruct about best position to facilitate drainage.
- Encourage increased fluid intake.
- Provide a high-humidity face mask or humidifier.

ADVOCATING ADHERENCE AND PREVENTION

- Instruct that TB is a communicable disease and that taking medications is the most effective way of preventing transmission.
- Instruct patient about hygienic measures, including mouth care, covering mouth and nose when coughing and sneezing, proper disposal of tissues, and hand washing.
- Clarify medications, schedule, and side effects.

MONITORING AND MANAGING
POTENTIAL COMPLICATIONS

- Collaborate with health care team to identify strategies to ensure adequate nutritional intake and availability of nutritious foods.
- Assess for side effects of medication therapy.
- Encourage liver and kidney function follow-up.
- Monitor sputum culture results to evaluate effectiveness of therapy.

- Teach patient to take medications on empty stomach or 1 hour before meals because food interferes with drug absorption.
- Teach patients taking INH to avoid foods containing tyramine and histamine (tuna fish, aged cheese, yeast extract).
- Inform patient that rifampin may discolor contact lenses and to wear eyeglasses.
- Instruct patient about risk of drug resistance if regimen is not followed continuously; failure to comply results in multidrug resistance.
- Caution about the spread of TB infection to nonpulmonary sites of the body (miliary TB), a consequence of late reactivation of dormant infection.

🏠 Promoting Home and Community-Based Care

Teaching Patients Self-Care
- Assess the ability of the patient to continue therapy at home.
- Instruct patient and family about infection control procedures.
- Teach and use universal precautions for body fluids, including sputum.
- Demonstrate and stress good hand-washing technique.
- Instruct patient to cover mouth when coughing; use disposable tissues if available, place in paper bag, and discard.

Continuing Care
- Evaluate patient's environment to identify other people who were potentially infected.
- Arrange follow-up screening for potentially infected contacts.
- Assess the patient's physical and psychological status and ability to adhere to the prescribed treatment.
- Reinforce previous teaching, and emphasize the importance of keeping scheduled appointments with the primary health care providers.

T

Evaluation

EXPECTED OUTCOMES
- Maintains a patent airway by managing secretions
- Demonstrates an adequate level of knowledge
- Adheres to treatment regimen by taking medications as prescribed
- Participates in preventive measures
- Maintains activity schedule
- Exhibits no complications
- Takes steps to minimize side effects

 Gerontologic Considerations

Elderly patients may have atypical manifestations, such as unusual behavior and altered mental status, fever, anorexia, and weight loss. TB is increasingly encountered in the nursing home population.

For more information, see Chapter 21 in Smeltzer and Bare: *Brunner and Suddarth's Textbook of Medical-Surgical Nursing,* 9th edition. Philadelphia: Lippincott Williams & Wilkins, 2000.

U

ULCERATIVE COLITIS

Ulcerative colitis is a recurrent ulcerative and inflammatory disease of the mucosal layer of the colon and rectum. It is a serious disease, accompanied by systemic complications and a high mortality rate. Eventually 10% to 15% of the patients develop carcinoma of the colon. It is characterized by multiple ulcerations, diffuse inflammations, and desquamation of the colonic epithelium, with alternating periods of exacerbation and remission. Ulcerative colitis most commonly affects white people, including people of Jewish heritage, and peaks in the third to fifth decade of life.

Clinical Manifestations
- Predominant symptoms: diarrhea, abdominal pain, intermittent tenesmus, ineffective straining at stool, and rectal bleeding
- Anorexia, weight loss, fever, vomiting, dehydration, cramping, and feeling an urgent need to defecate (may report passing 10 to 20 liquid stools daily)
- Hypocalcemia and anemia
- Rebound tenderness in right lower quadrant
- Skin lesions, eye lesions (uveitis), joint abnormalities, and liver disease

Diagnostic Evaluation
- Stool examination to rule out dysentery and test for blood
- Sigmoidoscopy and barium enema
- Blood studies

Medical Management

Medical treatment for both regional enteritis and ulcerative colitis is aimed at reducing inflammation, suppressing inappropriate immune responses, and providing rest for a diseased bowel, so that healing may take place.

Diet and Fluid Intake

- Oral fluids; low-residue, high-protein, high-calorie diets with supplemental vitamin therapy and iron replacement
- Correction of fluid and electrolyte imbalance by intravenous therapy
- Avoidance of foods that exacerbate diarrhea; avoidance of milk, cold foods, and smoking; total parenteral nutrition (TPN) as indicated

Pharmacologic Therapy

- Sedative, antidiarrheal, and antiperistaltic medications
- Sulfonamides: sulfasalazine (Azulfidine) or sulfisoxazole (Gantrisin), which are effective for mild or moderate inflammation
- Antibiotics for secondary infections
- Adrenocorticotropic hormone (ACTH) and corticosteroids
- Aminosalicylates (topical and oral)
- Immunosuppressive agents

Psychotherapy

Psychotherapy is aimed at determining the factors that distress the patient, coping with these factors, and attempting to resolve conflicts.

Surgical Management

When nonsurgical measures fail to relieve the severe symptoms of inflammatory bowel disease, surgery may be recommended (segmental, subtotal, or total colectomy). A fecal diversion may be needed, such as ileostomy, continent ileal reservoir (Kocks' pouch), or ileoanal anastomosis.

Nursing Management: The Patient With Inflammatory Bowel Disease

Assessment

HEALTH HISTORY

- Onset and duration of abdominal pain; presence of diarrhea, tenesmus, nausea, anorexia, weight loss
- Dietary pattern, including amounts of alcohol, caffeine, and nicotine used daily or weekly
- Family history of inflammatory bowel disease
- Allergies, especially to milk or lactose
- Bowel elimination patterns, including character, frequency, and presence of blood, pus, fat, or mucus
- Sleep pattern disturbances if diarrhea or pain occur at night

OBJECTIVE ASSESSMENT

- Auscultate for bowel sounds and their characteristics.
- Palpate for distention, tenderness, or pain.
- Inspect the skin for evidence of fistula tracts or symptoms of dehydration; inspect stool for blood.

Ulcerative Colitis

- Dominant sign is rectal bleeding.
- Distended abdomen with rebound tenderness may be present.

Regional Enteritis

- Most prominent symptom is intermittent pain associated with diarrhea that does not decrease with defecation.
- Pain usually is localized in the right lower quadrant.
- Abdominal tenderness noted on palpation.
- Periumbilical regional pain usually indicates involvement of terminal ileum.

Major Nursing Diagnoses

- Diarrhea related to the inflammatory process
- Pain related to increased peristalsis and gastrointestinal inflammation

- Fluid volume and electrolyte deficits related to anorexia, nausea, and diarrhea
- Anxiety related to impending surgery
- Ineffective individual coping related to repeated episodes of diarrhea
- Risk for impaired skin integrity related to malnutrition and diarrhea
- Risk for ineffective management of therapeutic regimen related to insufficient knowledge deficit concerning the process and management of the disease

Collaborative Problems/Potential Complications
- Cardiac dysrhythmias related to electrolyte depletion
- Gastrointestinal bleeding with fluid volume loss
- Perforation of the bowel
- Electrolyte imbalance

Planning and Goals
The major goals of the patient may include attainment of normal bowel elimination, relief of abdominal pain and cramping, prevention of fluid volume deficit, maintenance of optimal nutrition and weight, avoidance of fatigue, reduction of anxiety, effective coping, prevention of skin breakdown, acquisition of knowledge and understanding of the disease process and therapeutic regimen, and absence of potential complications.

Nursing Interventions
MAINTAINING NORMAL ELIMINATION PATTERNS
- Determine if there is a relationship between diarrhea and certain foods, activity, or emotional stress.
- Identify any precipitating factors as well as stool frequency, consistency, and amount.
- Provide ready access to bathroom or bedpan; keep environment clean and odor free.
- Administer antidiarrheal agents as prescribed, and record frequency and consistency of stools after therapy has started.
- Encourage bed rest to decrease peristalsis.

RELIEVING PAIN
- Describe character of pain (dull, burning, or cramplike) and its onset, pattern, and medication relief.
- Administer anticholinergic medications 30 minutes before a meal to decrease intestinal motility.
- Give analgesics as prescribed; reduce pain by position changes, local application of heat (as prescribed), diversional activities, and prevention of fatigue.

MAINTAINING FLUID BALANCE
- Keep accurate record of intake and output, including wound or fistula drainage.
- Monitor patient's weight daily.
- Assess for signs of fluid volume deficit: dry skin and mucous membranes, decreased skin turgor, oliguria, exhaustion, decreased temperature, increased hematocrit.
- Evaluate urine specific gravity, and note hypotension.
- Encourage oral intake; monitor intravenous flow rate.
- Initiate measures to decrease diarrhea: dietary restrictions, stress reduction, and antidiarrheal agents.

PROMOTING NUTRITIONAL MEASURES
- Use TPN when symptoms are severe.
- Maintain an accurate record of fluid intake and output and daily weight during TPN therapy; test for glucose daily.
- Give feedings high in protein, low in fat and residue after TPN therapy; note intolerance (eg, vomiting, diarrhea, distention).
- Provide small, frequent low-residue feedings if oral foods are tolerated.
- Restrict activities to conserve energy, reduce peristalsis, and meet calorie requirement.

PROMOTING REST
- Recommend intermittent rest periods during the day; schedule or restrict activities to conserve energy and reduce metabolic rate.

- Encourage activity within limits; advise bed rest with active or passive exercises for a patient who is febrile, has frequent stools, or is bleeding.

REDUCING ANXIETY

- Establish rapport by being attentive and displaying a calm, confident manner.
- Provide time for patient to ask questions and express feelings.
- Listen carefully and sensitively to nonverbal indicators of anxiety (restlessness, tense facial expressions).
- Tailor information about impending surgery to patient's level of understanding and desire for detail.

PROMOTING COPING SKILLS

- Give essential understanding and emotional support for isolated, helpless, and out-of-control feelings.
- Recognize that behavior may be affected by a number of factors unrelated to inherent emotional characteristics.
- Support patient's attempts to deal with stresses.
- Communicate that the patient's feelings are understood; encourage patient to talk and ventilate and to discuss any disturbing matters.
- Use stress-reduction measures: relaxation techniques, breathing exercises, and biofeedback.

PREVENTING SKIN BREAKDOWN

- Examine patient's skin, especially perianal skin.
- Provide perianal care after each bowel movement.
- Give care to reddened or irritated areas over bony prominences.
- Use pressure-relieving devices to avoid possible skin breakdown.
- Consult with a wound care specialist or enterostomal therapist as indicated.

MONITORING AND MANAGING
POTENTIAL COMPLICATIONS

- Monitor serum electrolyte levels; administer replacements.
- Report dysrhythmias or change in level of consciousness.

- Monitor rectal bleeding, and give blood and volume expanders.
- Monitor blood pressure; provide laboratory blood studies often.
- Monitor for indications of perforation: acute increase in abdominal pain, rigid abdomen, vomiting, or hypotension.
- Monitor for signs of obstruction and toxic megacolon: abdominal distention, decreased or absent bowel sounds, changes in mental status, fever, tachycardia, hypotension, dehydration, and electrolyte imbalance.

🏠 Promoting Home and Community-Based care

Teaching Patients Self-Care

- Assess need for additional information about medical management (medications, diet) and surgical interventions.
- Provide information about nutritional management (bland, low-residue, high-protein, high-calorie, and high-vitamin diet).
- Give rationale for using steroids and antiinflammatory, antibacterial, antidiarrheal, and antispasmodic agents.
- Emphasize importance of taking medications as prescribed and not abruptly discontinuing (especially the steroids because serious medical problems may result).
- Explain procedure and preoperative and postoperative care if surgery is required; review ileostomy care as necessary; obtain information from the National Foundation for Ileitis and Colitis.

U

Continuing Care

- Refer for home care nurse if nutritional status is compromised and patient is receiving TPN.
- Explain that disease can be controlled and patient can lead a healthy life between exacerbations.
- Encourage patient to rest as needed and modify activities according to energy levels during a flare-up; advise to limit tasks that impose strain on the lower

abdominal muscles and to sleep close to bathroom because of frequent diarrhea; suggest room deodorizers for odor control.

- Give information about medications and the need to take them on schedule while in home setting (eg, use of medication reminders—containers that separate pills according to day and time).
- Recommend low-residue, high-protein, high-calorie diet during an acute phase; encourage patient to keep a record of foods that irritate bowel and to eliminate them from diet; encourage intake of 8 glasses of water per day.
- Provide support for prolonged nature of disease because it is a strain on family life and financial resources, arrange for individual and family counseling as indicated.
- Provide time for patient to express fears and frustrations.

Evaluation

EXPECTED OUTCOMES
- Reports a decrease in frequency of diarrhea stools
- Experiences less pain
- Maintains fluid volume balance
- Attains optimal nutrition
- Maintains skin integrity
- Prevents fatigue
- Experiences less anxiety
- Copes successfully with diagnosis
- Acquires an understanding of the disease process
- Recovers without complications

For more information, see Chapter 35 in Smeltzer and Bare: *Brunner and Suddarth's Textbook of Medical-Surgical Nursing,* 9th edition. Philadelphia: Lippincott Williams & Wilkins, 2000.

UNCONSCIOUS PATIENT

Unconsciousness is a condition in which the patient is unresponsive to and unaware of environmental stimuli (usually for a short duration). Coma is a clinical state of unconsciousness in which the patient is unaware of self or the environment for prolonged periods (days to months, or even years). Akinetic mutism is a state of unresponsiveness to the environment in which the patient makes no movement or sound but sometimes has eyes open. A persistent vegetative state is one in which the patient is described as wakeful, without cognitive or affective mental function. The causes of unconsciousness may be neurologic (head injury, stroke), toxicologic (drug overdose, alcohol intoxication), or metabolic (hepatic or renal failure, diabetic ketoacidosis).

Diagnostic Evaluation
• Neurologic examination
• Laboratory tests: major chemical profile, serum ammonia, osmolality, prothrombin time, serum ketones, alcohol, drug and arterial blood gases (ABGs)

Medical Management
• The first priority is to obtain a patent and secure airway.
• Circulatory status (carotid pulse, heart rate and impulse, blood pressure) is assessed.
• Adequate oxygenation is maintained.
• An intravenous line is established to maintain fluid balance status.
• Nutritional support is provided (feeding tube or gastrostomy).

Nursing Management
Assessment
Assess for level of responsiveness (consciousness) by using the Glasgow Coma Scale.

U

- Evaluate pupil size, equality, and reaction to light; note movement of eyes.
- Assess facial symmetry and swallowing reflexes, and elicit deep tendon reflexes.
- Assess for purposeful or nonpurposeful responses: decorticate posturing (arms flexed, adducted, and internally rotated, and legs in extension) or decerebrate posturing (extremities extended and reflexes exaggerated).
- Rule out paralysis or stroke as cause of flaccidity.
- Examine body functions (circulation, respiration, elimination, fluid and electrolyte balance) in a systemic manner.
- Suspect a toxic or metabolic disorder if patient is comatose and pupillary light reflex is preserved.
- Assume that neurologic disease is present if patient is comatose and localized signs are severe.

Major Nursing Diagnoses
- Ineffective airway clearance related to inability to clear respiratory secretions
- Risk for fluid volume deficit related to inability to ingest fluids
- Altered oral mucous membranes related to mouth breathing, absence of pharyngeal reflex, and inability to ingest fluids
- Risk for impaired skin integrity related to immobility or restlessness
- Impaired tissue integrity of cornea related to diminished or absent corneal reflex
- Ineffective thermoregulation related to damage to hypothalamic center
- Altered bowel elimination (diarrhea or constipation) or urinary elimination (incontinence or retention) related to the unconscious state
- Altered family process related to sudden crisis of unconsciousness

Collaborative Problems/Potential Complications
- Respiratory distress or failure
- Pneumonia

- Pressure ulcer
- Aspiration

Planning and Goals

The goals of care during the unconscious period may include maintenance of a clear airway, attainment of fluid volume balance, achievement of intact oral mucous membranes, maintenance of normal skin integrity, absence of corneal irritation, attainment of thermoregulation, absence of urinary retention and infection, absence of diarrhea or fecal impaction, maintenance of intact family or support system, freedom from injury, and absence of complications.

Nursing Interventions

MAINTAINING THE AIRWAY
- Establish an adequate airway, and ensure ventilation.
- Position patient in a lateral or semiprone position; do not allow patient to remain on back.
- Remove secretions to reduce danger of aspiration; elevate head of bed to a 30-degree angle to prevent aspiration; provide frequent suctioning and oral hygiene.
- Auscultate chest every 8 hours for crackles, wheezes, or absence of breath sounds.
- Maintain patency of endotracheal tube or tracheostomy; monitor ABGs; maintain ventilator settings.
- Promote pulmonary hygiene with chest physiotherapy and postural drainage.

PROVIDING SAFETY
- Provide padded side rails for protection; maintain patient in raised position.
- Carry out every measure available and appropriate for calming and quieting a disturbed patient; avoid physical restraints if possible to prevent rise in intracranial pressure (ICP).

ATTAINING FLUID AND NUTRITIONAL BALANCE
- Assess for hydration status: examine mucous membranes; assess skin for tissue turgor.

- Meet fluid needs by giving required intravenous fluids and then nasogastric or gastrostomy feedings.
- Give intravenous fluids and blood transfusions slowly for patient with intracranial conditions.
- Never give oral fluids to a patient who cannot swallow; insert feeding tube for administration of enteral feedings.

MAINTAINING HEALTHY ORAL MUCOUS MEMBRANES

- Inspect mouth for dryness, inflammation, and presence of crusting; cleanse and rinse carefully to remove secretions and crust and keep membranes moist; apply petrolatum on lips.
- Assess sides of mouth and lips for ulceration if patient has an endotracheal tube. Move tube to opposite side of mouth daily.

MAINTAINING SKIN INTEGRITY

- Give special attention to a regular schedule of turning and repositioning to prevent ischemic necrosis over pressure areas.
- Give passive exercise of extremities to prevent contractures; use a splint or foam boots to prevent footdrop and eliminate pressure on toes.
- Keep hip joints and legs in proper alignment with supporting trochanter rolls.
- Position arms in abduction, fingers lightly flexed, and hands in slight supination.

MAINTAINING CORNEAL INTEGRITY

- Cleanse eyes with cotton balls moistened with sterile normal saline to remove debris and discharge.
- Instill artificial tears every 2 hours, as prescribed.
- Use cold compresses as prescribed for periocular edema after cranial surgery, and avoid contact with cornea.
- Use eye patches cautiously because of potential for further corneal abrasions.

ATTAINING THERMOREGULATION
- Adjust environment to promote normal body temperature.
- Use prescribed measures to treat hyperthermia: remove bedding, except light sheet, repeated antipyretics; avoid shivering, which may be due to chlorpromazine (Thorazine).

🚦 NURSING ALERT
Take body temperature rectally.

PREVENTING URINARY RETENTION
- Palpate bladder at intervals to determine whether urinary retention is present.
- Insert indwelling catheter if there are signs of urinary retention; observe for fever and cloudy urine; inspect urethral orifice for drainage.
- Use external penile catheter (condom catheter) for male patients and absorbent pads for female patients if they can urinate spontaneously.
- Initiate bladder training program as soon as conscious.
- Monitor frequently for skin irritation and breakdown; implement appropriate skin care.

PROMOTING BOWEL FUNCTION
- Evaluate abdominal distention by listening for bowel sounds and measuring girth of the abdomen.
- Monitor number and consistency of bowel movements; perform a rectal examination for signs of fecal impaction; patient may require enema every other day to empty lower colon.
- Enemas may be contraindicated if Valsalva maneuver increases a compromised ICP.
- Administer stool softeners and glycerin suppository as indicated.

U

SUPPORTING THE FAMILY
- Reinforce and clarify information about patient's condition to permit family members to mobilize their own adaptive capacities.

- Listen and encourage ventilation of feelings and concerns.
- Support family in decision-making process concerning posthospital management and placement.

PROMOTING SENSORY STIMULATION
- Provide continuing sensory stimulation to help patient overcome profound sensory deprivation.
- Make efforts to maintain usual day and night patterns of activity and sleep; orient patient to time and place every 8 hours.
- Touch and talk to patient; encourage family and friends to do the same; avoid making any negative comments about status in patient's presence.
- Introduce sounds from patient's home and workplace by means of a tape recorder.
- Read favorite books and provide familiar radio and television programs to enrich environment.

ATTAINING SELF-CARE
- Begin to teach, support, encourage, and supervise activities of daily living as soon as consciousness returns.

MONITORING AND MANAGING POTENTIAL COMPLICATIONS: PNEUMONIA
- Monitor vital signs and respiratory function for signs of respiratory failure or distress.
- Assess for adequate red blood cells to carry oxygen: total blood count and ABGs.
- Obtain cultures to identify organism for appropriate antibiotics if pneumonia develops.
- Monitor closely for evidence of impaired skin integrity, and implement strategies to prevent skin breakdown and pressure ulcers.
- Address factors that contribute to impaired skin integrity, and undertake strategies to promote healing, if pressure ulcers do develop.

Evaluation

EXPECTED OUTCOMES

- Maintains clear airway and demonstrates appropriate breath sounds
- Experiences no injuries
- Attains or maintains healthy oral mucous membranes
- Attains or maintains adequate fluid status
- Maintains normal skin integrity
- Has no corneal irritation
- Attains or maintains thermoregulation
- Has no urinary retention

For more information, see Chapter 57 in Smeltzer and Bare: *Brunner and Suddarth's Textbook of Medical-Surgical Nursing,* 9th edition. Philadelphia: Lippincott Williams & Wilkins, 2000.

UROLITHIASIS

Urolithiasis refers to stones (calculi) in the urinary tract. Stones are formed in the urinary tract when urinary concentrations of substances, such as calcium oxalate, calcium phosphate, and uric acid, increase. Calculi may vary in size from minute granular deposits to bladder stones the size of an orange. Certain factors favor formation of stones, including infection, urinary stasis, periods of immobility, and altered calcium metabolism (hypercalcemia and hypercalcuria). The problem occurs predominantly in the third to fifth decades and affects men more than women.

U

Clinical Manifestations

Manifestations depend on presence of obstruction, infection, and edema. Symptoms range from mild to excruciating pain and discomfort.

Stones in Renal Pelvis
- Intense, deep ache in the costovertebral region
- Hematuria and pyuria
- Pain that radiates anteriorly and downward toward bladder in female and toward testes in male
- Acute pain, nausea, vomiting, costovertebral area tenderness, (renal colic)
- Abdominal discomfort, diarrhea

Ureteral Colic (Stones Lodged in the Ureter)
- Acute, excruciating, colicky, wavelike pain, radiating down the thigh to the genitalia
- Frequent desire to void, but little urine passed; usually contains blood because of the abrasive action of the stone

Stones Lodged in Bladder
- Symptoms of irritation associated with urinary tract infection and hematuria
- Urinary retention, if stone obstructs bladder neck
- Possible sepsis if infection is present with stone

Diagnostic Evaluation
- Most stones are radiopaque and can be detected by radiograph
- Diagnosis is confirmed by kidney, ureter, and bladder (KUB) studies, intravenous urography, or retrograde pyelography.
- Chemical analysis is preformed to determine stone composition.

Medical Management
The basic goals are to eradicate the stone, determine the stone type, prevent nephron destruction, control infection, and relieve any obstruction that may be present.

Pharmacologic Therapy
- Analgesics (morphine or meperidine to prevent shock and syncope) and nonsteroidal antiinflammatory drugs (NSAIDs)

- Hot baths or application of moist heat to flank areas
- Increased fluid intake to assist in passage, unless vomiting
- Increased round-the-clock fluid intake to reduce urine concentration, dilute the urine, and ensure high urinary output

Stone Removal
- Cystoscopic examination and passage of small ureteral catheter
- Chemical analysis of stones for determination of composition

Nutrition and Medication Therapy
- Calcium stones: reduced dietary calcium, protein, and sodium; liberal fluid intake; medications to acidify urine, such as ammonium chloride, sodium cellulose phosphate (Calcibind), and thiazide diuretics if parathormone production is increased
- Phosphate stones: diet low in phosphorus; aluminum hydroxide gel
- Uric stones: low-purine and limited protein diet; allopurinol (Zyloprim); alkalinization of urine
- Cystine stones: low-protein diet; alkalinization of urine; penicillamine
- Oxalate stones: dilute urine; limited oxalate intake (green, leafy vegetables such as spinach, strawberries, rhubarb, wheat bran, chocolate, tea, and peanuts)

Methods of Stone Removal
- Extracorporeal shock wave lithotripsy (ESWL)
- Percutaneous nephrostomy; endourologic methods
- Electrohydraulic lithotripsy
- Ureteroscopy: stones fragmented with use of laser, electrohydraulic lithotripsy, or ultrasound, and then removed
- Chemolysis: stone dissolution—alternative for those who are poor risks for other therapy, refuse other methods, or have easily dissolved stones (struvite)

U

• Surgical removal: performed in only 1% to 2% of patients

Nursing Management

Assessment

• Assess for pain and discomfort, including severity, location, and any radiation of the pain.
• Assess for presence of associated symptoms, including nausea, vomiting, diarrhea, and abdominal distention.
• Observe for signs of urinary tract infection (chills, fever, dysuria, frequency, and hesitancy) and obstruction (frequent urination of small amounts, oliguria, or anuria).
• Observe urine for presence of blood; strain for stones or gravel.
• Focus history on factors that predispose to urinary tract stones or may have precipitated current episode of renal or ureteral colic.
• Assess patient's knowledge about renal stones and measures to prevent their occurrence or recurrence.

Major Nursing Diagnoses

• Pain related to inflammation, obstruction, and abrasion of the urinary tract
• Knowledge deficit regarding prevention of recurrence of renal stones

Collaborative Problems/Potential Complications

• Infection and sepsis (from urinary tract infection and pyelonephritis)
• Obstruction of the urinary tract by a stone or edema, with subsequent acute renal failure

Planning and Goals

The major goals of the patient may include relief of pain and discomfort, prevention of recurrence of renal stones, and prevention of complications.

Nursing Interventions

RELIEVING PAIN

- Use narcotic analgesics as prescribed.
- Encourage and assist patient to assume a position of comfort.
- Assist patient by ambulating to obtain some pain relief.
- Monitor pain closely and report promptly increases in severity.
- Prepare for treatment (eg, lithotripsy) if pain is unrelieved.

MONITORING AND MANAGING COMPLICATIONS: INFECTION AND OBSTRUCTION

- Instruct patient to report decreased urine volume and bloody or cloudy urine.
- Monitor total urine output and patterns of voiding.
- Encourage increased fluid intake and ambulation.
- Begin intravenous fluids if patient is unable to take adequate oral fluids.
- Observe patient constantly to detect the spontaneous passage of a stone.
- Strain urine through gauze.
- Crush any blood clots passed in urine, and inspect sides of urinal and bedpan for clinging stones.
- Instruct patient to report any increases in pain; administer analgesics.
- Monitor patient's vital signs for early signs of infection.
- Treat infections with antimicrobials before stone dissolution.

U

🏠 Promoting Home and Community-Based Care

Teaching Patients Self-Care

- Explain the causes of kidney stones and ways to prevent their recurrence.
- Encourage patient to maintain a high fluid intake—to drink enough to excrete 3000 to 4000 mL of urine every 24 hours.

- Instruct patient to avoid sudden increases in environmental temperatures and occupations and activities that produce excessive sweating and dehydration.
- Give detailed verbal and written information about specific foods.
- Explain prescribed medications and their actions and importance.

HOME CARE AND FOLLOW-UP AFTER ESWL.
- Instruct patient to increase fluid intake to assist passage of stone fragments (may take 6 weeks to several months after procedure).
- Instruct patient about signs and symptoms of complications: fever, decreasing urinary output, and pain.
- Inform patient that hematuria is anticipated but should disappear in 24 hours.
- Give appropriate dietary instruction according to composition of stones.
- Encourage regimen to avoid further stone formation; advise patient to adhere to prescribed diet.
- Teach patient to take sufficient fluids in the evening to prevent urine from becoming too concentrated at night.
- Recommend that patient have urine cultures every 1 to 2 months the first year and periodically thereafter.
- Recommend that recurrent urinary infection be treated vigorously.
- Encourage increased mobility whenever possible, and discourage ingestion of vitamins (especially vitamin D) and minerals.
- Instruct patient about signs and symptoms of complications appearing after surgical procedures that warrant physician notification.
- Emphasize to family and patient the importance of follow-up to assess kidney function and to ensure removal of all kidney stones.

Continuing Care
- Instruct patient to monitor and interpret urinary pH.
- Teach signs and symptoms of stone formation, obstruction, and infection; advise patient to report these to physician promptly.
- Explain the actions and importance of medications prescribed to prevent stone formation.

Evaluation
EXPECTED OUTCOMES
- Reports relief of pain
- Experiences no complications
- States increased knowledge of health-seeking behaviors to prevent recurrence

For more information, see Chapter 41 in Smeltzer and Bare: *Brunner and Suddarth's Textbook of Medical-Surgical Nursing,* 9th edition. Philadelphia: Lippincott Williams & Wilkins, 2000.

U

V

VEIN DISORDERS (VENOUS THROMBOSIS, THROMBOPHLEBITIS, PHLEBOTHROMBOSIS, AND DEEP VEIN THROMBOSIS [DVT])

Although the vein disorders described here do not necessarily present an identical pathology, for clinical purposes, these terms are often used interchangeably. The exact cause of *venous thrombosis* remains unclear, although three factors (Virchow's triad) are believed to play a significant role in its development: stasis of blood, injury to the vessel wall, and altered blood coagulation. *Thrombophlebitis* is an inflammation of the walls of the veins, often accompanied by the formation of a clot. When a clot develops initially in the veins as a result of stasis or hypercoagulability, but without inflammation, the process is referred to as *phlebothrombosis*. *Venous thrombosis* can occur in any vein but is most frequent in the veins of the lower extremities. Both superficial and deep veins of the legs may be affected. Damage to the lining of blood vessels creates a site for clot formation, and increased blood coagulability occurs in patients abruptly withdrawn from anticoagulant medications and occurs with oral contraceptive use and several blood dyscrasias. The danger associated with venous thrombosis is that parts of a clot can become detached and produce an embolic occlusion of the pulmonary blood vessels. Upper extremity venous thrombosis is less common than lower extremity.

Clinical Manifestations

- Half of all patients have no symptoms; signs and symptoms are nonspecific.
- Obstruction of the deep veins of the legs produces edema and swelling of the extremity.
- The skin over the affected leg may become warmer; superficial veins may become more prominent (cordlike venous segment).
- Bilateral swelling may be difficult to detect (lack of size difference).
- Tenderness occurs later and is detected by gently palpating the leg.
- Homans' sign (pain in the calf after sharp dorsiflexion of the foot) is not specific for DVT because it can be elicited in any painful condition of the calf.
- In some cases, signs of a pulmonary embolus are the first indication of DVT.
- Thrombus of superficial veins produces pain or tenderness, redness, and warmth in the involved area.
- In massive iliofemoral venous thrombosis (phlegmasia cerulea dolens), the entire extremity becomes massively swollen, tense, painful, and cool to touch.

Diagnostic Evaluation

- History revealing risk factors, such as varicose veins or neoplastic disease
- Doppler ultrasonography, impedance plethysmography, duplex imaging
- ^{251}I-labeled fibrinogen scanning, contrast phlebography (venography)

Medical Management

The objectives of management are to prevent the thrombus from growing and fragmenting, resolve the current thrombus, and prevent recurrence.

Therapeutic Anticoagulation

- Heparin is administered for 5 to 7 days by intermittent or continuous intravenous infusion; dosage is regulated by partial thromboplastin time (PTT), international normalized ratio (INR), and platelet counts. Low-molecular-weight heparin is given in one or two injections daily; it is more expensive than unfractionated heparin but safer.
- Oral anticoagulants (eg, warfarin [Coumadin]) are given with heparin therapy.
- Thrombolytic (fibrinolytic) therapy is given within the first 3 days after acute thrombosis. Streptokinase, urokinase, and tissue-type plasminogen activator are used.
- PTT, prothrombin time, hemoglobin, hematocrit, platelet count, and fibrinogen level are monitored frequently.
- Drug is discontinued if bleeding occurs and cannot be stopped.

Surgical Management

Thrombectomy is the treatment of choice when anticoagulant or thrombolytic therapy is contraindicated, the danger of pulmonary embolism is extreme, and permanent damage to the extremity will probably result. A vena cava filter may be placed.

Nursing Management

Assessment

- Assess patient carefully for early signs of venous disorders in lower extremities.
- Take history of varicose veins, hypercoagulation, neoplastic disease, cardiovascular disease, or recent major surgery or injury. Obese people, elderly people, and women taking oral contraceptives are at risk.
- Question patient about presence of leg pain, heaviness, and any functional impairment or edema.

- Inspect legs from groin to feet, noting asymmetry and measuring and recording calf circumference (one early indication of edema is engorgement of the space behind the ankle).
- Note any increase in temperature in the affected leg.
- Identify areas of tenderness and any thromboses.

Prevention
Prevention is dependent on identifying risk factors for thrombus and on educating the patient about appropriate interventions.

- Advise patient to remove elastic stockings for a brief interval at least twice daily and at night; inspect skin for signs of irritation; examine calves for possible tenderness; and report any skin changes or signs of tenderness.
- Intermittent pneumatic compression (IPC) devices can be used with elastic stockings for prevention of DVT; ensure that prescribed pressures are not exceeded and assess for comfort.
- Subcutaneous heparin is used in surgical patients.

Nursing Interventions
PROVIDING COMFORT
- Recommend bed rest, elevate the affected extremity, provide elastic stockings, and administer analgesics for pain.
- Advise bed rest for 5 to 7 days after diagnosis of DVT.
- Use elastic stocking when patient begins to ambulate; apply and monitor carefully to prevent rolling down to form a tourniquet (which restricts circulation).
- Encourage walking (better than standing or sitting for long periods).
- Recommend bed exercises, such as dorsiflexion of the foot against a footboard.
- Apply warm, moist packs to affected extremity to reduce discomfort.
- Provide additional relief for pain control with mild analgesics as prescribed.

V

POSITIONING THE BODY AND
ENCOURAGING EXERCISE

- Elevate feet and lower legs periodically above heart level when on bed rest.
- Perform active and passive leg exercises, particularly those involving calf muscles, to increase venous flow preoperatively and postoperatively.
- Provide early ambulation in preventing venous stasis.
- Encourage deep-breathing exercises because they produce increased negative pressure in the thorax, which assists in emptying the large veins.

 Promoting Home and Community-Based Care

Teaching Patients Self-Care

- Teach the patient how to apply elastic stockings.
- Instruct patient on the purpose and importance of medication (correct dosage at specific times) and need for scheduled blood tests to regulate medications.

 Gerontologic Considerations

Elderly patients may be unable to apply elastic stockings properly. Teach family member who is to assist the patient to apply the stockings so that they do not cause undue pressure on any part of the feet or legs.

For more information, see Chapter 28 in Smeltzer and Bare: *Brunner and Suddarth's Textbook of Medical-Surgical Nursing,* 9th edition. Philadelphia: Lippincott Williams & Wilkins, 2000.

INDEX